Deutsches Krebsforschungszentrum

Current Cancer Research

1995

Steinkopff Darmstadt
Springer New York

Cover photo:

Map of the cancer atlas "Atlas of Cancer Mortality in Central Europe" (IARC Scientific Publications No. 134, Lyon 1995)
The map shows the mortality rates in Germany, Poland, and other countries in central Europe from cancer of the trachea, bronchi and lung, which vary from one region to another (green: lowest, red: highest mortality rates)

ISBN 3-7985-0989-1
ISSN 0940-0745

Publisher:

Deutsches Krebsforschungszentrum
Im Neuenheimer Feld 280
D-69120 Heidelberg
Tel.: +62 21 / 42-0
Telex: 46 15 62 dkfz d
Telefax: +0 62 21 / 42-29 95

Editorial responsibility:

Presse- und Öffentlichkeitsarbeit
Hilke Stamatiadis-Smidt, M.A.

Coordination:

Elisabeth Hohensee, M.A.

Co-workers:

Dipl.-Biol. Susanne Glasmacher
Hans von Kalckreuth
Dr. Margund Mrozek
Dipl.-Biol. Ulrike Nell
Dipl.-Biochem. Martin Roos
Mareile Schulte
Dr. Michèl Schummer
Dr. Birgitt Sickenberger

Translation:

Stefanie von Kalckreuth, akad. gepr. Übers., Heidelberg
Angela Lahee, PhD, Oberflockenbach
Dipl.-Phys. Dirk Meenenga, B. Sc., Heidelberg

Lay-out:

Heidi Hnatek

Photos:

Josef Wiegand

Photos in the research reports by the authors or by members of the staff.

Fig. 2 Dr. Stefan Joos, Dr. Peter Lichter, Division of Organisation of Complex Genomes, with kind permission of Springer-Verlag, Heidelberg; fig. 3 Prof. Dr. Manfred Schwab, Division of Cytogenetics; fig. 4 Dr. Gabriela Möslein, Düsseldorf; figs. 5, 10 Priv.-Doz. Dr. Jürgen Kartenbeck, Division of Cell Biology, and Dr. Herbert Spring, Research Program Cell Differentiation and Carcinogenesis; figs. 6, 13 Cäcilia Kuhn, Division of Cell Biology; figs. 7, 34, 48, 55, 88, 89, 91, 123, 130, 132 Ulrich Soeder, Heidelberg; figs. 11, 12 Peter Lütkes, Heidelberg; fig. 25 with kind permission of ecomed-Verlagsgesellschaft mbH, Landsberg; figs. 26, 27, 28 with kind permission of Bayer AG, Leverkusen; fig. 29 with kind permission of Marc Greenblatt, National Cancer Institute, Bethesda, U.S.A.; figs. 35, 36 Dr. Gerd Moeckel, Division of Toxicology and Cancer Risk Factors; figs. 37, 38, 39 Prof. Dr. Neidhard Paweletz, Division of Cell Growth and Division; figs. 57, 59 Priv.-Doz. Dr. Hanswalter Zentgraf, Research Program Applied Tumor Virology; fig. 62 with kind permission of John Wiley & Sons, New York, U.S.A.; fig. 83 copyright Larry Landweber and the Internet Society; fig. 98 National Council for Research and Development, Jerusalem, Israel; fig. 99 Dagmar Welker, Heidelberg; fig. 126 b Heidenreich, Hannover; fig. 141 Stefan Kresin, Heidelberg

Printing:

Brühlsche Universitätsdruckerei, Giessen
Printed in Germany 1995

Chapter | Page

Cancer Research: Prospects for the Future

by Harald zur Hausen

For years now cancer research has been an area marked by rapid progress. In particular, we have reached a better understanding of cell biology and the mechanisms of carcinogenesis; further, our knowledge of cancer risk factors and patients at risk and how to identify them has grown substantially. Progress is less evident in cancer prevention, early detection, and therapy – although particularly in cancer treatment, new concepts now evolving as a consequence of our enhanced understanding of carcinogenesis are showing great promise.

In the field of cell biology it is primarily the processes of cell division that are better understood today. We are achieving increasing success in characterizing the components involved in these processes, namely those of inter- and intracellular signal transduction which control growth and differentiation.

Defects in the regulation of cell division often are due to changes in the DNA of specific genes of somatic cells. These changes are caused either by external influences (chemical or physical factors) or by viral genes that become integrated in the genome of the cell and remain there. In addition, epigenetic modifications (e.g., methylations), which can permanently alter gene functions, are also of relevance.

The identification of genes whose modification or functional failure leads to a defective control of cell growth, and the analysis of the resulting functional changes in associated signal chains is an area of cancer research that is today advancing very rapidly. The interplay of genome research, protein analyses, and functional research has proven particularly valuable in this area and has brought about fundamental changes in cancer research in the past decade.

Today, the analysis of cell surface molecules gives insight into changes of the "social conduct" of cells and into the way in which they make modified molecular structures identifiable for defense mechanisms. Without the rapid advance of cell biology and molecular biology we would never have attained our current level of knowledge about the mechanisms of carcinogenesis. In the case of certain types of cancer (colon cancer, cervical cancer) we are now beginning to understand the signal pathways whose disruption appears to be an essential prerequisite for invasive growth.

The knowledge of specific genetic changes increasingly allows us to identify patients with a particular risk of developing certain kinds of cancer, especially if the respective genes are already damaged in the germ line. Thus, these patients can be subjected to relevant and improved measures of early detection, which can significantly increase their chances of being cured.

Viruses as cancer-causing factors

In relation to cancer risk factors, particular progress has been made in the identification of infectious events taking part in carcinogenesis. Starting with the discovery of the Epstein-Barr virus 30 years ago, the identification of cancer-related types of papillomavirus in the case of anal cancer, genital cancer, cancer of the oral cavity, and skin cancer as well as the elucidation of the role of hepatitis viruses in the development of liver cell carcinoma have brought

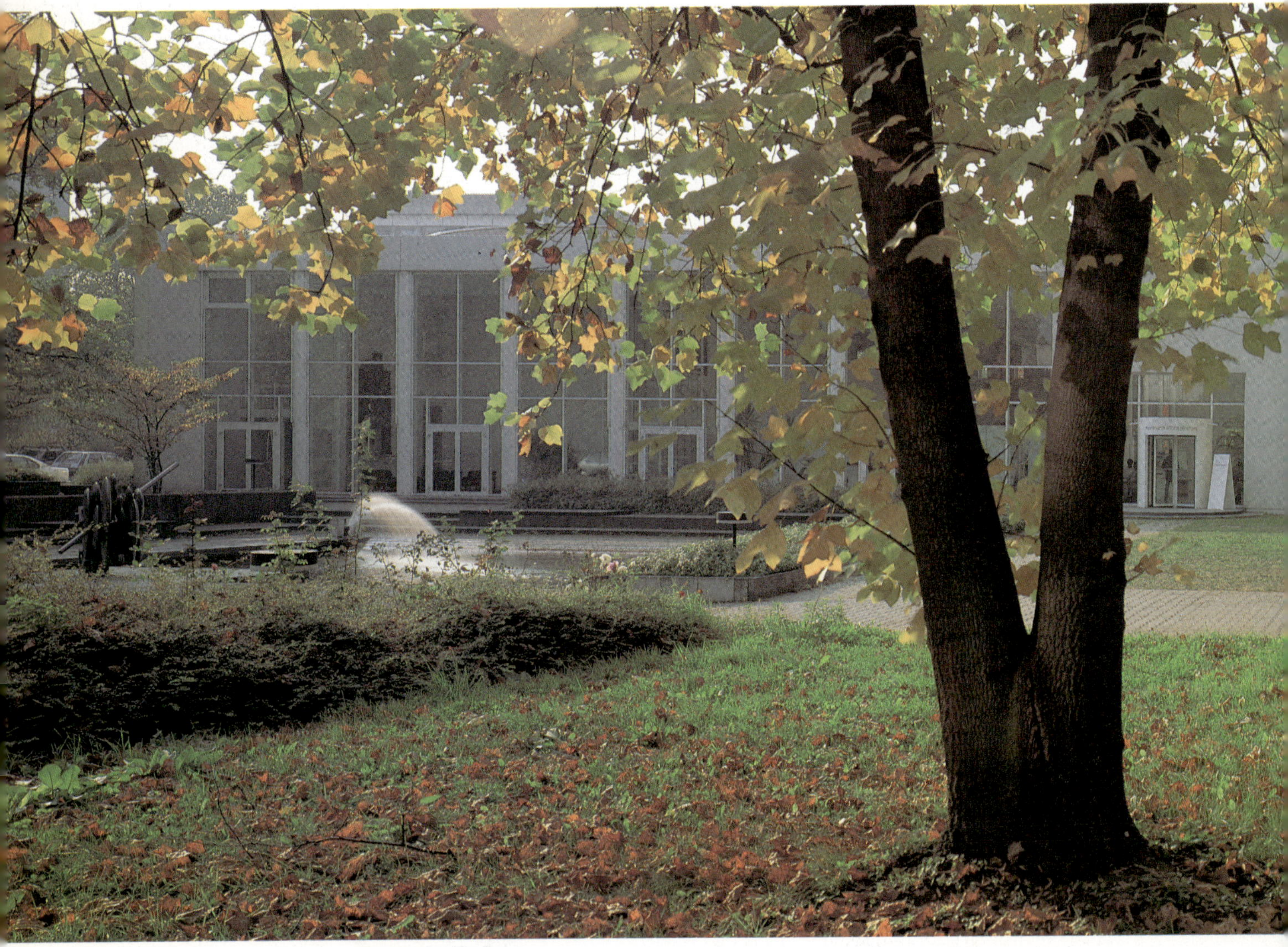

Fig. 1
Main entrance of the Deutsches Krebsforschungszentrum

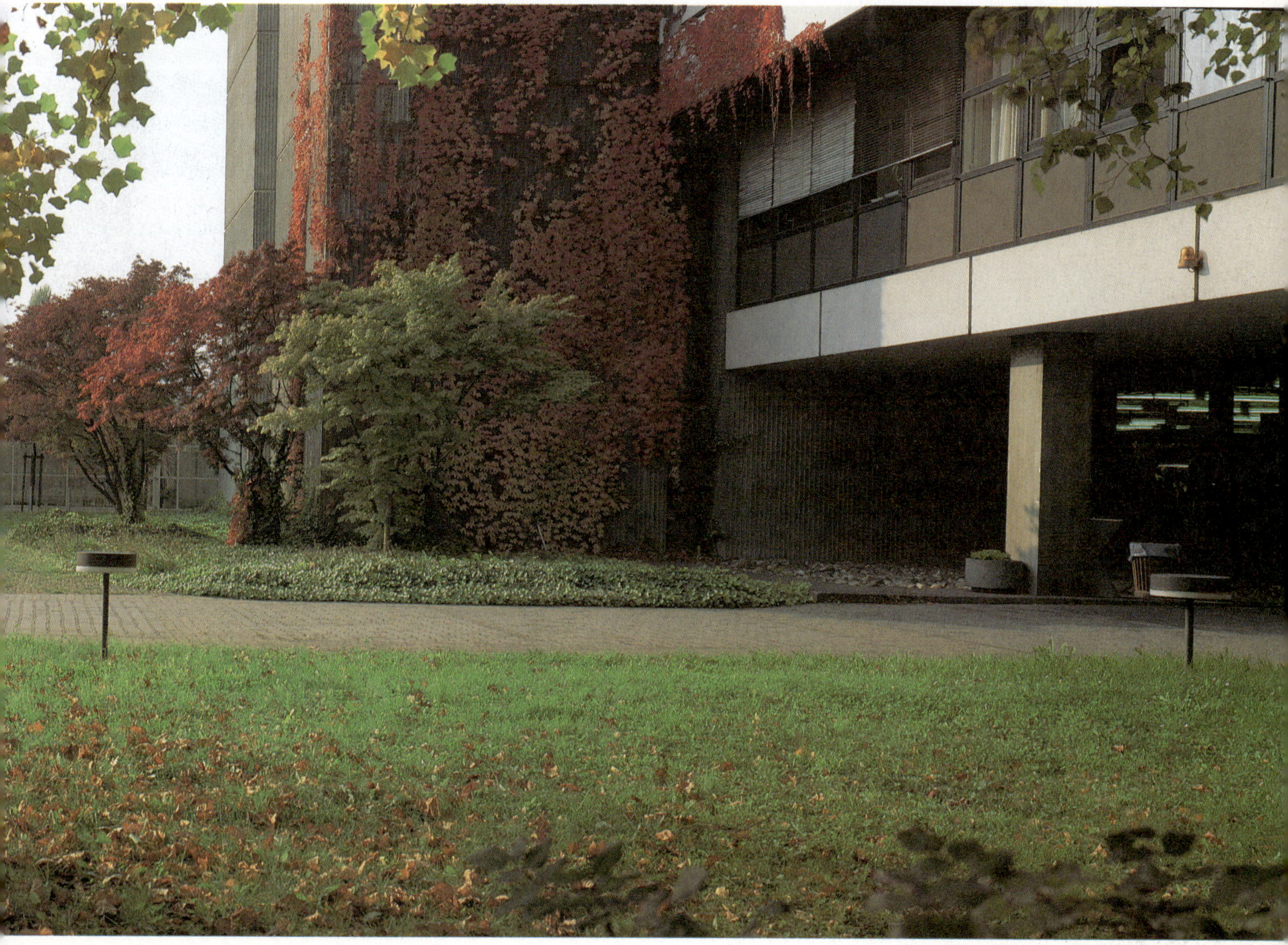

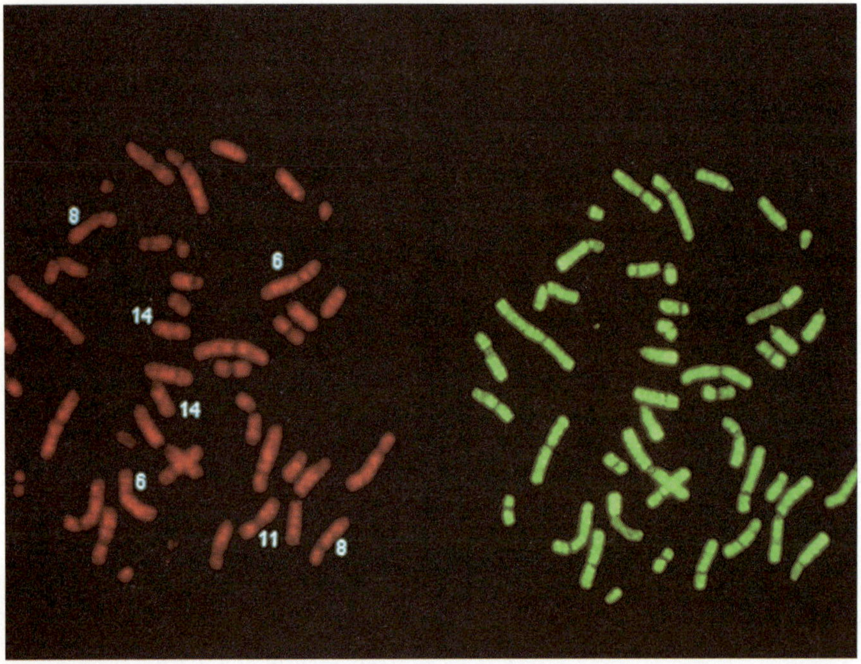

Fig. 2
The red-dyed fragments of the genetic material (DNA) of a healthy person attach to a set of chromosomes from normal cells and fluoresce evenly. The green-dyed DNA of a leukemia patient shows a patchy and uneven fluorescence pattern because specific gene segments on the chromosomes are missing or repeated

about what one could call a change of paradigms. Today, the role of viruses as cancer-causing factors is being investigated all over the world. In addition, the elucidation of the interaction of viruses with host cells and host organisms contributes substantially to the understanding of carcinogenesis.

Alongside viral agents, non-viral infections have come to the fore as cancer risk factors in the past few years. Examples are Helicobacter pylori in the case of gastric cancer and certain kinds of helminth infection (schistosoma and opisthorchis) in cancers of the bladder, rectum, and bile duct in specific geographic regions.

For cancer prevention, new avenues are continually being opened by the findings of molecular biology. Besides the possibilities of vaccine production in the case of viral infections, the development of methods for diagnosing genetically determined forms of cancer and the preventive examination of risk patients are gaining importance. Also, in more recent times a field of research called "chemoprevention" has become established. This refers to the prevention of the possible development of a cancer in a risk patient by medication.

In the field of diagnostics, the existing physico-technical diagnostic techniques (such as magnetic resonance tomography) have been refined and are contributing to an enhanced organ-specific diagnosis. In radiology, efforts to optimize existing therapies, to tailor them to each individual case (conformation precision radiotherapy, consideration of tumor form and tumor volume, etc.) and thereby to reduce side-effects have already benefitted patients. The refinement of imaging techniques, particularly of three dimensional methods, makes it possible to irradiate tumors more precisely, while sparing the healthy tissue. The applications of positron emission tomography, which are continuously being extended, today allow us to check the effectiveness of ongoing drug treatments and thus, if necessary, to change the therapy so as to prevent unnecessary side effects. The clinician today has available a set of instruments for optimizing and individualizing diagnosis and therapy which can be combined with new methods of therapy planning and follow-up. Cancer patients profit not only from this extension of the technical limits, but also from greater efforts (compared to 5 or 10 years ago) to maintain life quality, to improve aftercare, and to provide continuous information about cancer.

Preparatory works for gene therapy

In the long run, however, the decisive breakthroughs are to be expected from the growing use of immunological and molecular-biological methods of examination and treatment. The determina-

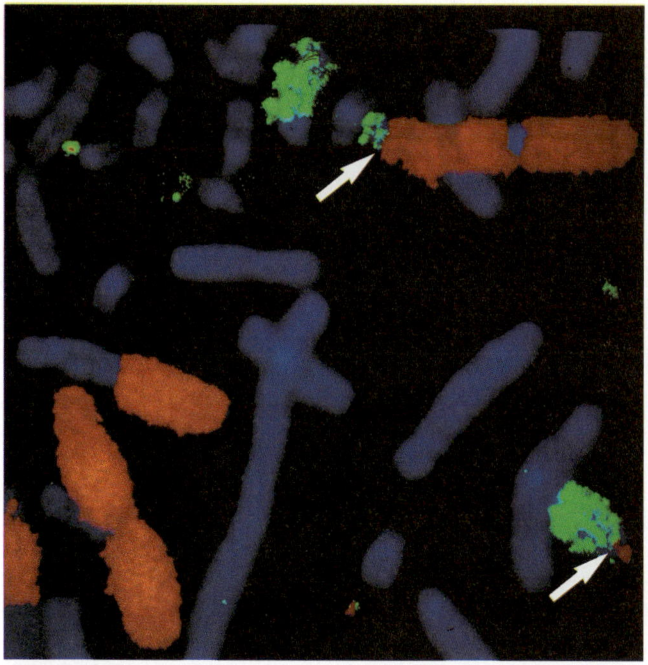

Fig. 3
Changes in the genetic material of a cancer cell of a neuroblastoma, a nerve cell tumor affecting children. A segment of chromosome 1 (red) has switched places with a segment of chromosome 15 (green). This damage is made visible by fluorescent DNA probes that attach to the genetic material. A gene situated on the breaking point on chromosome 1 may be involved in the development of neuroblastoma and possibly also in the pathogenesis of intestinal and breast cancers

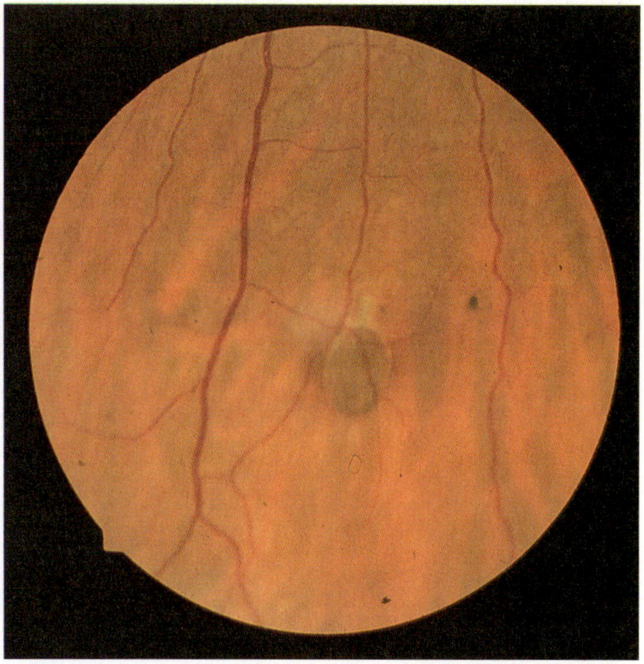

Fig. 4
Examination of the ocular fundus in the diagnosis of patients with familial adenomatous polyposis (FAP), a hereditary condition. The retina shows congenital alterations in affected individuals. FAP patients develop multiple benign polyps in the colon and rectum, which almost invariably turn malignant with time. Some years ago a gene was identified, which, if defective, is responsible for the development of the polyps

tion of further tumor markers has made considerable progress in the past few years. As mentioned before, gene-diagnostic methods are increasingly finding their way into clinical practice. Nevertheless, cancer therapy, like cancer diagnostics, can hardly do without standard treatments (surgery, radiotherapy, and chemotherapy) even in the long run. Their optimization thus remains a worthwhile goal. And, since they are indispensable for reducing the mass of advanced tumors, they will foreseeably also play a certain role in the use of new methods of gene technology which promise to be successful primarily in the case of relatively small cell numbers.

Several concepts from basic research in molecular biology, from immunological and virological preparatory studies are today almost ready for clinical use and some are presently undergoing clinical or preclinical testing. Under the banner "gene therapy" a worldwide search is in progress for suitable carrier molecules and gene transfer systems, which in the next few years is expected to lead to advances in cancer treatment, too.

The Deutsches Krebsforschungszentrum has made highly-valued contributions to all of the above-mentioned areas on an international scale and has published its results in leading specialist journals.

In cell biology the molecular principles of cell architecture have been thoroughly analyzed and the modifications accompanying tumor growth have been

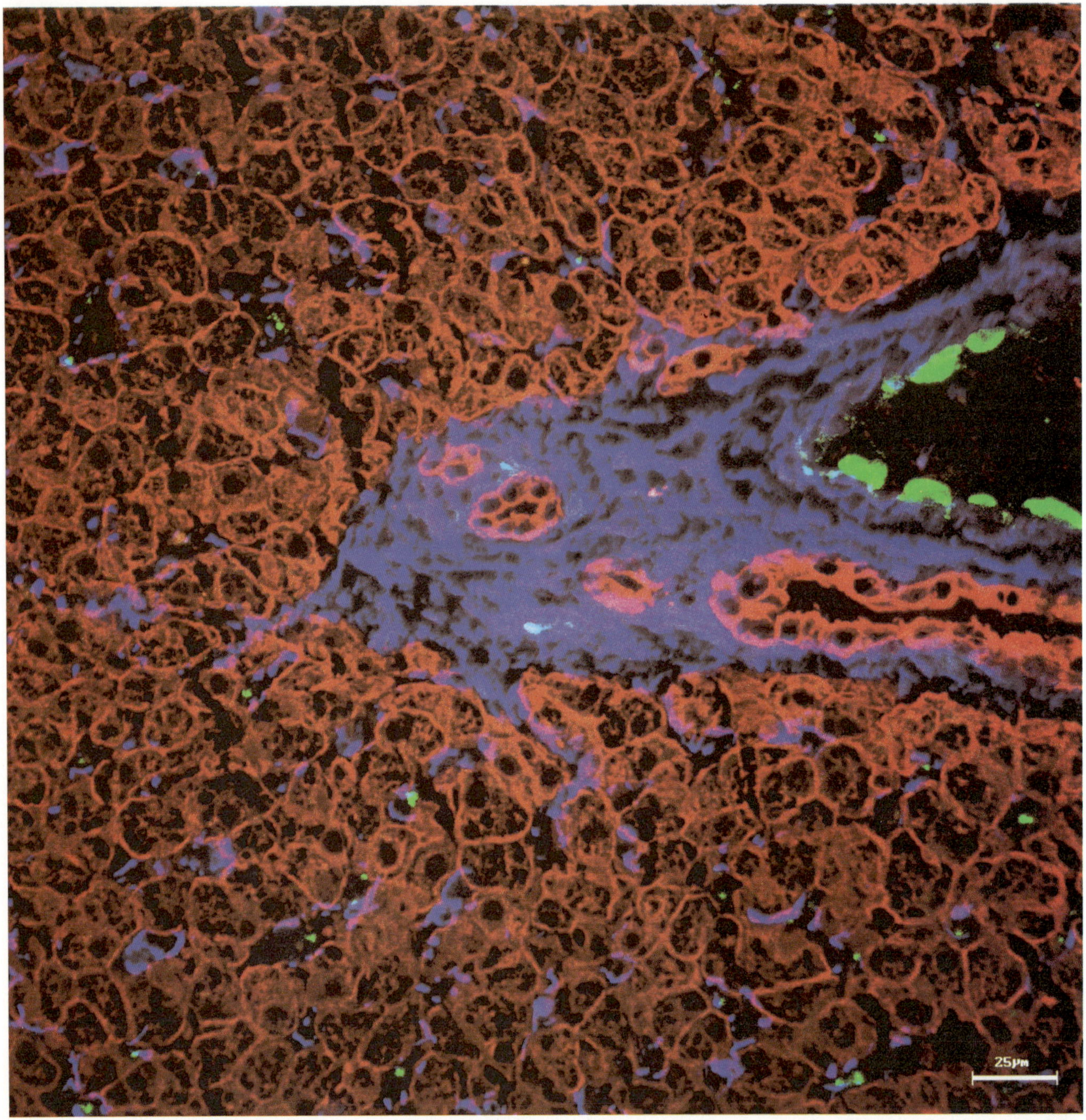
25μm

characterized. This has had manifold consequences for diagnostics, particularly for the detection of unidentified primary tumors by characterizing the cytoskeleton proteins of metastases. Among other things, these investigations led to the identification of a monoclonal antibody (CYFRA 21–1) that can be used for early detection of a specific protein molecule in the blood of patients suffering from small-cell lung carcinoma.

There is growing evidence to suggest that specific cell-surface molecules ("junction proteins"), previously identified in the Center, play a role as tumor suppressor genes. In this area of research, the basic principles of hormone-mediated gene regulation have been investigated and additional tumor suppressor genes have been characterized.

Formerly unknown functional molecules of the human immune system have been discovered by scientists from the Deutsches Krebsforschungszentrum and their biochemical/molecular-biological characteristics and their function have been investigated. In this context, the so-called CD44 protein, which makes lymphocytes able to move through the body, should be mentioned. It is by "copying" this mechanism that tumor cells become mobile and start metastasizing.

Important accomplishments in immunology

Immunological research in the Center has yielded fundamental contributions to the phenomenon of immune tolerance, describing it as a multi-step development, and explaining it on the basis of cell apoptosis. Analyses of the mechanism of disruption of this tolerance in tumors, and the production of bispecific antibodies for treating lymphomas and leukemias are further components of these efforts. In addition, research is being performed on the redox regulation of transcription factors, whose practical role in AIDS infections is being investigated via the administration of N-acetylcysteine. Substantial contributions to the presentation of antigenic domains and efforts aimed at the allogenation of tumor cells by virus infections round off the picture of immunologically oriented research at the Center.

Fig. 5
Fluorescent antibodies are used to label different cell types in liver tissue with the aim of identifying the type of tumor. An exact classification is critical in treatment planning

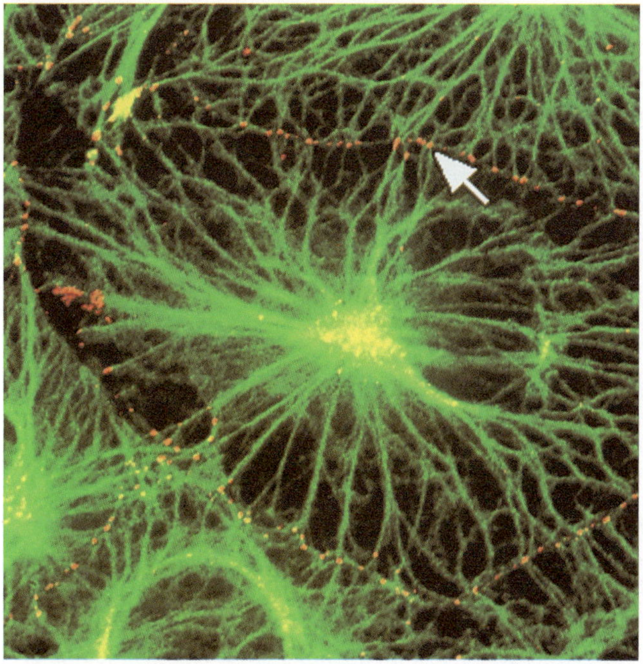

Fig. 6
Fluorescent antibodies are used to make the cytoskeleton, the basic structure of a cell, clearly visible. Fragments of the cytoskeleton circulating in the bloodstream can also be detected with this method. Because the cytoskeleton of each cell type has its own characteristic protein composition, which is retained despite mutation, it reveals its origin even if the mutated cell has left its usual tissue environment

Virological research at the Deutsches Krebsforschungszentrum has led to the identification of the main types of papillomavirus that contribute to the development of genital cancers (HPV 6, 11, 16, 18) and cancers of the skin and the nasopharynx (HPV 41, 57). The causal connection between infection with HPV and cervical cancer, the second most frequent cancer in women worldwide, has been conclusively proven; furthermore, the basic principles of the molecular pathogenesis of this cancer, which is mainly due to HPV 16 and 18, have been elucidated. The sensitizing effect of infections with certain parvoviruses on tumors under radio- or chemotherapy as well as the differentiation of tumor cells caused by these infections were established in the Center, as were the fundamentals of a gene therapy using the capsids of these viruses. Two interdisciplinary work groups for the development of such a gene therapy and a particularly positively assessed special research program on AIDS make the picture complete.

Research efforts aimed at the chromosomal localization of genes by light-microscope analysis of hybridization reactions as well as studies on human DNA and cDNA banks have been crowned with great success. The identification of leukemic cells on the basis of rearrangements of genes and the contribution to the identification of the Huntington gene, which causes a disease called Saint Vitus' dance, were important milestones of this development. It is complemented by intensive sequence analyses, which include, for example, nearly all 70 types of papillomavirus that have been identified to date, and by a comprehensive research program in molecular biophysics, which has turned the Deutsches Krebsforschungszentrum into the national node of the Genome Program of the European Union. Within this framework it cooperates closely with other data networks.

Numerous significant research results have been achieved in the area of tissue-specific regulation via cytokines and mediators of low molecular weight, the characterization of mitosis-specific proteins, and the characterization of modifications of the cell surface accompanying AIDS infections and cancer.

Due to one division head leaving the Center and the retirement of another, the traditionally strong area of registering cancer-causing and cancer-promoting substances is now being pursued less vigorously. This is not so much because of its relevance for cancer research, but more as a consequence of a stronger focus on fields of research that are less well represented in other research facilities, such as in industry and academia.

As far as research programs with immediate clinical orientation are concerned, we should, above all, mention the advances in magnetic resonance tomography and positron emission tomography, which have not only improved methodologies and practical clinical applications, but have also brought about close clinical cooperations between Heidelberg University and the Deutsches Krebsforschungszentrum.

Reinforcing clinical cooperation

From the above, the main focuses of research at the Deutsches Krebsforschungszentrum of the last few years are apparent. They can be summarized under the headings cell biology, immunology, and virology; in addition, genome research is developing into a further focal area. The existing clinical program in the field of radiological diagnostics and therapy will be substantially expanded by the clinical cooperation units in the areas of hematology/oncology, and dermatology with oncological orientation, which is planned to be established within the university hospitals of Heidelberg/Mannheim.

An important area, and for the most part newly developing, is the epidemiological and toxicological registration of cancer risk factors – an area which has already been given a solid foundation thanks to the establishment of the division of epidemiology and which has now received further strong support from the newly staffed Division of Toxicology and Cancer Risk Factors. In the future, it is planned to reinforce this focus with activities in the field of cancer prevention.

Although this brief outline covers most of the main existing and evolving research interests of the Center, it should be pointed out that in addition to these, interdisciplinary activities play an important role and are indispensable for the Center. These include, in particular, central activities in the fields of pathology, bioinformatics, and data processing, in spectroscopic techniques, and in other specific synthetic and analytical research. It should also be mentioned that a broad infrastructure ensures a smooth flow of the scientific work.

Finally, in order to secure the future of a scientifically active research center it remains a permanent task to take up newly evolving research ideas and methods, to provide a framework for new concepts, and to give original ideas a chance of being put into practice. About 10% of the research funds are reserved as "risk capital" for such ideas, the effectivity of which is regularly being assessed.

National and international collaboration

A discussion of the main areas of our research program is not complete without a reference to the international and national network of which our activities are a part.

The international standing of the Center is confirmed by the frequency of publications in international specialist journals, by reports on the Center for example in the American, French, and Italian specialist press, and also by the

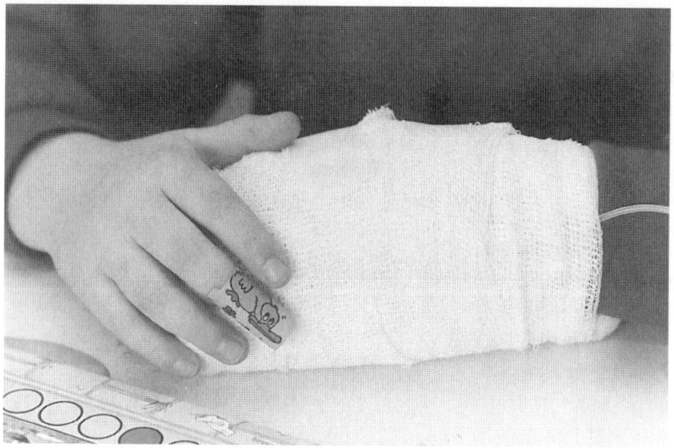

Fig. 7
Approximately 70 to 80% of the children with acute lymphoblastic leukemia, the most common form of leukemia during childhood and adolescence, can today be expected to be cured by chemotherapy. The Deutsches Krebsforschungszentrum and the Pediatric Clinic of the Heidelberg University Hospital have embarked on a clinical cooperation program with the aim of developing new therapeutic regimens

joint publication of the Center's journal "einblick" with the Imperial Cancer Research Fund (ICRF) in London. Long-standing cooperations with scientists in the United States and Japan, with the National Council for Research and Development in Israel, and with scientific institutions in many other countries serve to illustrate this international orientation. The establishment of a work unit of the French research organization INSERM (Institut de la Santé et de la Recherche Médicale) at the Deutsches Krebsforschungszentrum bears witness to the increasing attraction of our Center for international cooperations. Further support for this claim is provided by the large numbers of visiting scientists at the Center over the past 3 years (1993:168; 1992:154; 1991:167).

On the national level, the recent founding of the "Association for Clinical-Biomedical Research" (Verbund Klinisch-Biomedizinische Forschung, KBF) has marked an important step in strengthening clinically oriented research efforts. The association is designed to specifically promote cooperation projects between groups from the participating research facilities and clinical partners and to provide funds enabling scientifically active clinicians to visit member institutions.

Interested laypersons, cancer patients, and their families can obtain information about the current state of the art in the clinical application of the above-mentioned new diagnostic and therapeutic concepts from the telephone cancer information service KID (Krebsinformationsdienst). This service aims to make transparent and available the ever-growing fund of knowledge about cancer and the factors leading to the development of cancer, their relevance for new prospects in the battle against cancer, the processes of establishing and optimizing standard procedures, and the possibilities offered within our health-care system. Now, we have come full circle from basic research, clinical research and application, to man, who is at the center of all efforts.

Prof. Dr. Dres. h.c. Harald zur Hausen
Chairman and Scientific Member of the Management Board of the Deutsches Krebsforschungszentrum

A Framework for Biomedical Research in Germany

by Reinhard Grunwald

Every one is agreed: For a highly industrialized country such as Germany, research is of utmost importance. Is this view reflected in a sustained support of research, or is it paid only lipservice?

Via the direct influence on gene regulation and function, it has become possible since 1990 to carry out "gene repair," a procedure contributing to revolutionary progress in therapy. Remembering that the path from research to the development of a new medication spans 10 to 15 years, it is clear that the seed sown at the beginning of the 1990s will only bear fruit – or, indeed, prove to be barren – in the first decade of the new millenia. Are those of us in biomedical research and development already on a similar course to that of energy research, where German concepts for nuclear power plants can no longer be realized and where German engineering know-how is in danger of being lost? Prophets of doom are raising their voices: for German biomedical research and industry, they say, it is no longer 5 minutes to 12, but already 5 minutes past the hour. The American competition does not seem to take its German counterpart seriously, or indeed even recognize its existence: "Young researchers with initiative and who are prepared to take risks are scarcely to be found"; even the renowned European pharmaceutical companies "do not provide a suitable platform for biotechnology: Their 'dusty old chemists' make sure that the new graduates' enthusiasm and desire for activity is rapidly dissipated" (Art Brouwer, AMGEN Europe).

More than enough analyses have been made of the situation in Germany. Numerous good suggestions lie unheeded in the filing cabinets of the ministries that commissioned them; for example, the recommendations made in 1992 by the "Basic Research Commission" concerning the support of basic research by the Federal Ministry of Research and Technology. Good bases for decisions lie at hand. But, from the standpoint of biomedical research, decisions are not being made energetically enough.

The division of labor between Europe and the Federal Republic of Germany

Since the Maastricht Treaty, European research funding has a new basis. In contrast to the previous, almost exclusively industry-oriented, support of research, the European Union now has the possibility, according to a comprehensive general clause on research, to provide support where it judges there to be a need. The relevance of strengthening and improving the competitiveness of European commercial enterprises still remains clearly at the forefront; nonetheless, the more "independent" research, previously confined to a few areas – including nuclear physics–, is likely to increase considerably. This is already apparent in the 4th European Framework Program for the Support of Research, which shows considerable growth rate, not least in the area of biomedical research. It is to be hoped, and efforts must be made to ensure, that German research organizations and institutes make good use of the new European funding possibilities. It is thereby important that they are supported with equal skill and energy by the Federal Government, as is the case for their Italian, French, and English partners. However, the national programs should no longer be initiated without a clear view of European programs. It is important to avoid a game of mutual hide-and-seek behind the relevant European or nationally upheld subsidiarity principle in which support can only be obtained for work that is not already receiving support from another source. An idea that should be further pursued is that, via the Coordinating Agency of German Science Organizations (KoWi), not only should an information bridgehead be established in Brussels, but that from there the interplay of the national and European partners should be actively encouraged. A dead end would be met if with the Europeanization of research a revival of "experimental dinosaurs" that were previously unfinanceable at the national level was tried. What is needed is networking and collaboration in all areas, from basic research through to large-scale experiments.

The division of labor between the Federal Government and the German States

Observers from abroad are somewhat surprised to see how the Germans are increasingly frustrating their own efforts. Does it make sense, one is asked in the USA, to have 16 cultural ministries in Germany? Those in the know can surely make positive claims for decentralization, likewise for regionalization and for the preservation of self-supporting traditions. But faced with the question of whether it makes sense, for example, to have 17 laws – including the federal law – regulating travel expenses, or to have a collective agreement for employees which, in the meantime, could hardly have become more absurd (the detailed regulations go so far as to pertain to individual crew members of river dredgers), then one has to answer with a definite "no". We are also experiencing the after-effects of the controversy surrounding the politics of nuclear technology. The attempts of the politicians to please as many people as possible meant that important demands made by scientists were ignored, purely because they appeared to be unpopular. This is also true in the areas of biotechnology and genetic engineering, and in relation to the need for animal experiments. The fact that many contemporary therapies – modern heart surgery is but one – would not exist were it not for prior animal experiments is slow to sink in, despite intensive efforts on the part of science to inform; and, in comparison to their international competitors, the scientists are already subjected to a host of controls and reports. The simplification of the genetic engineering law which was recently passed would not have been necessary were it not for the over-zealous regulations prescribed in the original young law.

What is to be done?

A foremost and decisive element for research is that the basis for a good education in Germany is maintained and improved. At present, the "competition to attract the best" is largely overshadowed by the efforts to fend off the massive onrush of students. This is also true in biomedical research which has to rapidly define and pursue new goals. The education of a highly qualified young generation of scientists is clearly an "extremely important asset for the community" in the sense of the rules for professional entry drawn up by the Federal Constitutional Court, which enable access to the highest-level education to be limited to the best qualified. The impetus necessary to change the univer-sity regulations has to come predominantly from the individual German states.

Research in two worlds – Commercial versus government-supported research

In Germany there is a traditional division between commercial, particularly industrial, research, and the government-supported research sector. Funding of research that does not aim to serve an immediate application is a matter for the government. Everything that is application-oriented and can bring commercial profit is the domain of industry. Since the pharmaceutical industry in Germany developed from the chemical industry, and since "biological upstarts" like AMGEN and GENENTECH are practically nonexistent here, the disadvantages of this "research in two worlds" are sorely felt: As long as the industrial research laboratories were concerned mainly with analyzing and synthesizing new materials, transfer from the laboratories into production was possible within the one firm. Only in exceptional cases were external purchases necessary in addition. Materials not developed internally were regarded as dangerous and as "not invented here". The businessmen's argument suggested itself: "Why didn't our own expensive research effort come up with that?" In the USA in particular, but also in Japan, a different division of labor has emerged. Research divisions within individual companies have declined, while, at the same time, cooperations

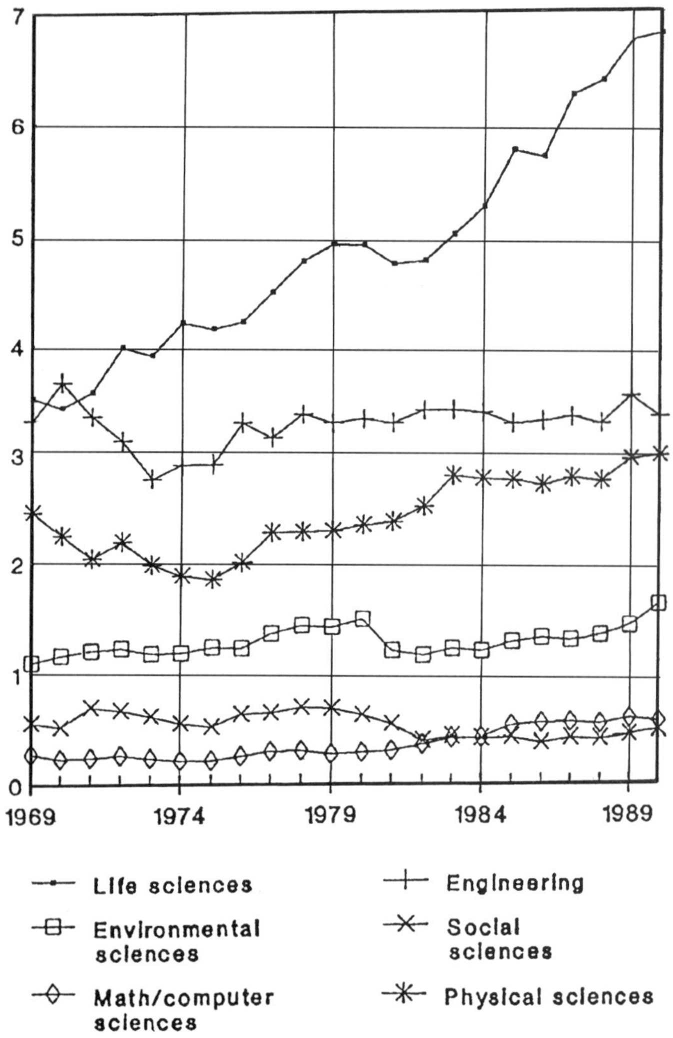

NOTE: Research includes both basic and applied. Fields not included in this figure collectively accounted for $1.1 billion (4.9 percent) of all federally funded research in 1990. Figures were converted to constant 1982 dollars using the GNP Implicit Price Deflator. 1990 figures are estimates.

SOURCE: National Science Foundation, *Federal Funds for Research and Development, Detailed Historical Tables: Fiscal Years 1955-1990* (Washington, DC: 1990), table 25; and National Science Foundation, *Selected Data on Federal Funds for Research and Development: Fiscal Years 1989, 1990 and 1991* (Washington, DC: December 1990), table 1.

Fig. 8
National Science Foundation figures on research financed by federal funds in the United States. The graph shows the development from 1969 to 1989 (in billion US dollars)

with university institutes and non-university research centers have been extended. German companies have taken up the scheme and, since the 1970s and especially 1980s, to a large extent they have transferred their biologically oriented pharmaceutical research particularly to the USA. What is most painful is not the sensation-causing award of large individual research grants made to US-American research institutes by Swiss and German companies, but far more the exodus from Germany of this extremely promising research itself. If one speaks to representatives of the German pharmaceutical industry, one rapidly learns of the efforts made to attract them to potential locations in America. They are wooed by regional representatives – sometimes even the mayor or governor – whereas in Germany they receive no encouragement. This is, of course, not the only reason for the exodus: The US market is by far the largest pharmaceutical market, and it is clearly an advantage to manufacture where one wants to sell, and likewise to do research where one wants to manufacture. However, pharmaceutical companies act internationally and particularly their research could be located anywhere in the world.

This awkward situation has been exacerbated by the hesitancy of government-funded research to become more actively involved in the application oriented sector. In fact both sides were rather inflexible: Industry clung for a long time to the model of contract re-

Fig. 9
In a Delphi Study published in 1993 experts assessed the quality of German research and development with respect to other countries. The United States is seen as being far ahead in the fields of medicine and life sciences (German Federal Ministry for Research and Technology, German Delphi Report on Trends in Science and Technology)

International Comparison of the Research and Development Levels

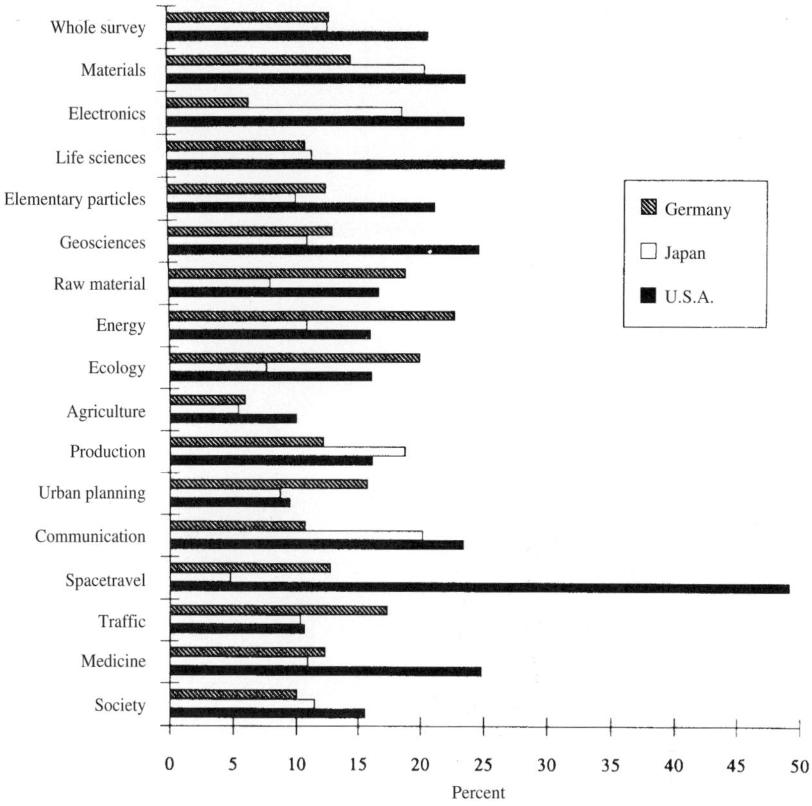

search and to attempts to use government-funded research institutes as extensions of the work benches in their own laboratories. This concept of simultaneous engineering across institutional borderlines has to be practiced in Germany – perhaps the Genome Project can become a good model for such a joint activity involving groups from industry, universities and other research centers and agencies.

The necessary course of action is clear for all to see: By means of a regular dialog at all levels, one needs to encourage feedback effects between the commercial sector and the government-funded research areas. Although on the one hand it is not sufficient for boards of directors to meet for "strategy discussions," individual collaborations between laboratories alone can be equally unproductive. What needs to become standard practice is the selective exchange of personnel and the presentation of results for the other partner – for example, in the form of workshops covering subjects of mutual interest or, even more attractive, joint projects. The new generation of young scientists has a right to adequate employment. It would be absurd and economically dangerous to let these well-trained young people go to work for our competitors abroad, and have them make there the discoveries for which they were educated in Germany. The aim of our cooperation politics must be to produce "wanderers between the worlds". The plea for a flexible scientific career has thus far fallen on deaf ears in Germany. Why shouldn't we have far more part-time lecturers in the universities whose other professional activities are in the commercial sector? And why shouldn't a great many more managers in industry be active in the government – funded research area? To realize this, one naturally needs a set of rules different from the existing law on sideline occupations. Carl Djerassi has made corresponding suggestions for the U.S.A. The privilege of patent law according to which an individual professor can himself decide whether or not to let patent his discovery should be replaced by a set of rules under which the university becomes owner of the discovery, including, of course, an appropriate share of the revenues for the inventor(s). Some successful schemes of this type are already practiced, for example, by the Max-Planck Society and at the Deutsches Krebsforschungszentrum: The income from externally exploiting the invention is distributed in three equal parts to the inventor, his institute, and the society or research center. This

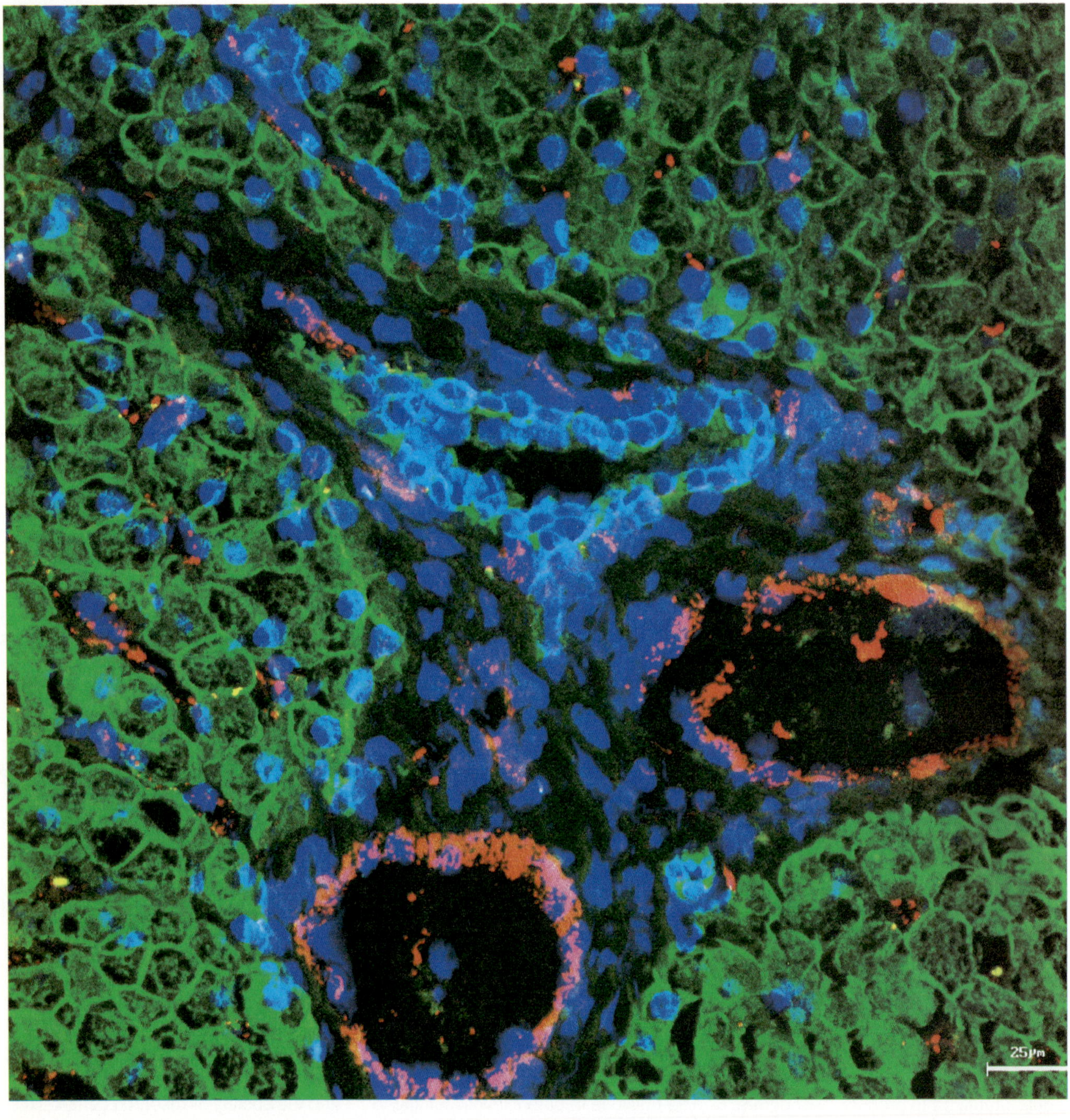
25µm

ensures a fairer representation of interests in a procedure which aims to encourage the exploitation of research results. The organizations assigned to look after the exploitation, Garching Innovation for the Max-Planck Society and the patent departments of the Fraunhofer Society and of a growing number of universities, should be used more intensively to further develop the dialog with the commercial sector. On a regional scale, the existing collaboration of universities and research centers with chambers of industry and commerce could be extended. Selective information events could improve the cooperation between the government-funded and commercial research areas.

Deutsches Krebsforschungszentrum

The problems and potential solutions outlined above are all encountered in the microcosm which is the operational level of the Deutsches Krebsforschungszentrum.

Funding

Since the government funding of institutions is no longer growing to match the increase in their tasks, project financing has become ever more important: Additional funding goes not to the Deutsches Krebsforschungszentrum as a whole, but is used to support certain individual activities. In this the European Union is taking on an increasingly important role, whereas support from the Federal Ministries and from the German Research Society (DFG) is tending rather to stagnate. As far as support through cooperations with industry is concerned, the Deutsches Krebsforschungszentrum sees good potential especially in relation to small and medium-sized firms. Here, too, the process of Europeanization is beginning to make itself more strongly felt. Cooperations with firms from abroad have increased significantly in number and value. The Center attaches particular importance to its collaboration with the Institut National de la Santé et de la Recherche Médicale (INSERM), the French medical research organization. The first INSERM unit outside France began work in 1993 at the Center under the leadership of the Belgian Professor Jean Rommelaere. It is jointly financed by INSERM and the Deutsches Krebsforschungszentrum. Another traditionally very important collaboration is that with the National Council for Research and Development (NCRD) of Israel, and, with growing importance of late, with the German-Israeli Foundation for Scientific Research and Development (GIF). Collaborations with the USA, in particular with the National Institutes of Health, especially with the National Institute of Cancer, but also with universities, have always been of great significance for the Deutsches Krebsforschungszentrum.

By introducing new forms of collaboration the Center hopes not only to encourage synergy effects, but also to tap new sources of funding. For example, joint projects involving non-university research centers and university hospitals have been initiated by the Association for Clinical-Biomedical Research (Klinisch-Biomedizinischer Verbund, KBF), itself co-founded in part by the Deutsches Krebsforschungszentrum. These projects are supported by funds from the Federal Ministry of Research and Technology. The clinical cooperation units, which are being jointly established by the Center, the Heidelberg University Hospital, and the Mannheim City Hospital, receive the majority of their funding from the health services.

The Deutsches Krebsforschungszentrum is concerned to obtain its financial resources not only by virtue of its existence as a National Research Center. It is successfully finding other sources of support, in which private donations represent an increasingly important part.

Personnel

A research center's most important resource is its personnel. Thus the policy of the Deutsches Krebsforschungszentrum aims to attract the best scientists, to offer them optimum working facilities, and, through intensive efforts for the up-and-coming generation, to ensure that top scientists continue to attract other top scientists to the Center.

At the most senior level, posts such as head of department are generally filled in a joint appointment procedure with the University of Heidelberg. When taking up a senior management post at the Deutsches Krebsforschungszentrum a scientist is simultaneously appointed by the state of Baden-Württemberg to a professorship at the University of Heidelberg. There, he must give a certain amount of instruction, but is otherwise given leave to carry out research at the Center. Since the appointment procedures tend to be very time-consuming, often lasting more than a year, the Deutsches Krebsforschungszentrum occasionally appoints particularly promising young scientists to temporary po-

Fig. 10
Fluorescent antibody labeling of different cell types in liver tissue – an important breakthrough in tumor diagnosis by methos of molecular biology

sitions that are not associated with a professorship, for example, to departmental head for a period of 5 years.

A whole spectrum of measures are pursued to attract and encourage the young generation into science. These begin at high school level in the form of information events, and also include practicals for the regional winners in the competition "Jugend forscht" ("Youth researches"). Many students carry out the work for their diploma theses at the Center. The support of doctoral students ranks particulary high: At present more than 200 young scientists are working on their doctoral projects at the Center. The period as a post-doc, i.e., the stage immediately following completion of the doctorate, is frequently one of the most productive phases and is also decisive for a scientist's career. Here it is decided whether the future holds a working life in science or a career in another field. The Deutsches Krebsforschungszentrum attempts to create appropriate opportunities for self-development, in particular by arranging research stays abroad. An example is the AIDS-scholarship program, which enables young scientists to spend 2 years at a renowned research center abroad and thereafter supports them for a further 3 years in Germany. At present, there are 55 post-docs working at the Center. Before a scientist is awarded a permanent contract, his work and his potential are evaluated by a "Tenure Commission" consisting of top-ranking scientists, who make recommendations to the Center's Management Board.

These personnel policies give the Deutsches Krebsforschungszentrum an unusual personnel structure. Of the present 1569 staff members, only 771 are permanent employees with the other 798 have temporary contracts. If one takes into account that technical support functions and laboratory infrastructure require good continuity in order that the necessary knowledge and skills remain available – also in matters of safety, radiation protection, biological safety, and not least animal protection – then it becomes clear that a decisive element in the flexibility is preserved by means of a carefully graded system of appointment, especially for scientists.

Performance-related allocation of resources

The distribution of resources in this system is of great importance. Space, money, and personnel must be allocated according to transparent, i.e., predictable and comprehensible, procedures. The decisive role in this is played by peer review, i.e., the assessment of experts by experts. The Forschungsschwerpunkte (Research Programs) of the Deutsches Krebsforschungszentrum are subjected to an international evaluation every 5 years. The result is supplemented by that of the biennial internal visits, in which the individual divisions present their work to the other staff at the Center. Based on these results, the Management Board, together with the Coordinators of the Research Programs, determine each year the priorities for the use of resources in the forthcoming fiscal year. There is general acceptance of this performance-related allocation of resources, which in fact has led to quite clear differences in the amounts awarded to the various units. Cross-section commissions of the Scientific Council, determined essentially by scientists, advise the Management Board on such diverse topics as allocation of staff, promotion, and financial matters, through to the procurement of equipment. These commissions have an important integrative function in that they bring the internal expert knowledge to bear as a preliminary to decision making.

Summary

The Deutsches Krebsforschungszentrum is optimistic that it will retain its flexibility in the future. The internal prerequisites for this are good: Following intensive discussions and without external pressure, the Center has modified its structure from an essentially hierarchical institute organization to a program-oriented structure based on Research Programs.

For its utilization of resources the Center has devised rules which enable it to set priorities. Finally, it is exploring various new avenues, particularly in relation to international networking and to funding. It works with a highly motivated staff who are willing to undergo a regular assessment of their work according to international standards.

Based on its broad experience of national and international collaboration, the Deutsches Krebsforschungszentrum offers numerous possibilities for cooperations both with the commercial sector and with government-funded research areas. It is willing to remain active in the front line of cancer research and expects in these efforts the full support of all those involved.

Dr. Reinhard Grunwald

Administrative Member of the Management Board of the Deutsches Krebsforschungszentrum

Mission and Structure of the Deutsches Krebsforschungszentrum

The Deutsches Krebsforschungszentrum (DKFZ) was founded in 1964 on the initiative of the Heidelberg surgeon Prof. Dr. h.c. K. H. Bauer, who died in 1978 at the age of 86. It was constituted as a foundation of public law on the decision of the Government of the State of Baden-Württemberg. Since 1975, it has been one of the major national research institutions. On the basis of § 91b of the German Basic Law, it is financed by the German Federal Government (Ministry for Education, Science, Research and Technology: 90%) and by the State of Baden-Württemberg (Ministry for Science and Research: 10%).

In accordance with its Statutes and Articles, it is the task of the Center to engage in cancer research. As a consequence of this general formulation, the question as to whether all of the Center's research projects really entail "cancer research", a term which every discipline defines differently, is a question that must be reconsidered on occasion. In a center with a multidisciplinary structure, the discussion about the contents of the research programs never ceases, and the "equilibrium of forces" must always be re-established. This balancing process is a continuous one; it is sustained by new discoveries, the importance and weighing of which must be determined in the context of the statutory objectives. The necessary balance takes into account the interests of all the scientists, who inevitably consider the problem of cancer from different methodological approaches and assign them different priorities in competition for financial resources. On the other hand, the benefit which scientists, for the solution of their research problems, gain from consultation and collaboration with a large number of experts from all other fields relevant to cancer research is exceedingly great and cannot be provided by any other organizational form.

Four years ago the Deutsches Krebsforschungszentrum was given a new structure. The former institutes were replaced by subject-oriented Research Programs, which are represented by Coordinators and are regularly limited to a period of six years. Depending on results, this period can be extended. Alongside the existing permanent divisions, temporary divisions with a time limit of, as a rule, five years have been established. The aim of this is to provide young scientists aged between 30 and 35 with an opportunity to assume responsible tasks in the management of an independent research unit. Thus, the rapid developments in cancer research are better taken into account. When a line of research turns into an essential part of the respective Research Program, the divisional head can be appointed on a permanent basis.

The new, flexible structure of the Deutsches Krebsforschungszentrum also fosters the exchange of experience among scientists of different disciplines. Moreover, it provides possibilities for a quick reorientation once a research task can be regarded as fulfilled.

The complex problems of cancer research and therapy involve the biological, natural, and social sciences. They can only be successfully tackled in close collaboration with scientists from all these disciplines on a national and international level and by the concentration of available research capacities.

In May 1994, seven years after the first one, a second meeting of all scientists occupying leading positions at the Deutsches Krebsforschungszentrum took place at Reisensburg castle. At

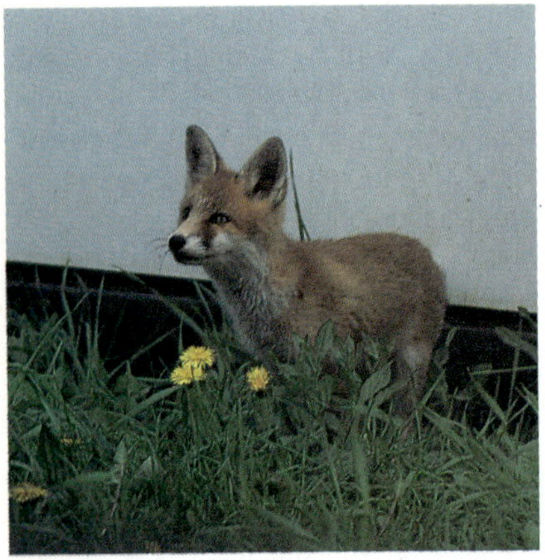

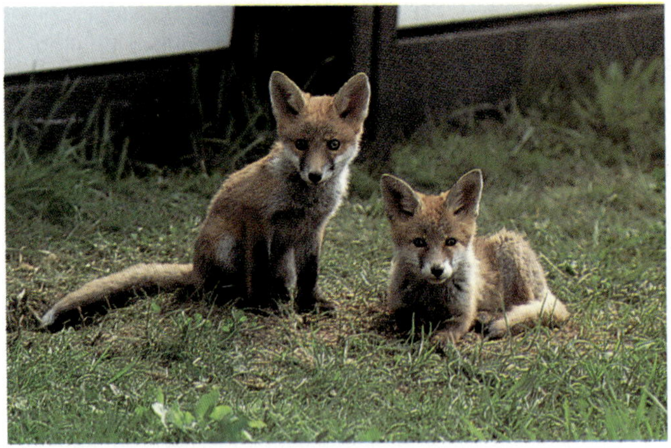

Fig. 11, 12
A vixen has set up home for her cubs under a prefab laboratory belonging to the Deutsches Krebsforschungszentrum in Heidelberg's Technology Park

this meeting, the future prospects and orientation of the Center's research program were developed and discussed. Objectives and priorities for the next decade were defined, which are presented in the introductory article by Professor Harald zur Hausen.

It is the objective of the Center's research program to make a tangible contribution to the understanding of carcinogenesis, to the identification of cancer risk factors, and to the prevention, diagnosis, and therapy of cancer. The multitude of human cancers is an indication of the difficulties of scientific analysis.

Taking into consideration the multitude of methods and approaches in cancer research, the Center's programs focus on eight multi-disciplinary priorities:

- Cell Differentiation and Carcinogenesis
- Tumor Cell Regulation
- Cancer Risk Factors and Prevention
- Diagnostics and Experimental Therapy
- Radiological Diagnostics and Therapy
- Applied Tumor Virology
- Tumor Immunology
- Bioinformatics.

In 1993, the concepts concerning joint clinical cooperation units developed in cooperation with the University Hospitals of Heidelberg/Mannheim were given concrete form. The positions of the heads of the research units at the Outpatient Clinic and at the Pediatric Clinic of the University of Heidelberg were filled in 1994. A third oncological-dermatological research unit in cooperation with Mannheim Hospitals is in preparation. This cooperation unit is planned to deal with new approaches in the treatment of skin cancer, while the units at Heidelberg University Hospitals are focused on new concepts in the diagnosis and therapy of leukemias and lymphomas.

The clinical research groups will be established at the University Clinic for a period of five years. The physicians and scientists of the Deutsches Krebsforschungszentrum will provide the clinical treatment, whereas the Clinic will provide the beds and the clinical infrastructure. The Deutsches Krebsforschungszentrum will take over any costs which are not covered by the patients' health insurances.

Research

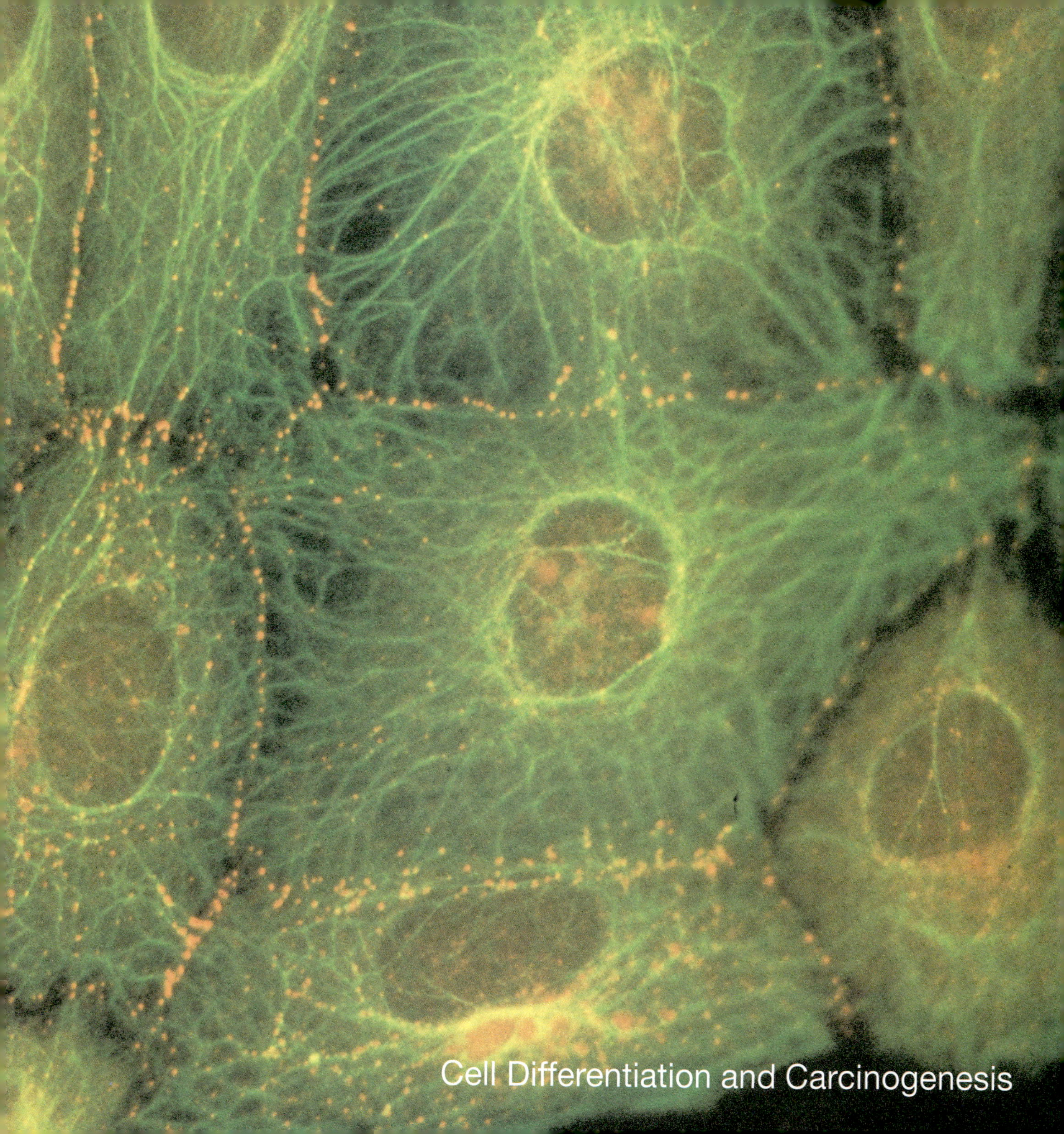
Cell Differentiation and Carcinogenesis

2

Cell Differentiation and Carcinogenesis

The confrontation of scientists in basic research with the problem of cancer has yielded a multitude of new findings and new approaches in theory and experimental research in recent years. While the selection of promising research approaches in the past tended to be somewhat fortuitous and accidental, i.e., was based on isolated observations of differences between normal and malignant cells, in recent years it has also become possible to investigate the origin, diagnosis as well as possible prevention and therapy of cancer diseases with well-defined aims, following basic principles of cell and molecular biology.

Changes in the genome or in the expression of specific genes in somatic cells are in many cases responsible for the early events of carcinogenesis, leading to fundamental disturbances in the social and growth behavior of cells. In functional terms, two different principles of tumorigenesis can be distinguished: 1) enhanced activity of oncogenes may lead to uncontrolled growth; 2) the failure of genes suppressing cell transformation, the tumor suppressor genes, may have the same effect. The research Program Cell Differentiation and Carcinogenesis therefore directs special attention at finding and analyzing those genes and their products that might play a role in carcinogenesis. Cell biological and molecular biological methods are used to find genetic probes for specific chromosome changes, for gene mutations or for integrated viral genes which may be applied in tumor diagnostics as well as possibly in the prevention of cancer, such as the identification of patients at risk.

Another line research is directed at the examination of disturbances in gene expression and in the synthesis of certain gene products. Differences in gene expression between normal and transformed cells, between resting and proliferating cells, and between cells in various states of differentiation are detected using appropriate nucleic acid probes or monoclonal antibodies against specific gene products. „Cell typing“ by the microscopic identification of marker molecules characteristic for the specific state of differentiation contributes to the correct diagnosis of tumors and in many cases allows the detection of primary and metastatic tumors as well as the identification of the initial tumor from which a metastasis has spread. In addition, the research program examines the biological function of the proteins and hormones involved in the regulation of gene expression and the growth and metastatic spread of certain kinds of cancer.

Embryonic development of an organism including the controls of cell division and tissue formation provides the master plan for the normal and healthy correlations of cell proliferation and differentiation. An understanding of these elementary life process will therefore point the way for future experimental cancer research. Consequently, a division Molecular Embryology has recently been established in the research program to study fundamental processes in embryonic development.

Coordinator of the Research Program:
Prof. Dr. Werner W. Franke

Divisions and their heads:

Cell Biology:
Prof. Dr. Werner W. Franke

Molecular Biology of the Cell I:
Prof. Dr. Günther Schütz

Molecular Biology of the Cell II:
Prof. Dr. Ingrid Grummt

Developmental Genetics:
Prof. Dr. Bernard Mechler

Cytogenetics:
Prof. Dr. Manfred Schwab

Molecular Embryology:
Dr. Christof Niehrs

Biophysics of Macromolecules:
Prof. Dr. Jörg Langowski

2.1 Cadherins and Carcinomas

by Stephan Schäfer and Werner W. Franke

Temporally and spatially controlled cell-to-cell contact sites are of fundamental importance to the embryonic development of tissues and organs and their correct functioning. Disturbed cell contact sites in the skin, due to the deposition of antibodies directed against cell adhesion structures, result for instance in the development of diseases of the pemphigus type, which are characterized by the formation of blisters in the skin. Dysfunction of cell-to-cell contact sites also causes metastasis in malignant tumor growth. Tumors are classified according to their site of origin into carcinomas (originating from epithelial tissue) and sarcomas (derived from the mesenchyme). Some of the commonest cancers, affecting the bronchi, gastrointestinal tract, urogenital tract, and epidermis (outermost layer of the skin), are carcinomas. Carcinomas originate from any epithelia or epithelium-derived organs whose cells are linked via calcium-dependent cell adhesion molecules (cadherins). A knowledge of the molecular components of cell-to-cell contact structures and the mechanisms underlying pathologically altered cell adhesion is a prerequisite to understanding a whole series of clinical pictures, notably tumor growth and the formation of secondaries.

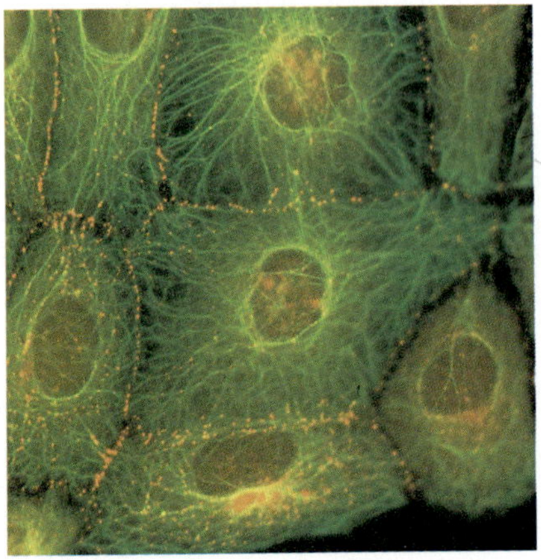

Fig. 13
The intermediary filaments (green lines) in the cytoskeleton build a complex network which embeds the nucleus in the center and is attached on the periphery to the desmosomes (orange dots) of the cell membrane

Structure and function of epithelial cell-to-cell contact sites

Mammalian tissues are classified into two main groups according to their site of genesis during embryonic development. Mesenchymal tissues (for instance connective tissue, cartilage, bone, musculature) are derived from the middle germ layer (mesoderm) of the embryo. Epithelial tissues develop from the inner and outer germ layers (ectoderm and endoderm) and consist of joined cells whose primary function is to line the outer and inner surfaces of the body (respiratory tract, gastrointestinal tract, urogenital tract) and which also make up internal organs such as the pancreas, liver, and kidneys.

Mechanical cohesion of most mesenchymal tissues is maintained indirectly via the intercellular substance between the cells. Epithelial tissues are stabilized via direct cell-to-cell contact sites, i.e. specialized regions on plasma membranes of adjacent cells that are classified in three groups on the basis of their difference in structure and function:

(1) In gap junctions, channels (connexons) permit the exchange of low molecular-weight substances between

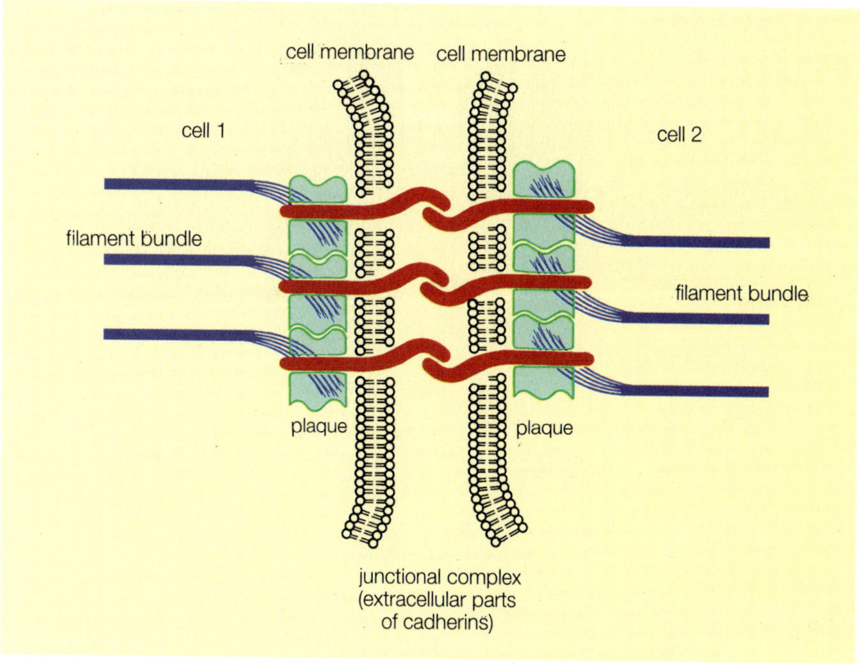

Fig. 14
Schematic representation of intercellular adherent junctions

apposed cells through their plasma membranes, resulting in functional couplings.

(2) Tight junctions form a barrier to the penetration of substances between adjacent cells, for instance in preventing the uncontrolled entry of substances from the diet into the organism by sealing the space between cells on the internal intestinal surface.

(3) The „adherens" type of cell-to-cell contact sites, which is discussed in this article, mediates mechanical adhesion between adjacent cells and is represented in epithelial tissues in the form of two subtypes, intermediate junctions and desmosomes. The common structural principle of the two types are transmembraneous proteins which belong to the family of calcium-dependent cell adhesion molecules (cadherins). They bind with their extracellular molecular domain to the cadherin domain of the adjacent cell. A plaque protein complex associated to the intracellular cadherin domain (visible as a submembraneous plaque with an electron microscope) serves to anchor filaments of the cytoskeleton (Fig. 14).

Depending on the type of membrane attachment site, intermediate junctions are described as zonula adhaerens, fascia adheraens, or, punctum adhaerens. Classical cadherins (i. e. E-cadherin and N-cadherin) guarantee cell cohesion by homotypic association of their extracellular domains. They are intracellularly coupled to actin filaments via an anchor protein complex comprising catenins, vinculin, and a-actinin.

Desmosomes are disc-like membrane contact sites with a diameter of 0,1-0,5 micrometer, containing the two desmosomal cadherins desmocollin and desmoglein. While the structure and size of desmocollin is similar to that of classical cadherins (molecular size of approximately 750 amino acids), desmoglein has more than a thousand amino acids. The desmosomal anchor protein complex consisting of plakoglobin and desmoplakin serves as an anchoring site for intermediate filaments with a diameter (7-12 nanometers) between that of actin filaments (5-6 nanometers) and that of microtubuli (20-25 nanometers). Plakoglobin is the only plaque protein occurring in both intermediate junctions and desmosomes.

The epidermis (surface layer of the skin), a tissue subjected to considerable mechanical strain, has a particularly large number of cell-to-cell contact sites. More than 50 percent and more of the plasma membrane area is occupied by desmosomes. The epidermis is a multilayer keratinizing squamous epithelium, i.e. it consists of multiple layers of squamous cells piled up on each other. The keratinizing upper layers (stratum corneum) protect the body from mechanical, chemical and radiation impacts. The hardly penetrable horny layer protects from pathogens. Cells transformed into horny flakes are peeled off the surface and are continuously reproduced by the germinative layers (stratum germinativum).

The single-layer cylindrical epithelium lining the gastrointestinal tract mainly consists of so-called brush border cells (enterocytes) which are responsible for

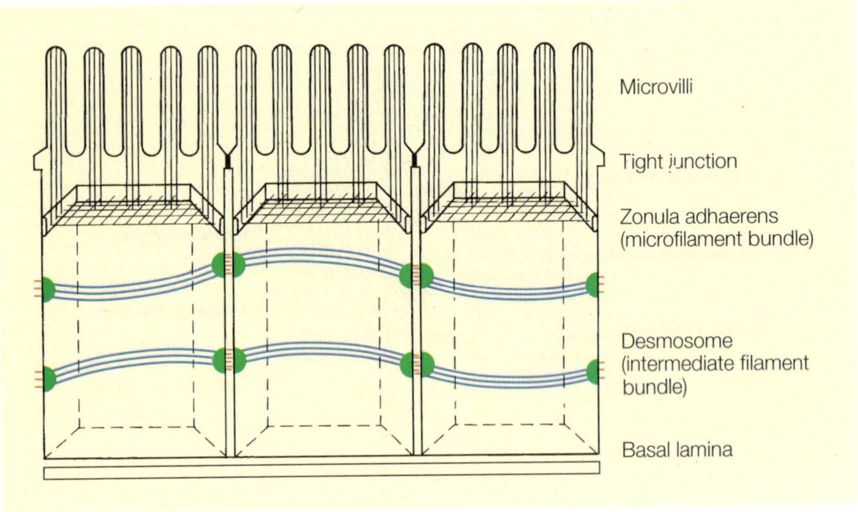

Fig. 15
Intercellular junctions linking epithelial cells in the small intestine

the secretion of digestive fluids and the uptake of food. Following a short life of 0.5 to 3 days they are expelled into the intestine (daily epithelial cell loss in humans amounts to approximately 250 grams). Stem cells in the lower region of the crypts, i.e. small, pitlike tubular recesses of the intestinal epithelium in the intestinal mucous membrane, replenish the supply of short-lived brush border cells by continuous reproduction.

While the two cell adhesion and filament systems are similarly located in the multilayer epithelium of the epidermis, they are organized differently in the epithelial cells lining the gastrointestinal tract. Below the tight junction a zonula adhaerens (intermediate junction) encloses the upper cell pole in a belt-like manner. The actin filament network interlinked with the cadherin belt serves as an anchoring site for actin filaments of microvilli. By contrast, the desmosomal intermediate filament complex appears as a system of mechanical struts running through all cells to protect them from the shear forces arising during intestinal peristalsis (Fig. 15).

The distinct functions of basal, proliferating cells on the one hand and suprabasal cells eventually forming horny flakes of the epidermis on the other hand correlate with the expression pattern of classical cadherins, with P-cadherin being restricted to basal cell layers and E-cadherin occurring in all cell layers.

Three genotypically distinct desmogleins and desmocollins have been identified among desmosomal cadherins. The different isoforms of desmosomal cadherins show tissue type specific expression patterns. Desmoglein-2 and desmocollin-2 are formed in all tissues containing desmosomes. Multilayer epithelia also contain the desmoglein and desmocollin isoforms 1 and 3.

Regulation of cadherin-mediated cell adhesion

The binding of a cadherin molecule to a cadherin molecule of an adjacent cell can be seen as an association of two binding domains with a complementary steric structure and loading pattern. Calcium appears to promote the formation of the adhesive structure by deposition in calcium-binding sites of the extracellular domain. In cell cultures calcium withdrawal from the culture medium results in the dissolution of cell-to-cell contact sites and a separation of cells.

Intracellular binding of cadherins to submembranous plaque proteins is a further important prerequisite to the establishment of functioning cell-to-cell contact sites. Plaque proteins connect the intracellular domains of the cadherins to the microfilament cytoskeleton and indirectly enhance the association of extracellular binding domains. In cell cultures withdrawal of plaque proteins from cell-to-cell contact sites by the artificial introduction of cadherins without functioning extracellular domains suppresses the formation of both intermediate junctions and desmosomes.

Classical cadherins form complexes with catenins via their cytoplasmatic domains, which connect to the actin filament network. Catenin function can be controlled by chemical modification. Cell culture experiments indicate that the adhesion of phosphoric acid (phosphorylation) to tyrosine residues results in a dissociation of the cadherin-catenin complex from the actin filament network with a simultaneous loss of the cell-to-cell contact sites.

The number of cadherin molecules in the cell membrane is the crucial factor in determining the stability of cell contact sites. Reduction in the cadherin content by decreased synthesis or increased breakdown weakens cell-to-cell contact sites. For instance, the transformation of tightly joined ectodermal epithelial cells into loosely joined mesodermal cells during early mammalian embryogenesis is associated with the loss of E-cadherin. Conversely fibroblasts which do not establish extensive cell-to-cell contact sites under normal cell culture conditions form compact colonies with extensive cell-to-cell contact sites following artificial introduction of E-cadherin.

Finally the splitting-off of the extracellular binding domain by proteases may also result in reduced cell adhesiveness. Organ cultures from embryonic retinal tissue lose cell-to-cell contact sites during retinal differentiation by cleavage and release of the extracellular N-cadherin domains.

The role of cadherins in tumorigenesis and the formation of secondaries

In regenerative epithelial tissues, such as the epidermis or intestinal mucosa, a stem cell population capable of division provides the permanent replacement of cells lost due to normal function. A system comprising cell cycle regulator proteins in the cell nucleus and cytoplasm provides the temporal coordination of processes involved in cell division. The growth cycle of stem cells is adapted to cell loss by integration and implementation of stimulatory and inhibitory signals from the extracellular environment. Uncontrolled growth is the cause of malignant tumors, the development of which can be illustrated by the example of carcinoma of the colon. Epithelial growth is locally decoupled and cell replacement from the malignantly multiplying cell population exceeds the loss of differentiated cells. Mucosal growth results in the formation of polyps. Normal (intestinal) epithelium grows on a basal membrane made up of a collagen fiber network with deposited glycoproteins which functions as a cell pad. Carcinoma cells locally dissolve the basal membrane and invade the subepithelial tissue (aggressive infiltration of the environment). Invasion into the blood and lymph vessels of the intestinal wall finally results in the spread of tumor cells to other organs and the development of secondary growths.

Cell-to-cell contact sites are important for the development and spreading of malignant epithelial tumors in various respects. Adenomatous polyposis coli (APC) is a hereditary disease in which a mutation of the APC gene frequently results in the development of colon cancer from multiple colon polyps. The APC gene product is capable of binding β-catenin and as a complex with β-catenin possibly transmits growth inhibitory signals.

Plaque proteins (catenins, α-actinin, vinculin) act as tumor suppressors. The term „tumor suppressor gene“ was originally coined from the observation that tumor cells lost their malignant properties following experimental fusion with normally multiplying cells, showing that „tumor suppressors“ from the genome of healthy cells normalized cell growth. This led to the identification of a whole series of genes with tumor-suppressing properties.

The PC9 cell line derived from a lung carcinoma does not form α-catenin and, despite the presence of E-cadherins, exhibits a profoundly downregulated cell aggregation profile. Experimental reconstruction of the cell's a-catenin content restitutes epithelial growth morphology. Breast cancers presenting a loss of α-catenin show diffuse growth without the formation of cell-to-cell contact sites between the carcinoma cells.

On the basis of the expression of classical cadherins carcinomas can be classified in four groups: in addition to cancers with a normal cadherin distribution pattern there are cancers with locally reduced cadherin formation. Complete cadherin loss and the formation of aberrant, nonfunctioning cadherin molecules lead to a loss of cell adhesion. This, in turn, results in undifferentiated cell morphology, which means that originally columnar ephitelium cells take on the shape of spindles. Carcinomas of the stomach with nonfunctioning E-cadherin diffusely invade adjacent tissue and are more likely to spread via the blood and lymph vessels.

All carcinomas studied so far produce desmoglein-2 and desmocollin-2. Desmoglein-1 only occurs in cancers of the squamous epithelia while desmoglein-3 is also formed in adenocarcinomas which originate from the glandular epithelium. The expression pattern of desmosomal cadherins in carcinomas is similar to that of the tissue of origin, meaning that the unknown site of origin of a primary tumor can in theory be identified by examining the desmoglein / desmocollin pattern in metastatic tissue.

Despite the cited examples of disturbed intercellular adhesion, the majority of carcinomas produce compact tumors with well developed intermediate junctions and desmosomes. Further studies are required to find out the mechanism by which cancer cells leave the primary tumor via the blood or lymph vessels to form remote metastases.

Dr. Stephan Schäfer
Prof. Dr. Werner W. Franke
Division of Cell Biology

In cooperation with

Priv.-Doz. Dr. Roland Moll
Institute of Pathology,
University of Mainz

Prof. Dr. Heinz Höfler
Institute of Pathology,
GSF-Research Center for Environment and Health,
Neuherberg, Munich

Selected Publications

Schwarz, M.M., Owaribe, K., Kartenbeck, J., Franke, W.W.: Desmosomes and Hemidesomsomes: Constitutive Molecular Components. Ann. Rev. Cell Biol. 6, 461–491 (1990)

Becker, K.-F., Atkinson, M., Reich, U., Huang, H.-H., Nekarda, H., Siewert, J.R., Höfler H.: Exon Skipping in the E-Cadherin Gene Transcript in Metastatic Human Gastric Carcinomas. Human Mol. Genetics 2, 803–804 (1993)

Moll, R., Mitze, M., Frixen, U.H., Birchmeier, W.: Differential Loss of E-Cadherin Expression in Infiltrating Ductal and Lobular Breast Carcinomas. American J. Pathol. 143, 1731–1742 (1993)

Schäfer, S., Trojanovsky, S.M., Heid, H., Eshkind, L.G., Koch, P.J., Franke W.W.: Cytoskeletal Architecture and Epithelial Differentiation: Molecular Determinants of Cell Interaction and Cytoskeletal Filament Anchorage. C. R. Acad. Sci. Paris, Sciences de la vie/Life sciences 316, 1316–1323 (1993)

Schäfer, S., Koch, P.J., Franke, W.W.: Identification of the Ubiquitous Human Desmoglein, Dsg2, and the Expression Catalogue of the Desmoglein Subfamily of Desmosomal Cadherins. Exp. Cell Res. 201, 391–399 (1994)

2.2 Drosophila as an Animal Model System for Identifying Tumor Suppressor Genes and Analyzing Their Function

by Dennis Strand, Istvan Török, and Bernard M. Mechler

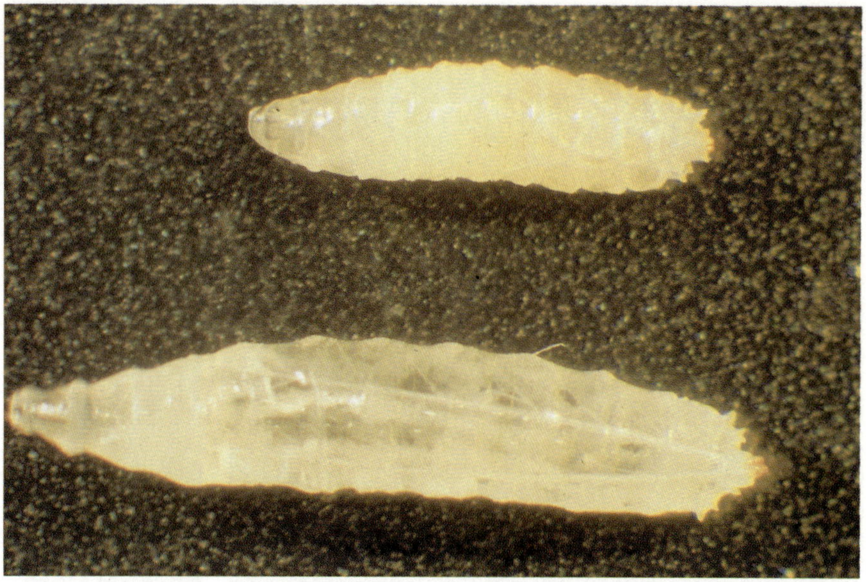

Fig. 16
Wild-type fruit fly (Drosophila) larva (above) and a giant larva containing a defective tumor suppressor gene – the first to be genetically identified and cloned

Cancer is generally considered as a failure in the normal progression of differentiation. As a result, the cancer cells escape the mechanism controlling normal growth, and they proliferate. When the growth of cancer cells reaches a critical threshold, complex syndromes arise and lead ultimately to the death of the organism.

A genetic basis for cancer is now firmly established and includes the discovery of proto-oncogenes, whose activation or altered expression promote cell division, and tumor suppressor genes, whose inactivation or loss disrupt the process of normal differentiation and subsequent death and endow the cell with a proliferative advantage.

In human, cancer is viewed as a dynamic process driven by the accumulation of a series of genetic alterations rather than by the occurrence of a single genetic defect (a noteworthy exception of this, however, is the retinoblastoma syndrome involving defects at a single genetic locus on chromosome 13q). Each genetic alteration confers a genetically altered daughter cell with a selective growth advantage, but in order to become fully malignant a cell must sustain damages in several cancer genes which should occur in a relatively preferred order. The first changes spur the growth of the cell by deregulating intracellular mechanisms of growth control whereas the later changes impair homeostatis, affecting such processes as hormonal communication, immune surveillance, regulation of angiogenesis, tumor invasion and metastasis, and result in the expansion of the number of tumor cells and their dispersion in the whole organism.

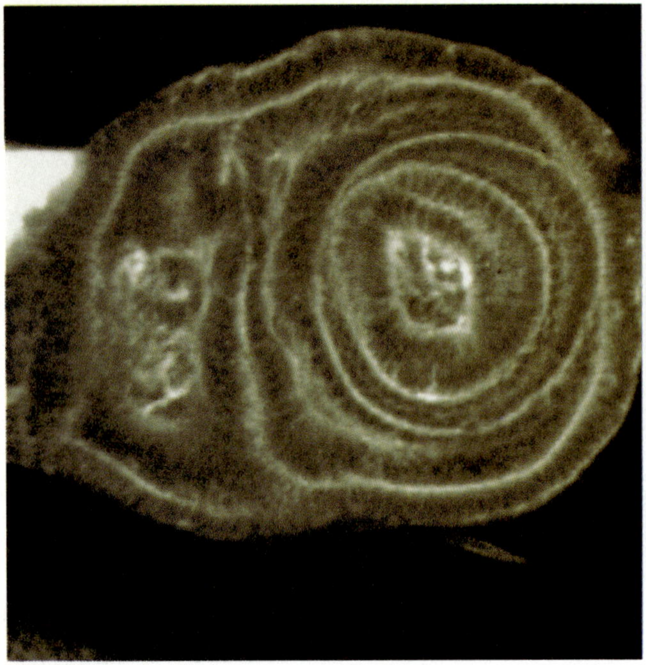

Fig. 17
Pupation of Drosophila larva is regulated by hormones via the imaginal disk. The figure depicts a normal imaginal disk

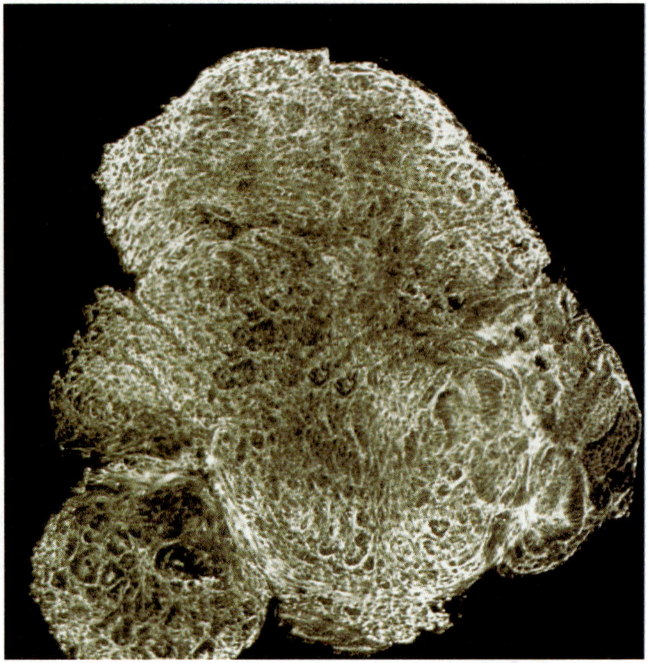

Fig. 18
The imaginal disk is infiltrated with tumors and no longer functions properly

Identification of some of the human genes associated with the early onset of tumor development has been successfully achieved by analyzing mutations in the germ lines of persons with well recognized forms of hereditary cancer. Eight human cancer predisposing genes have been isolated so far, and for 10 other heritable cancer states the relevant genes have been mapped but not cloned. However, the number of cancer predisposing genes may be much larger, with present estimates of about 50 or more. The identification of these genes is presently hampered by their poor penetrance and the difficulty to map them on precise genetic loci. Furthermore, other human cancer genes may never be identified as inheritable traits because germline mutations at some sites may be lethal to embryos. Thus it is important to study genes controlling cell proliferation and tumorigenesis in an animal model system more suitable for genetic investigations.

The importance of mutations in cancer formation has been genetically well documented in the fruitfly Drosophila. Over the past two decades Drosophila has become the organism of choice for molecular and genetic investigations of eukaryotic biology. Its emergence as an animal model system is closely related to the rapid advances in recombinant DNA technology and a wealth of knowledge in classical genetics and embryology accumulated over more then 80 years of exponentially growing studies. More than 100 000 scientific articles have been published on Drosophila since the first recorded publication dating from 1684. Further advantages of Drosophila are the size and complexity of its genome which are intermediate between those of prokaryotes and mammals, its relatively short life span and ease of rearing in the laboratory. Such a combination makes Drosophila particularly good for investingating the genes which control cell proliferation and differentiation, for evaluating in the whole organism the importance of these genes in terms of cancer, and for elucidating the function of these genes. In Drosophila, more than 60 genes controlling excessive cell proliferation have been so far identified by mutations.

When and where do tumors arise in Drosophila

The fruitfly has two distinct phases of development combined in one life cycle: embryonic development, which gives rise to larval organization, and larval-pupal development, which produces the definitive adult organization following a breakdown of larval tissues during metamorphosis. During these two developmental phases, Drosophila displays a very precise program of cell proliferation. Embryogenesis begins with a phase of rapid nuclear divisions. Thirteen rapid cycles of synchronous nuclear divisions occur at approximately 10-min intervals. Then the nuclei migrate to the cortex and becomes cellularized at the interphase of cycle 14. From this developmental phase the cell cycle lengthens and a few divisions occur in complex mitotic domains according to a specific temporal program which is coordinated by a complex pattern of gene expression and leads to the morphogenesis of specific tissues within the embryo. After 24 hours, the embryo hatches and contains about 50 000 cells which can be subdivided into two classes, those that form the larval tissues and grow by expansion of the cell volume with endoreplication of DNA in the absence of mitoses, and those that will constitute the imaginal cells and form the adult organism. These cells resume their proliferation from the middle of the first larval instar and continue to divide throughout the three larval instars up to the beginning of metamorphosis, arresting as terminal differentiation occurs. In the adult, only the germline cells and their associated gonadial tissues are actively dividing.

Manifestion of cell overproliferation can become noticeable at the end of both major periods of cell proliferation: late embryogenesis and larval-pupal transition phase. Mutations giving rise to tumorous growth have been identified at the end of either one or the other period of cell proliferation but it is much easier to detect mutations giving rise to tumors occurring at the end of the larval development. In particular, the mutant animals are easily recognized because the growth of the tumorous tissues is accompanied by developmental arrest. As a consequence, the larval life of the mutant animals is prolonged over several days and the tumorous tissues can reach a considerable mass which is readily observed upon dissection. Currently, mutations giving rise to tissue overgrowth during larval development have been identified in more than 60 different genes.

The tissues which can become tumorous are made of cells from the presumptive adult organs which are actively dividing during the larval development. These tissues are 1) the larval brain hemispheres that will constitute the adult optic centers; 2) the imaginal discs that will form the adult cuticle; 3) the hematopoietic organs, and 4) the germline.

Drosophila tumors can be classified into two broad categories: neoplasia and hyperplasia. The difference between both types of overgrowth is particularly visible in the case of the imaginal discs which form distinct groups of undifferentiated cells present in the larvae and give rise to various parts of the adult cuticle during metamorphosis. Throughout the larval life, the imaginals are growing and forming folded sacs of epithelia which are made of a monolayer of columnar cells.

In the imaginal discs neoplasia is characterized by a massive proliferation of cells which completely disrupt the mono-layered epithelial structure of the discs. The tumorous cells lose their cell polarity and expand in all directions giving rises to amorphic masses of tissues. By constrast, hyperplasia is characterized by proliferation of the imaginal cells which maintain, however, a columnar shape with a normal apical-basal polarity. During the prolonged larval life the hyperplastic discs can grow to several times their normal size and keep a folding pattern.

How many genes can cause tissue overgrowth in Drosophila?

All the genes so far identified in Drosophila are recessive determinants of tissue overgrowth and are classified as tumor suppressor genes, for their normal function is to control cell proliferation and/or cell differentiation. In Drosophila demonstration of tumor suppression has been shown by introducing an intact allele of a cloned tumor suppressor gene into the genome of homozygous mutated animals and by showing restoration of a normal growth and development.

Mutagenesis screens and analysis of spontaneously occurring mutations have allowed the identification of a series of genes controlling tissue over-

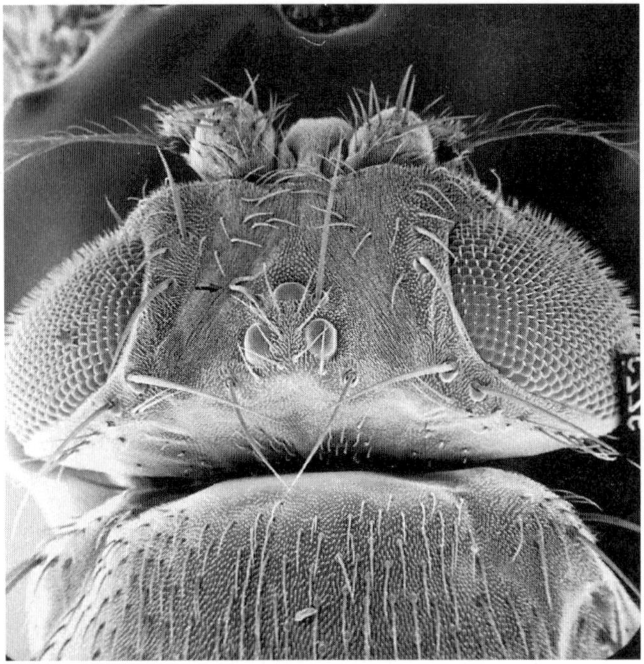

Fig. 19 a
The result of a mutation late in the development of the insect: deformed ocellar setae on the head of the fly (scanning electron microscopic image, 1:130 magnification)

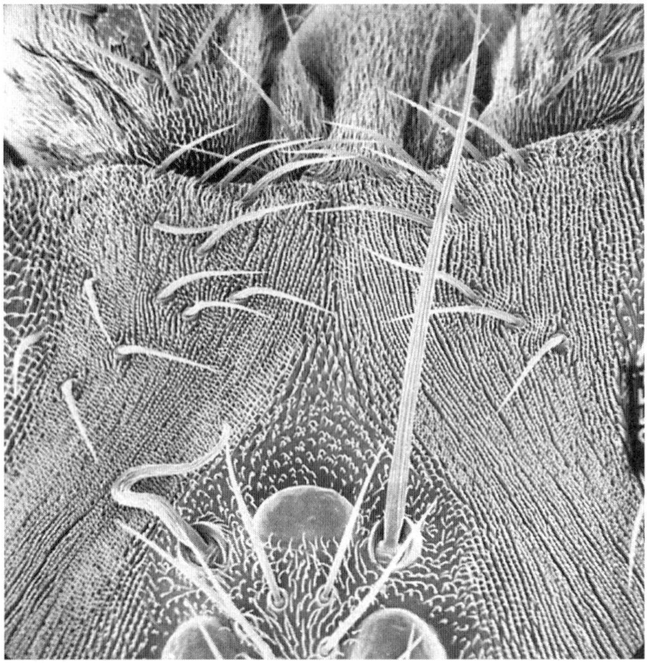

Fig. 19 b
1:390 magnification

growth. More than 60 genes causing tissue overgrowth are presently known in Drosophila. Their identification has occurred erratically over the last 25 years and, until recently, no systematic search for mutations giving rise to tumors has been undertaken. However, the recent development of synthetic P-element transposons has provided new tools for gene tagging and direct molecular cloning of genes of interest. Through this apporach a saturation mutagenesis of the second chromosome of Drosophila has been conducted by our cooperation partner at the Biological Research Center of the Hungarian Academy of Sciences at Szeged and has led to the identification of 17 new tumor suppressor genes bringing to 23 the total number of known tumor suppressor genes on the second chromosome. Based on the number of mutant alleles recovered for each gene, it is possible to estimate the total number of tumor suppressor genes to be more than 100. These findings indicate that numerous genes may prevent cell overproliferation during the development of Drosophila.

One of the major efforts of our group is to molecularly isolate these genes in collaboration with other European groups organized in an EC-network.

Oho31, a new tumor suppressor gene involved in nuclear cytoplasmic interaction

From the collection of P-element induced mutations, we have successfully cloned the oho31 (overgrown hematopoietic organs at chromosomal position 31A) gene. Mutations in the oho-31 gene cause overgrowth of the hematopoietic organs and excessive cell proliferation in the imaginal discs during larval development. The oho31 gene encodes a protein of 522 amino acids displaying strong similarities with the sequence of three other proteins. Sequence similarity is extensive with the

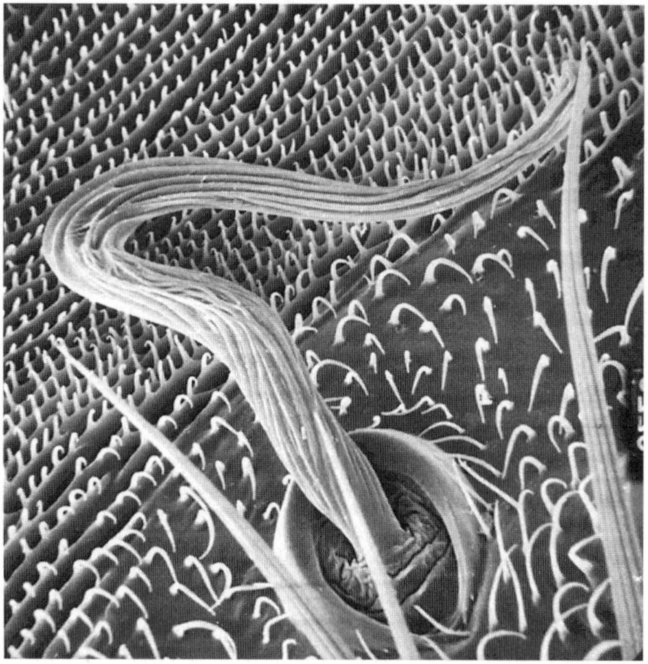

Fig. 19c
1:600 magnification

yeast SRP1 protein identified as a suppressor of temperature-sensitive mutations in RNA polymerase 1 as well as with two mammalian proteins, namely, the human RCH1 and mouse mSRP1 proteins which were recently identified through their interaction with the RAG-1 recombination-activating protein. The sequence similarity extends over the entire length of the four proteins and is more pronounced in their central region made of eight degenerate 42-amino-acid repeats. Spatio-temporal analysis of the expression of the oho31 protein revealed that this protein is usually present in the cytoplasm, but migrates rapidly in the nucleus, apparently at the beginning of each mitosis. In yeast, the homolog to the oho31 protein, the SRP1 protein, was recently found to interact with proteins of the nucleopore complexes as well as with other non-related proteins, indicating the SRP1 protein may be involved in RNA or protein transport between the nucleus and the cytoplasm or conversely. Our findings indicate that the disruption of a shuttling system between the cytoplasm and the nucleus can be the cause of tumor formation. This represents a novel mechanism in growth regulation.

Elucidation of the function of the lethal(2)giant larvae tumor suppressor gene

The other major objective of our group is to elucidate the function of the lethal (2)giant larvae (l(2)gl) gene, the first genetically identified and molecularly cloned tumor suppressor gene and to characterize the proteins which specifically interact with the l(2)gl gene product.

Homozygous l(2)gl mutations lead to neoplastic transformation of the neuroblasts and ganglion mother cells of the adult optic centers in the larval brain and neoplasia of the imaginal discs. In the mutant animals, these neoplasms first become visible at the end of the third larval instar, although an abnormal pattern of growth can be detected earlier during larval development. These neoplasms continue to grow during the prolonged life of the mutant larvae and the neoplastic brain hemispheres and imaginal discs can reach several times their normal size.

Using techniques of molecular biology, we have cloned the l(2)gl gene and subjected it to molecular analysis.This approach has unequivocally shown that the tumorous phenotype results from a lack of gene function. Moreover, we have been able to prevent tumorigenesis by introducing a normal copy of this gene into the genome of l(2)gl deficient animals. Such successful "rescue" experiments demonstrate that the l(2)gl gene has characteristics of a tumor suppressor gene.

The l(2)gl gene was shown to encode a protein of 1161 amino acids in length with an estimated molecular weight of 127 kdaltons and therefore designated as p127. Immunohistochemical and biochemical investigations have revealed that the p127 protein participates to a cytoskeleton network which is dispersed in the cytoplasm and undercoats the plasma membranes at lateral junctions. Gel filtration techniques have further shown that the p127 protein is always recovered in high molecular weight complexes of sizes ranging between 500 and 1000 kdaltons in molecular weight. These complexes are made of homo-oligomerized p127 protein, but also contain other proteins which specifically bind to p127. In particular, the p127 complexes display *in vitro* a strong autokinase activity, phosphorylating specifically p127 at serine residues and resulting from the presence of a tightly associated kinase. Purification of several proteins bound specifically to the p127 has been achieved by two different procedures of affinity chromatography. Among the most abundant proteins present in these complexes, we have first concentrated our efforts on a protein displaying an apparent molecular weight of 200 kdaltons. Proteolytic peptides of this protein have been isolated and microsequenced. This analysis has revealed that this protein corresponds to nonmuscle myosin type II heavy chain, a component of the cytoplasmic network of microfilaments which contains also actin and plays important roles in cell locomotion, cell shape and structure. Further confirmation of the direct interaction between p127 and myosin was obtained by showing that 32P-labelled p127 protein can specifically bind to immobilized myosin proteins. Present investigations are directed towards the identification of the other components of the p127 complexes and the elucidation of their function in the regulation of cell proliferation.

Recent isolation of a human homolog to l(2)gl and its cytogenetical localization on chromosome 17p1.1 will certainly trigger research for elucidating whether the human homolog to the Drosophila gene may play a similar role in human disease involving excessive cell proliferation such as cancer.

Dr. Dennis Strand
Dr. Istvan Török
Prof. Dr. Bernard M. Mechler
Division of Developmental Genetics

Participating scientists

Kirsten Hartenstein
Daniela Herrmann
Ioannis Iliopoulos
Rainer Jakobs
Andreas Kalmes
Cécilia de Lorenzo
Gunter Merdes
Beate Neumann
Dr. Heide Schenkel
Thomas Schwinn-Arnold
Armin Weinzierl-Hinum

In collaboration with

Dr. Istvan Kiss
Gabriella Tick
Dr. Tibor Török
Biological Research Center,
Hungarian Academy of Sciences,
Szeged, Hungary

Dr. Ivan Raska
Institute of Experimental Medicine,
Academy of Sciences
of Czech Republic,
Prague, Czech Republic

Prof. Dr. Antonio García-Bellido
Consejo Superior de Investigaciones Cientificas,
Centro Biologia Molecular,
Universidad Autónoma de Madrid, Spain

Selected publications

Török, I., Hartenstein, K., Kalmes, A., Schmitt, R., Strand, D., Mechler, B.M.: The l(2)gl homologue of Drosophila pseudoobscura suppresses tumorigenicity in transgenic Drosophila melanogaster. Oncogene 8, 1537–1549 (1993)

Mechler, B.M.: Genes in control of cell proliferation and tumorigenesis in Drosophila. In: The Legacy of Cell Fusion. Siamon Gordon (ed.). Oxford Science Publications, Oxford, New York, Tokyo, 183–198 (1994)

Mechler, B. M.: Wenn ein Gen fehlt – Die Rolle der Tumorsuppressorgene bei der Krebsentstehung. In: Heidelberger Jahrbücher XXXVIII. Universitäts-Gesellschaft Heidelberg (ed.). Springer-Verlag, Berlin, Heidelberg, New York (1994)

Strand, D., Jakobs, R., Merdes, G., Neumann, B., Kalmes, A., Heid, H., Husmann, I., Mechler, B.M.: The Drosophila l(2)gl tumor suppressor protein forms homo-oligomers and is associated with nonmuscle myosin II heavy chain. J. Cell Biol. 127 (5), 1361–1373 (1994)

Strand, D., Raska, I., Mechler, B.M.: The Drosophila l(2)gl tumor suppressor protein is a component of the cytoskeleton. J. Cell Biol. 127 (5), 1345–1360 (1994)

2.3 Cell Growth and Regulation of Gene Activity

by Ingrid Grummt

The sole explanation for the huge diversity of life on earth is the remarkable degree of variation inherent in deoxyribonucleic acid (DNA), the genetic material of every living organism. The genetic information encoded in DNA is stored in genes, ready to be retrieved on demand in a process known as gene expression. The genetic information is first transcribed from DNA into complementary ribonucleic acid (RNA). Thus, an RNA copy of the gene is produced, providing the basis on which the actual gene product, i.e., a protein, is manufactured. Human DNA contains all the information needed to encode for roughly 100 000 different gene products. However, only a portion of this multitude of genes, representing the genome of a living organism, is expressed in all cells and at all times. These active genes include the so-called "house-keeping genes," responsible for cellular metabolism, energy supply, or the skeleton of the cell. In contrast, the action of many other genes is restricted to certain developmental stages or to individual tissues, their task being to take care that the different types of cells carry out different functions. This "differential gene expression" provides the molecular basis for the development of diverse tissues and organs, such as the skin or the liver. They not only differ in their external shape but also carry out different functions and are hence responsible for the necessary division of labor within a multicellular living organism.

As a prerequisite for controlling the activity of various genes in developmental and differentiating processes of cells, highly efficient control mechanisms are required, regulating gene expression and hence adapting the synthesis of different cellular proteins to cell demand. The various regulation processes are initiated and coordinated by signals from outside the cell. In this context, signals transmitted from cell to cell, together with other factors, play an important role in multicellular organisms. If certain signal paths or regulation centers fail, the cell is damaged irrevocably, resulting in cell death or, alternatively, transformation into a cancer cell. Thus, cancer is a disease that ultimately results from gene damage or errors in the expression of specific genes. This is the reason why elucidation of the fundamental mechanisms regulating the switching on and off of individual genes or whole gene families has been the chief focus of cancer research for a number of years now.

Genome regions where gene activities are manipulated in a positive or a negative way, depending on the cell reproduction rate, are indispensable to an analysis of the role of transcription control in the process of regulating complex biological processes. This manipulation is brought about by changing the activity of specific proteins that are required for overwriting the information encoded in genes. In this way detailed regulation of transcription of specified genes is achieved, enabling the cell to react quickly and effectively to a great number of environmental challenges. Therefore, scientists are now devoting their attention to understanding the complex processes by which signals from the outside get into the cell nucleus and how they control gene activities. Study of these processes includes the identification and characterization of the particular function of the proteins required for gene identification and transcription, and on another level, elucidation of the transmission paths of signals responsible for the adaptation of gene activities to the physiological state of the cells.

The enzyme that transcribes the information encoded in DNA into complementary RNA is called DNA-dependent RNA polymerase. RNA polymerase receives the signals for transcribing a gene from the "gene control center," known as the gene promoter. Promoters are short DNA sections, comprising a few hundred base pairs, from which transcription of a gene is regulated. Promoters normally contain a sequence which marks the beginning of a gene, and several clearly delineated elements with control functions. These regulatory elements receive specific signals from the inside and the outside of the cell and pass them on to the RNA polymerase. The signal then initiates or suppresses the activity of the particular gene.

The regulatory sequences within the promoter region function by binding specific proteins called "transcription factors". Depending on the physiologic state of the cells, they bring about cell- and tissue-specific changes in the expression of genes that are positively controlled, i.e., enhanced, or negatively controlled, i.e., suppressed, by the respective promoter. A vast array of regulatory sequences and transcription factors exists in the cell. Different combinations and arrangements of individual DNA elements identified by different transcription factors ultimately result in a chronologically coordinated, individual transcription program for each gene.

The genes coding for ribosomal ribonucleic acid (rRNA) are a suitable object for the elucidation of the molecular mechanisms coupling gene activity and cell growth. rRNA is an important constituent of ribosomes, the protein synthesizing factories of the cell. In the process of a single cell division, more than a million ribosomes need to be produced. This fact explains the vast quantities of this ribonucleic acid synthesized by the cell. The higher the growth rate of a tissue, the greater the number of proteins that has to be produced. This also results in an increase in demand for ribosomes and ribosomal RNA. rRNA synthesis accounts for almost 50% of the transcription activity of multiplying cells. In contrast, rRNA-synthesis activity is dramatically reduced in differentiated cells with a low rate of division.

Our research is directed at understanding the processes that, firstly, cause intensive rRNA-gene transcription and, secondly, adapt the rRNA promoter activity to the rate of cell growth. To achieve this aim, we first have to purify the proteins involved in promoter identification and in the transcription process, and analyze their structures and functions. This is a very difficult task since the transcription factors required for rRNA-gene transcription occur in the cell only in minute quantities and are furthermore highly sensitive. To have any chance of identifying these factors from the great number of cellular proteins, of isolating them, and of subsequently analyzing their functions in vitro, the purification of large quantities of these proteins is indispensable. Typi-

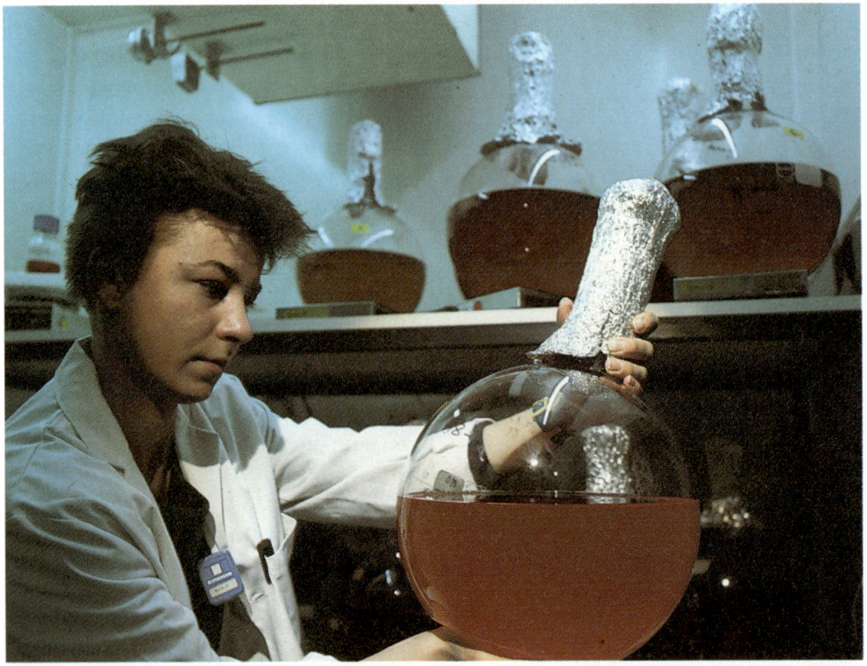

Fig. 20
It takes several liters of cultivated cells to make a few millionths of a gram of transcription factor

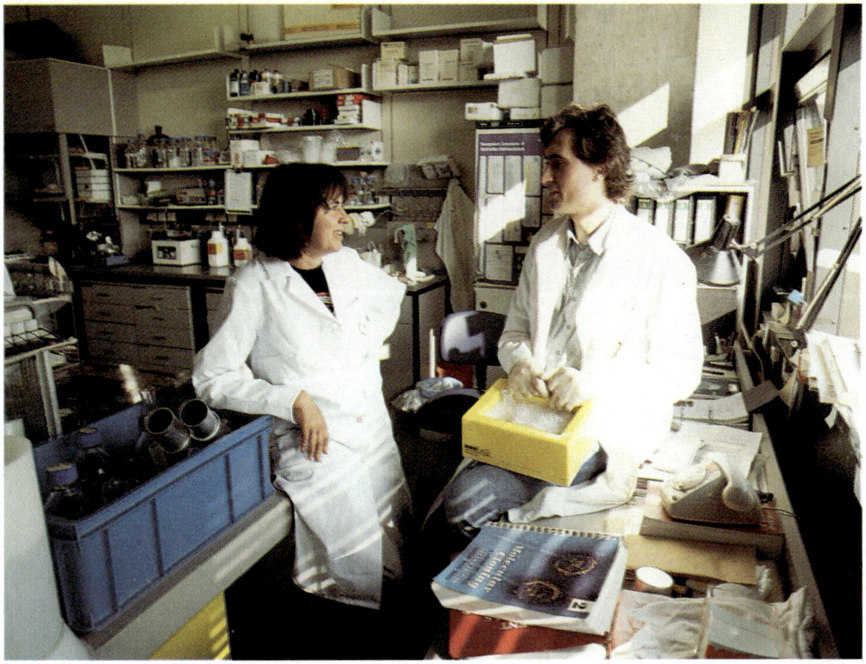

Fig. 21
Prof. Ingrid Grummt on her morning laboratory round

cally, we start working with 300 to 500 liters of cultivated cells. This volume corresponds to approximately 500 billion cells. However, as little as a few millionths of a gram of the RNA-polymerase enzyme and of the transcription factors required for rRNA synthesis are produced. Purification is effected by multiple chromatographs connected in series in which proteins are separated on the basis of different chemical properties, such as charge, size or solubility. Since these proteins lose their biological activity at room temperature, the whole purification procedure is carried out in the cold storage room at a temperature of 4° C.

We successfully developed the first cell-free system in which the mechanism and the regulation of rRNA-gene transcription can be studied using highly purified protein factors. The system contains, in a saline solution simulating the inside of the cell, the rRNA-gene matrix, the four RNA constituents, and RNA polymerase. In addition, five other transcription factors responsible for the selection of the beginning and/or the end of the gene by RNA polymerase are required. If the individual components are added in the right proportions, ribonucleic acid is synthesized in the test tube, representing an identical copy of the cellular ribosomal RNA. We can now analyze in detail the mode of action of this artificially constructed transcription system. There is still a long way to go before we are able to understand the complex process of gene expression and its regulation. However, we now have the tools to directly study the individual steps in the transcription process under experimental conditions and have a useful model for investigating the basic molecular processes implicated in carcinogenesis.

Prof. Dr. Ingrid Grummt
Division of Molecular Biology of the Cell II

Participating staff

Dirk Eberhard
Bettina Erny
Dr. Anne Kuhn
Andreas Schnapp
Gisela Schnapp

Selected publications

Kuhn, A., Grummt, I.: Dual role of the nucleolar transcription factor UBF: Transactivator and antirepressor. Proc. Natl. Acad. Sci. USA 89, 7340–7344 (1992)

Schnapp, A., Grummt, I.: Transcription complex formation at the mouse rDNA promoter involves the stepwise association of four transcription factors and RNA polymerase I. J. Biol. Chem. 266, 24588–24595 (1992)

Eberhard, D., Tora, L., Egly, J.M., Grummt, I.: A TBP-containing multisubunit complex (TIF-IB) confers promoter specificity to murine RNA polymerase I. Nucl. Acids Res. 21, 4180–4186 (1993)

Schnapp, A., Schnapp, G., Erny, B., Grummt, I.: Function of the growth-regulated factor TIF-IA in initiation complex formation at the murine rDNA promoter. Mol. Cell. Biol. 13, 6723–6732 (1993)

Schnapp, G., Santori, F., Carles, C., Riva, M., Grummt, I.: The HMG-box containing nucleolar transcription factor UBF interacts with a specific subunit of RNA polymerase I. EMBO J. 13, 190–199 (1994)

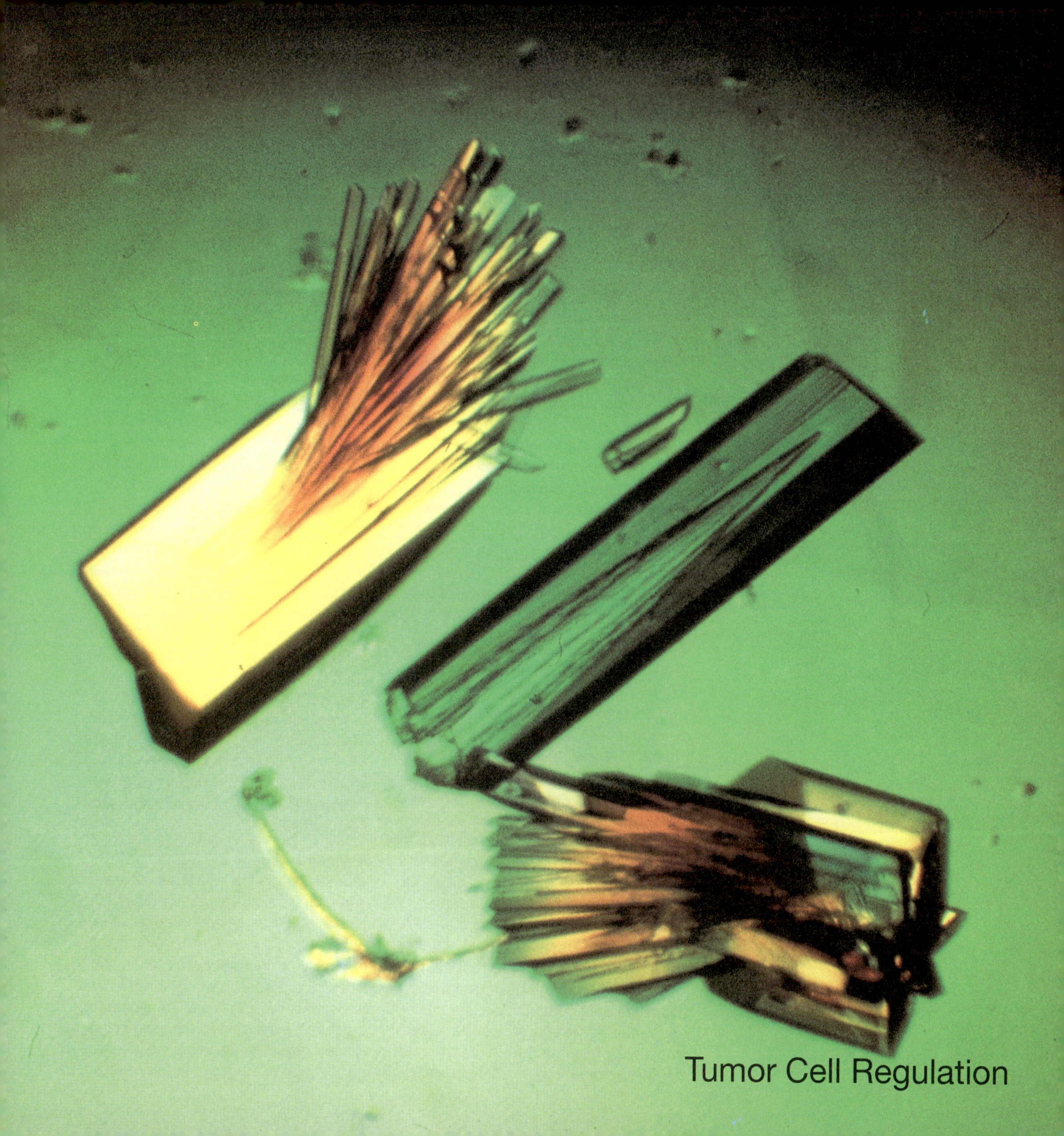

Tumor Cell Regulation

3

Tumor Cell Regulation

Today, cancer is thought of as resulting from the accumulation of genetic damages that occur accidentally or are due to external factors. The result is a permanently disturbed communication among the cells and between the tumor tissue and the organism, becoming evident by chaotic and destructive growth and senseless functioning.

Communication between cells and body tissues is mainly based upon the continuous exchange of chemical signals: Depending on their place of origin of effect, these can be characterized as hormones, neurotransmitters, cytokines, mediators, or growth factors. Each cell of the human body is able to emit and receive such signals and thus is in permanent contact with all other cells of the organism. This extremely complex system of communication ensures that all parts of the body behave coherently and cooperatively as if they were following a predefined plan.

Signals are emitted, received and interpreted. The recipient gives each received signal a meaning, which, in general, is a prompt to act. For this purpose, the cells have several complex chains of chemical reactions by which signals can be detected, modulated, modified, and passed on into the interior of the cell or even the nucleus. At their point of destination, they affect, for example, the activities of enzymes and genes, the structure of the cellular skeleton, the permeability of the cellular membrane, and thus the entire behavior of the cell. The intracellular signal transmission channels are retroactive and interlinked and thus constitute an extraordinarily complex "cellular nervous system". Presently, cellular signal transmission is, apart from the action of the genes, one of the most intensively studied areas in biomedical research, especially because it is now known that the majority of all genetic defects resulting in cancer or other diseases manifest themselves as a disturbed signal transmission.

Cellular signal transmission is one of the foci of the work done in the Research Program Tumor Cell Regulation. Several working groups are studying cellular signal molecules, in particular, the peptide hormones (growth factors) which promote or inhibit cell division and which have been proven to be directly and in many ways related to tumor growth. Other studies concentrate on short-lived mediators which are generated by tissues locally and only for short periods of time. Here, the work is focusing on the large group of eicosanoid-type mediators (such as prostaglandins, thromboxans, leucotriens, lipoxins). These highly active substances are involved in the regulation of almost all tissue and bodily functions. However, their role in pathological processes such as cancer is not yet understood. The detection of these short-lived signal molecules requires a great amount of funding to cover technical expenses. For this purpose, the Research Program's very efficient Division of Spectroscopy disposes of the latest analytical methods.

A second focus of the Research Program's work is the investigation of the intracellular signal transmission mechanisms, i.e., the cellular "interpretation apparatus". The key process is the biochemical protein phosphorylation and its involvement with proteinkinases and phosphatases. This reaction, comparable to electrochemical impulses in the nervous system, seems to be the standard signal of intracellular information transmission. Several working groups of the Research Program "Tumor Cell Regulation" are studying the isolation and characterization of protein kinases and their role in physiological and pathophysiological processes.

A third research project is investigating one of the central problems of experimental cancer research, the regulation of cell division. The complexity of the research requires the combined use of microscopic, cell-biologic, biochemical and molecular-biological methods and thus calls for an intensive collaboration, both among the Research Program's divisions, as well as with other Research Programs of the Deutsches Krebsforschungszentrum. Since the aforementioned intracellular signals and the cellular signal transmission mechanisms assigned to them (such as protein phosphorylation) directly or indirectly (by altering cell differentiation) affect the regulation of cell division, the Research Program's main projects are closely collaborated.

All these studies aim at deepening our knowledge of molecular processes whose disturbance results in the development and growth of tumors. It is hoped and expected that, on this basis, new preventive therapeutic approaches can be developed and that the search for risk factors can be improved. It is conceivable that the development of a tumor can be stopped or even reversed by purposely changing intracellular communication processes at specific stages, such as growth, supply with nutrients, or formation of metastases. This concept has already been realized successfully in other fields of medicine, such as in psychopharmaceutical and cardiovascular medicine. As far as cancer is concerned, aspirin and related drugs provide a current example since they have been shown to prevent the development of colorectal tumors in man. These drugs selectively influence intercellular communication by inhibiting the formation of chemical messengers such as the prostaglandins. Many of the cytostatics used in clinical practice today are limited in their applicability since they have serious side-effects. New methods may make it possible to better control these side-effects by purposely altering the intracellular signal transmission, and thus broadening the range of application and the success of existing cancer drugs.

Each year, in January, the Research Program Tumor Cell Regulation organizes a 1-day Colloquium on recent developments in the investigation of cellular signalling.

Coordinator of the Research Program:
Prof. Dr. Friedrich Marks

Divisions and their heads:

Pathochemistry:
Prof. Dr. Volker Kinzel

Biochemistry of the Cell:
Prof. Dr. Dieter Werner

Biochemistry of Tissue-Specific Regulation:
Prof. Dr. Friedrich Marks

Differentiation and Carcinogenesis in vitro:
Prof. Dr. Norbert Fusenig

Biochemistry of Tumors:
Prof. Dr. Dietrich Keppler

Molecular Biology of Mitosis:
Prof. Dr. Herwig Ponstingl

Project groups and their heads:

Biochemical Cell Physiology:
Prof. Dr. Walter Pyerin

3.1 Protein Kinases – The Crystal Structure Sheds Light on the Mechanism of a Key Pacemaker in Cellular Control

by Dirk Bossemeyer und Volker Kinzel

Protein kinases have been called "life's pacemakers". They are actually a family of enzymes that catalyze the phosphorylation of proteins. The discovery of this reaction by Edmond Fischer and Edwin Krebs was recognized in 1992 when they were awarded the Nobel Prize for Medicine.

Enzymes are bio-catalysts that are able to speed-up the rate of chemical reactions within cells. Through this function they make life possible, since without them the necessary chemistry would proceed far too slowly. Just like chemical catalysts, enzymes emerge unchanged from the biochemical reactions they control. Biochemical reactions are distinguished by the fact that atoms in the cell that are organized in specific groups are handled as a unit. Such a unit is the phosphoryl group. Within it, four oxygen atoms are assembled around a central phosphorous atom. Within the cellular environment this group is negatively charged, and thus displays an acidic character.

In itself, protein phosphorylation is a fairly simple chemical reaction. The phosphoryl group from adenosine triphosphate is transferred to a protein. The catalyst for this reaction is always a protein kinase. Now, proteins are the main components through which life is expressed in organisms and in cells. Their phosphorylation would be of no further interest if it were not for the fact that it has serious and far-reaching consequences for the protein concerned. The biological activity of a protein can be altered at a stroke by this means, even turned on or off. This is especially easy to see with enzymes, whose activity can be measured.

The function of a protein is ultimately dependent on its three-dimensional shape, or conformation, which is in turn genetically determined by the sequence in which its building blocks, the amino acids, are strung together. Phosphorylation changes this shape as well as the proteins's charge. In this way the function of the protein is altered. The direct consequences of phosphorylation can be propagated right through the affected protein and alter its interactions with other macromolecules or even its solubility within the cell.

One final important point should be emphasized. Through removal of the phosphoryl group – dephosphorylation – the protein can be returned to its original state. Not only does it adopt its previous structure again, but it can once again carry out its previous function. The process is thus completely reversible and behaves like a switch.

This switch is an essential element in the signals that control living systems. In fact, protein kinases and reversible phosphorylation are a key factor in the multiple signal cascades within a cell. In many cases several protein kinases are connected in a series, or even paralleled to one another. Since even such basic processes as cell division cannot take place without reversible protein phosphorylation, the term "life's pacemakers" for the catalysts responsible, the protein kinases, is hardly an exaggeration. We know as well that improperly regulated protein kinases can promote the development of certain types of cancer.

How do these switches function; that is to say, how do protein kinases work? Due to the enormous variety of protein kinases, it would seem a hopeless task at first to find a general answer to this question. Relatively small protein kinases exist next to quite large members

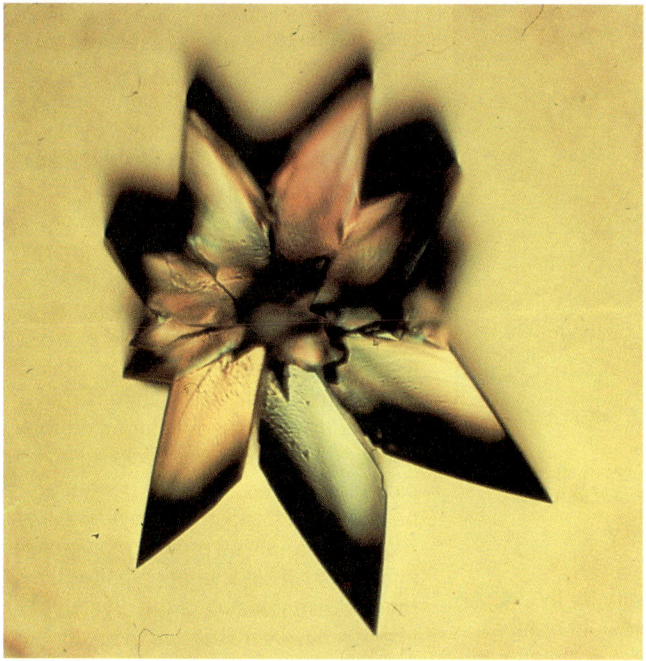

Fig. 22
Crystals of protein kinase A, a key cellular enzyme

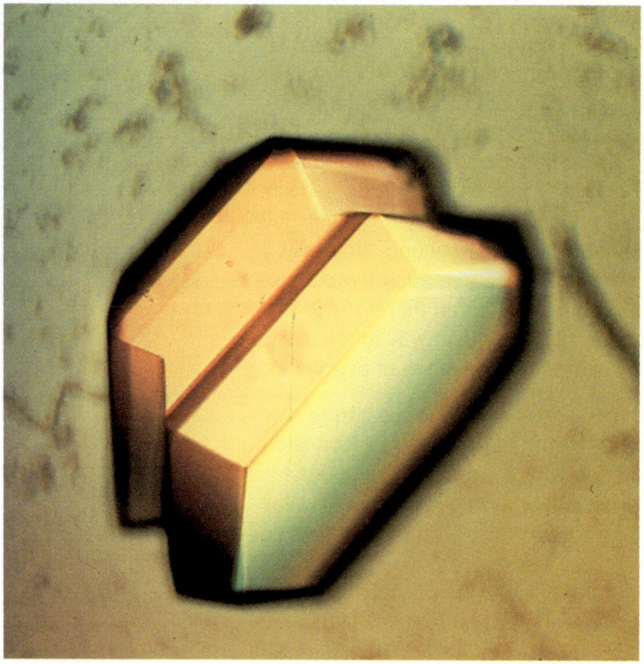

Fig. 23
High-quality ordered crystals are required to elucidate the three-dimensional structure of protein kinase A. Knowledge of the structure enables the enzyme's mechanism of action to be investigated. Active substances can then be developed, which alter the metabolic mechanisms in the cell, e.g., in cancer cells

of this enzyme family; some protein kinases are anchored in the cell membrane while others exist in solution in the cytoplasm; we know of protein kinases that are regulated by nucleotides, others through lipids, and still others through specific proteins or ions. If, however, one compares the genetically determined amino acid sequence of these protein kinases, it becomes apparant that all protein kinases known to date show a close resemblance in certain areas and are, in respect to some elements, fully identical. This conserved area of the proteins is the "catalytic heart" of all protein kinases. It consists of about 250 amino acid residues. The other molecular domains of the various protein kinases are totally different from one another; they serve a wide variety of functions but have nothing to do directly with the process of catalysis.

The ideal situation for studying the process of catalysis would naturally be if one could obtain the catalytic heart in pure form. Fortunately, this ideal situation exists – at least approximately. With the catalytic subunit of the cAMP-dependent protein kinase we have, in effect, the prototype protein kinase. About 70% of the 350 amino acid residues of the catalytic subunit are devoted to the catalysis of phosphoryl transfer to proteins. This protein kinase occurs in large amounts in skeletal and heart muscle and can be isolated from these in a highly pure form. The exact analysis of its structure and mechanism can serve as an example to gain information about the entire protein kinase family.

The goal of structural analysis is to understand the catalytic mechanism in detail at the atomic level. One must picture protein kinases, like other proteins, as quite flexible entities that can change their form in a pre-programmed way in order to carry out their function – molecules that work like machines. Their innate structural fluctuations are externally controlled by the molecules that bind to them. In the case of protein kinase these are, among others, adenosine triphosphate as the phosphoryl donor and substrate proteins as the phosphoryl acceptor. Normally, the transfer of the phosphoryl group takes place very rapidly and the protein kinase molecule can carry out many such transfers within a second. Naturally, one cannot observe such a rapid process directly. It must therefore be observed in an indirect way in order to reconstruct the sequence of events.

Just as the protein kinase can recognize the protein to be phosphorylated at a special binding site, so also must this substrate protein display certain structural characteristics in order to be recognized by the enzyme. Proteins should, after all, be phosphorylated specifically, not at random. These recognition sites differ for different protein kinases. In the case of the catalytic subunit of cAMP-dependent protein kinase the substrate is chiefly recognized through two positively charged (so-called basic) amino acid residues lying at a particular distance from the amino acid that will function as phosphoryl receptor. In this case the phosphoryl group binds to the hydroxyl group of the amino acid serine. If the basic amino acids are present, but the hydroxyl group at the correct position is not, then the protein kinase binds to the protein but cannot phosphorylate it. Such proteins with “defective” recognition sites are called pseudo-substrates and act as inhibitors of protein kinases. The enzyme has, in effect, been duped.

Particular features of the protein substrate or pseudo-substrate induce a series of specific structural changes in the protein kinase, as discovered by Jennifer Reed in our group. These changes

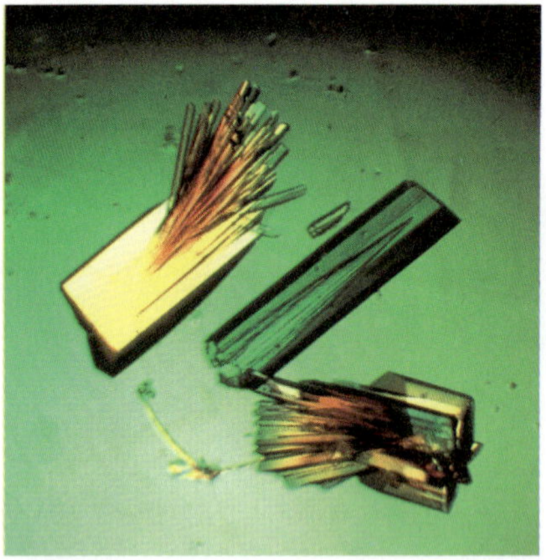

Fig. 24
Trillions of protein molecules must congregate to form a single crystal with a facet length of 0.5 to 1 millimeter

are apparantly necessary for the activation of the catalytic center. In order to examine the enzyme in the state in which it is catalytically active, a way must be found to “freeze” it in this position. This is achieved by a trick. The protein kinase is fobbed off with pseudosubstrates – with a molecular analog of adenosine triphosphate and with a protein pseudosubstrate. Both bind at the intended site of the protein kinase and induce certain structural alterations necessary for catalysis, but the reaction is blocked. The phosphoryl group cannot be detached from the imitation adenosine triphosphate and the pseudosubstrate cannot be phosphorylated; the protein kinase remains frozen in the catalytic state and is now available for exact structural analysis; provided – and that is the next difficulty – that it can be crystallized in this form.

X-ray crystallography is currently the only method by which the structure of protein kinase can be visualized in atomic detail. Direct observation methods, such as light- or electron-microscopy, do not show enough particulars. In a light microscope, one can see objects down to the size of cellular organelles (nucleii, mitochondria). Thanks to the shorter wavelengths used in electron microscopy, this method can distinguish large proteins or complexes of many small proteins. As useful as both techniqes are, they are clearly inadequate for determining the functional mechanism of an enzyme. Here, we turn to short wavelength x-rays which, in contrast to light and electrons, have the unfortunate disadvantage that they cannot be gathered and focused into a picture. However, an x-ray beam can be scattered through the several billion regularly organized protein molecules in a crystal. This scattering pattern, a reversed impression of the crystal lattice, displays variations in intensity that are caused by interference from the atoms of the protein molecule. A mathematical technique is substituted for an optical lens in order to calculate the spatial position of the atoms in the crystal from this interference pattern and, in this way, to construct a realistic picture of the protein. Details at the resolution of chemical bonds can be distinguished by this method. In order to organize molecules of protein kinase into a crystal, a solution of extremely pure protein is concentrated to the point of supersaturation. This methodology is not too different from the way in which salt or sugar is crystallized. Since, however, protein kinase consists of about four thousand atoms, it is quite large compared to the diatomic salt molecule, and in cumbersome and extremely sensitive as well. For this reason such a supersaturation only leads to a high quality crystal when the conditions are most carefully selected.

A protein kinase crystal of this type produced by us, "frozen" in the state that allows catalytic activity, offers the opportunity for a look at the smallest details of its interior and shows the enzyme just before catalysis; at the point, so to speak, of transferring the phosphoryl group. We can thus observe the way in which the protein phosphorylation switch operates mechanically and in what manner protein kinase fills its role as catalyst of this chemical reaction. By definition, a catalyst does not itself take part in a reaction, but lowers the activation energy involved. In the first step the reactants, that is, the final phosphoryl group of adenosinetriphosphate and the hydroxyl group of the protein to be phosphorylated (the substrate), are brought into close proximity. A deep cleft divides the protein kinase molecule into a smaller and a larger segment. This cleft, which can be opened and closed, offers a perfectly fitting shell for the adenosine triphosphate, which is almost totally enclosed by the protein. Only the terminal phosphoryl group remains exposed at the opening of the cleft. The substrate, or in this case the pseudosubstrate, is bound directly in front of the cleft opening in such a way that the phosphoryl-accepting hydroxyl group lies directly opposite the terminal phosphoryl group of the adenosine triphosphate. This is aided by binding sites on the protein kinase surface, negatively charged amino acids that attract the two positively charged residues of the recognition site. The simultaneous docking of the adenosine triphosphate and the pseudosubstrate affect the structure of the protein kinase. It induces an improvement of all contacts (induced fit), so that the two molecules together bind a hundredfold more closely to the protein kinase than either alone. This reciprocal, synergistic binding reenforcement was already known through biochemical methods, but now it can be understood at the structural level.

This forced spatial proximity of the reaction partners is not in itself sufficient to bring about phosphoryl transfer. The protein kinase affords, in addition, an environment in its catalytic center that simplifies the initiation of the chemical reaction. The tools the protein kinase uses are those very amino acids from which it is built. The charged amino acids in the catalytic center are especially important. A negatively charged amino acid residue pulls away the positive hydrogen atom of the phosphoryl-accepting hydroxyl group – leaving behind a negatively charged hydroxyl oxygen with a strong tendency to bind to the phosphorous atom of the phosphoryl group. However, since the oxygen atoms of the phosphoryl group also carry a negative charge, the approach of the hydroxyl oxygen is held off by the repulsion from these oxygen atoms. Negatively charged amino acids in the catalytic center position a positively charged magnesium ion in such a way that it binds to the phosphoryl oxygens. A further phosphoryl oxygen atom is neutralized by a positively charged amino acid. The hydroxyl oxygen can thus bind to the phosphorous atom and a transition state occurs in which the phosphorous atom probably binds five oxygen atoms at once. The ensuing break between the phosphoryl group and the remaining adenosine diphosphate dramatically alters the conditions at the active site. All at once the transferred phosphoryl group is surrounded by a series of repelling electrostatic forces, especially those from the phosphoryl group of the newly-formed adenosine diphosphate. In this way, the freshly phosphorylated protein is expelled from the protein kinase and can take on its altered function in the cell. This much can be deduced from the "snapshot" of a single structural state available from the crystal structure. Additional crystal structures of other structural states of the enzyme with accompanying experiments are necessary, however, in order to answer the many questions remaining open and to fully understand the picture of the complex mechanism of a protein kinase.

As well as the possibility of developing a general model of catalysis, the crystal structure of a protein offers further valuable hints and information. The enormous influence protein phosphorylation exerts on cellular processes places the precise control of protein kinase activity at a premium. We have already spoken of the inhibition of protein kinase by fooling it with a pseudosubstrate. Nature has anticipated research in the use of this principle of regulation. Protein kinases are often themselves the substrate for a phosphorylation reaction, for example. Thus there are specific positions at which some protein kinases (for example, those with a receptor function in the outer membrane) must be phosphorylated in order to be active. Other protein kinases, such as the cell-cycle-regulating, cyclin-dependent protein kinases, are inactive as long as they are phosphorylated at specific positions. They are activated by protein phosphatases that remove the phosphoryl group. Thanks to the crystal structure, the inhibition mechanism can already be seen is for some of these phosphorylations.

As well as the common factors that unite all protein kinases, among which the principle catalytic mechanism is numbered, there are also considerable differences between the individual members that one might hope to use advantageously once their crystal structure is understood. In addition to an understanding of their regulation and substrate recognition, one is offered a plethora of starting points for directed modification of particular protein kinases through techniques ranging from site-directed mutagenesis to computer-supported construction of therapeutically active substances.

Dr. Dirk Bossemeyer
Prof. Dr. Volker Kinzel
Division of Pathochemistry

Participating scientist
Norbert König

In collaboration with
Prof. Dr. Herwig Ponstingl
Division of Molecular Biology of Mitosis

Prof. Dr. Robert Huber
Dr. Richard A. Engh
Max-Planck-Institut für Biochemie, Martinsried

Selected Publications

Krebs, E.G., Fischer, E.H.: The phosphorylase b to a converting enzyme of rabbit skeletal muscle. Biochimica Biophysica Acta 20, 150–157 (1956)

Walsh, D.A., Perkins, J. P., Krebs, E. G.: An adenosine 3′, 5′-monophosphate dependent protein kinase from rabbit muscle. J. Biol. Chem. 243, 3763–3765 (1968)

Reed, J., Kinzel, V., Kemp, B., Cheng, H.C., Walsh, D.A.: Circular dichroic evidence for an ordered sequence of ligand/binding site interactions in the catalytic reaction of the cAMP-dependent protein kinase. Biochemistry 24, 2967–2973 (1985)

Knighton, D.R., Zheng, J., Ten Eyck, L.F., Ashford, V.A., Xuong, N.-H., Taylor, S.S., Sowadski, J.M.: Crystal structure of the catalytic subunit of cyclic adenosine monophosphate-dependent protein kinase. Science 253, 407–414 (1991)

Bossemeyer, D., Engh, R.A., Kinzel, V., Ponstingl, H., Huber, R.: Phosphotransferase and substrate binding mechanism of the cAMP-dependent protein kinase catalytic subunit from porcine heart as deduced from the 2.0 Å structure of the complex Mn^{2+}adenylyl imidodiphosphate and inhibitor peptide PKI (5-24). EMBO Journal 12, 894–859 (1993)

3.2 Aspirin: A Pain Reliever that Prevents Cancer?

by Gerhard Fürstenberger and Friedrich Marks

The 10th of October 1887 proved, in retrospect, to be a lucky day for Bayer AG. That was the day that chemist Felix Hoffmann synthesized acetylsalicylic acid in a chemically pure form. This analgesic and antipyretic drug with the trade name aspirin was to become a world-wide success. Approximately 16000 tons, i.e., 80 billion tablets, are consumed annually in the USA alone. Aspirin is the "refined" form of an old substance with similar properties, salicylic acid, itself a chemical derivative of salicin, a component of the bark of the willow tree (Salix) also known for its analgetic and antipyretic properties.

As early as the fifth century BC, the bark of the willow tree was recommended in the Corpus Hippocraticum by Greek physicians as a remedy against aches and fever. Later on, the abbess Hildegard of Bingen, (1098–1179) recommended the use of willow and poplar extracts. In 1763, the Reverend Edmund Stone in England again drew attention to the curative properties of the willow, which had been forgotten in the meantime. In 1828, Johann Andreas Buchner first isolated salicin, and in 1838, the Italian chemist Raffaele Piria produced salicylic acid from it. However, the complicated procedures required to isolate the precursor salicin from plants proved a barrier to the wide clinical use of salicylic acid. Despite this, Hermann Kolbe succeeded in producing the substance synthetically in the laboratory as early as 1859. After the development of mass production techniques in 1874, salicylic acid became established in hospitals and, despite its revolting smell and its many side-effects, was successfully used to treat acute inflammations, rheumatism, and gout until its displacement by its acetyl derivative, aspirin.

The development of aspirin is an exciting chapter of medical history. This is even more true of the discovery of its many and various effects. Further surprising properties of aspirin, which has become famous as an analgesic and antipyretic, have recently come to light, prompting the British daily "The Times" to call it "the sexiest drug of our age". In October 1985, the U.S. Food and Drug Administration (FDA) reported that daily ingestion of aspirin by patients having suffered a myocardial infarction reduced their risk of a second infarction by one-fifth. Another evaluation in 1988, including 22000 physicians as volunteers, showed that the regular intake of aspirin reduced the risk of myocardial infarction by almost 50%. Furthermore, a study published in 1991 proved that aspirin given immediately following a myocardial infarction reduced mortality by 23%. Other epidemiological studies showed a 23% decrease in the risk of stroke. Clinical studies revealed a decrease in the risk of developing venous thromboses and/or pulmonary embolism following surgery by 39% and 64% respectively.

In 1988, another page was turned in the aspirin success story. Again, epidemiological evaluations and controlled clinical studies turned the attention of doctors to a new attribute of aspirin and related substances – so-called non-steroidal anti-inflammatory drugs (NSAID) – namely, the propensity of these drugs given in regular doses to slow down or prevent the development of tumors in the intestine and to reduce the risk of developing and dying of intestinal cancer, one of the most common cancers, by more than 50%. This

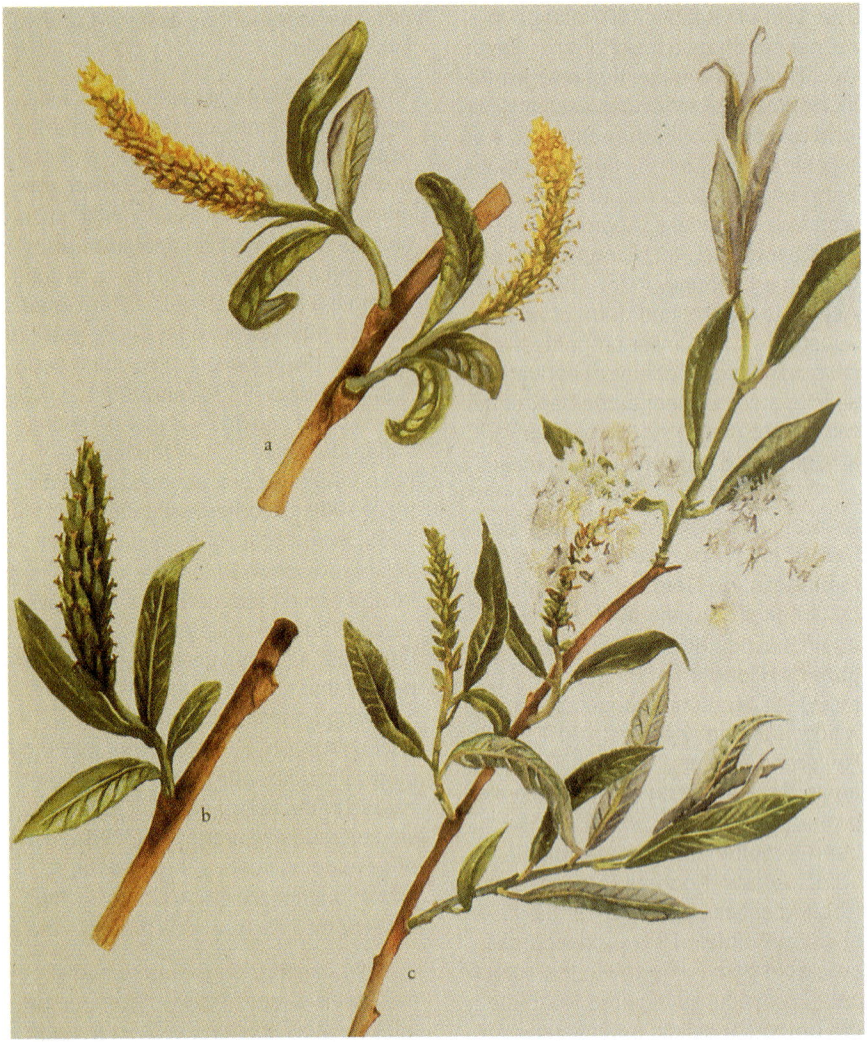

Fig. 25
The Salix alba willow bears male (upper left) and female (right) catkins. The figure below shows a leafy fruit-bearing twig during the seed-ripening season. Salicin, the basis for salicylic acid, was first extracted from Salix alba

applies especially to the group of at-risk patients suffering from familial polyposis. This is a hereditary disease in which large numbers of intestinal polyps occur, which are benign at the beginning, but have a strong tendency to become malignant. Aspirin and other NSAIDs seem to be able to inhibit or prevent a crucial process in the development of tumors in the intestine. Interestingly, these inhibitory effects of NSAIDs were very similar to those seen in intestinal cancer tests in laboratory animals.

Is there a common explanation for the manifold effects of aspirin? For three-quarters of a century we trusted in the pain-relieving and antipyretic effects of the drugs without understanding the underlying mechanism. This was only changed by work published in the 1970s by the British pharmacologist John Vane, who was awarded the Nobel prize for medicine together with the two Swedes Sune K. Bergström and Bengt I. Samuelsson. All three researchers were concerned with certain endogenous substances, the prostaglandins. Prostaglandins are highly efficient hormones, occurring throughout the tissues and body fluids, which are not stored in cells but are made available only on demand. This happens by enzymatic oxidation of arachidonic acid, a fatty acid contained in cellular membranes. Vane had observed that tissue injury triggered prostaglandin production. In addition, it was shown that certain prostaglandins caused or influenced typical inflammatory symptoms accompanied by tissue irritation and injury, such as reddening and warmth due to dilatation of blood vessels, swelling caused by a change in the permeability of cell walls, and fever. Vane proved that aspirin and related NSAID halted biosynthesis of these inflammation-promoting prostaglandins by inhibition of the enzyme prostaglandin synthase responsible for converting arachidonic acid into prostaglandins.

The multi-stage pathway of prostaglandin biosynthesis had in the meantime been elucidated in Samuelsson's laboratory. Vane's findings gave a satisfactory explanation for the inflammation-inhibitory and analgetic effects of aspirin and NSAIDs. The full details of the mechanisms by which prostaglandins cause an inflammatory reaction are still unknown, however. Moreover, prostaglandin synthesis seems to be only one of several ways in which aspirin acts on cells.

However, prostaglandins not only function as endogenous mediators of inflammation but have many different physiological functions including, for instance, the control of hydrochloric acid production in the gastric mucous membrane and excretion of salts and water in the kidneys. If prostaglandin synthesis is inhibited, by aspirin for instance, this results in overproduction of gastric juice, which may in turn lead to irritation of the gastric mucous membrane, bleeding, and peptic ulcers. Renal function may also be impaired. These and the rare but sometimes life-threatening hypersensitivity reactions of allergy sufferers are serious side-effects of acetylsalicylic acid.

Vane's prostaglandin concept also explains aspirin's preventive effects in coronary heart disease. Aspirin inhibits clumping (aggregation) of blood platelets and prevents constriction of vessels, both important steps in blood coagulation. At the onset of coagulation the platelets synthesize thromboxane B_2, a prostaglandin-related substance with potent vasoconstricting and platelet-aggregating effects. Its antagonist is prostacyclin (prostaglandin I_2) which is formed in endothelial cells, the cells lining the walls of blood vessels. The two substances complement each other in the healthy organism. Aspirin and similar substances inhibit synthesis of both thromboxane and prostacyclin, albeit to a different extent. Carefully selected doses of aspirin may suppress the release of thromboxane without completely blocking the synthesis of prostacyclin at the same time. The reason for this is that, although aspirin inactivates prostaglandin synthase in both cases, endothelial cells start producing the enzyme again, whereas blood platelets do not. This is the basis of the world-wide use of aspirin today in the prevention of stroke and myocardial infarction.

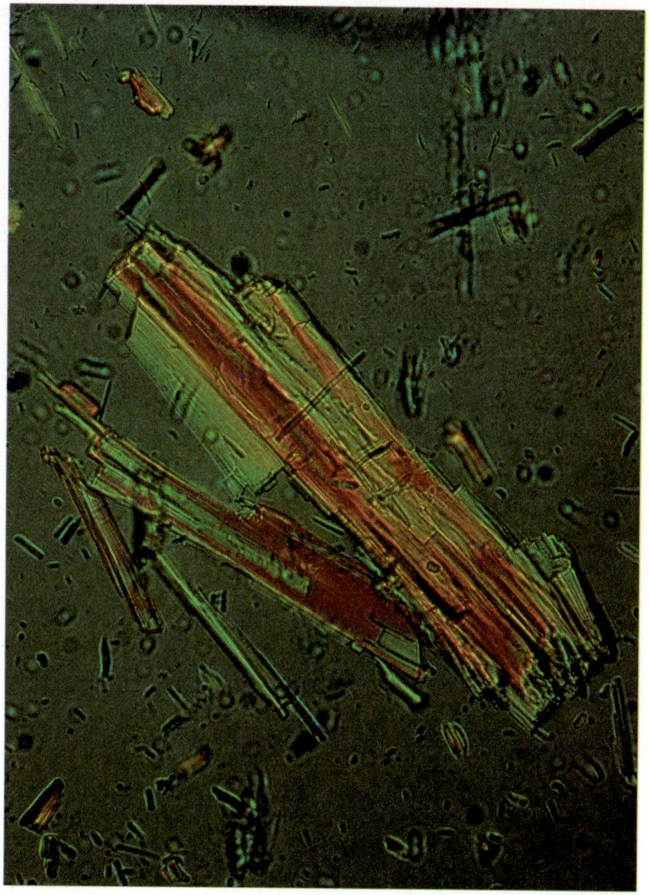

Fig. 26
Tiny crystals of acetylsalicylic acid under a microscope. In polarized light they show up in all colors of the rainbow. To the naked eye the crystals are just a white powder

Is there a link between the cancer-inhibitory action of NSAIDs and prostaglandins? It is a fact that intestinal cancerous tissue in humans produces excessive doses of a prostaglandin which is thought to impair the body's immune system. Aspirin and similar substances might overcome this immune suppression and strengthen the body's own defenses against tumor cells. At the same time, NSAIDs seem to stimulate the re-

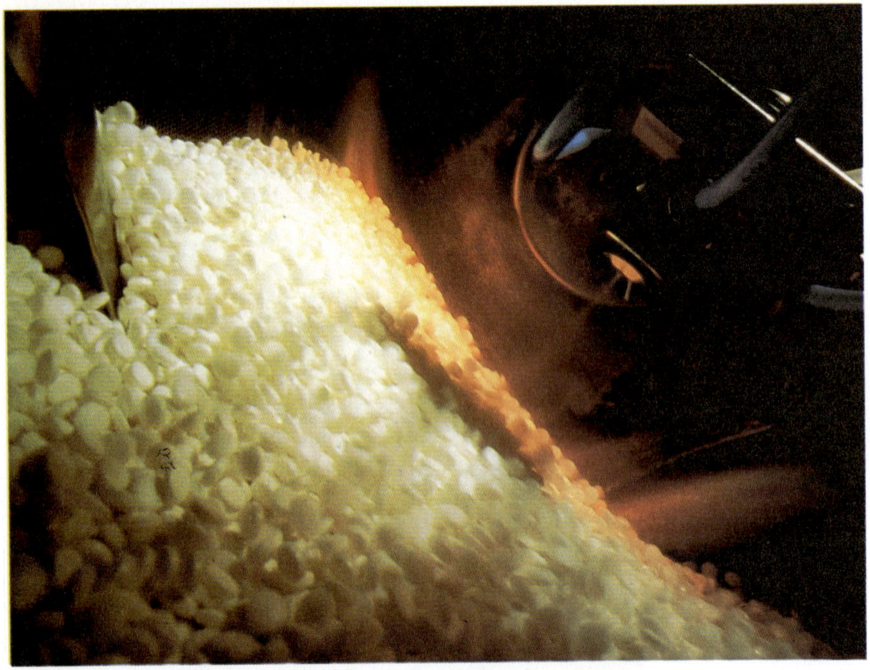

Fig. 27
Over 40 000 metric tons of acetylsalicylic acid are made into tablets worldwide every year. The picture shows a protective acrylic resin coating being sprayed on after tableting

lease of interleukin-2 and gamma interferon from immune cells. Both these hormones activate the immune system. Whether such a strengthening of the immune system contributes considerably to the cancer-preventive effect of NSAIDs is questionable. There are many factors pointing to a much more direct association between prostaglandins and carcinogenesis. Prostaglandin synthase not only catalyzes the conversion of arachidonic acid to prostaglandins, but is also capable of changing carcinogenic substances chemically so as to damage the cell's genetic material. Furthermore, malondialdehyde, a degradation product of prostaglandins produced in the body, has proved to be a substance with a gene-damaging (mutagenic) and carcinogenic potential. Malondialdehyde triggers, for example, the conversion of methylcytosine to thymine in the genetic material (DNA). This mutation is especially prevalent in the tumor suppressor gene p53 in intestinal tumors in humans. p53 thereby loses its capability to inhibit cancer growth. In addition, free radicals occur during prostaglandin synthesis; these are extremely aggressive compounds suspected of inducing cancer by causing gene mutations.

Since the mid-1970s, our group has elucidated connections between prostaglandins and the genesis of tumors in animal studies, in particular in the so-called multi-stage carcinogenesis model whereby carcinogens are applied to mouse skin and tumor formation is subdivided into at least three stages which are examined separately. In the first step, initiation, tumor cells are produced on the outer skin (epidermis) by applying a minimal dose of a carcinogenic substance, but which do not develop into tumors at the beginning. Only in the second step, tumor promotion, does sustained stimulation of cell division – either by injury or with the help of a chemical tumor promoter – lead to the formation of papillomas. These are benign tumors, some of which develop into malignant tumors without further external stimulation in the third step in the sequence, tumor progression. The genetic damage occurring at initiation is well known, and mainly affects the genes of the ras family. These genes play a key role for the cell in recognizing and processing endogenous signals controlling cell division. Tumor promotion is also closely related with cell division, permanent stimulation of excessive tissue growth being a prerequisite. However, disturbances occurring during this process do not seem to be associated with gene mutations. In contrast to this, genetic damage is necessary for the transformation of a benign into a malignant tumor. This damage manifests itself as alterations in chromosomes and individual genes, enhancing the effects of foregoing ras mutations taking place at initiation and, at the same time, inactivating the tumor suppressor gene p53. How this additional damage to the genetic material occurs is unknown. Since these lesions obviously occur "by themselves", the cause may lie in the papilloma cells. Could excessive prostaglandin production and the associated side-effects be implicated? Aspirin's action against intestinal cancer in humans points in that direction as do the results of animal experiments.

In our animal model carcinomas developed from papillomas which, however, only developed following promotion. This shows that the development of skin cancer in mice depends on tumor promotion and may be stopped by inhibition of this step in the sequence. Aspirin and related NSAIDs have proved to be especially potent inhibitory substances. At the same time, we demonstrated that the formation of prostaglandins in skin cells is a prerequisite of tumor promotion.

The striking thing is the close similarity between the development of intestinal cancer in humans and the experimental initiation of skin cancer in this animal model: in both cases the carcinomas develop from benign tumors, i.e., papillomas and/or polyps. In both cases the development of the tumor correlates with the same genetic damage, such as ras, p53, and chromosomal mutations. In both cases aspirin and other NSAIDs have an inhibitory effect. In intestinal cancer bile acids are suspected of functioning as tumor promoters; and it is a fact that their inflammatory and cell-division promoting properties are very similar to those of tumor promoters used in animal studies. Thus, artificially induced skin cancer in mice seems to be a useful model to examine tumor development in humans. It permits the elucidation of a variety of unsolved questions which clinical observations may not be able to answer, but which are critically important to understanding the process of how cancer develops and to improving preventive and therapeutic measures. For instance, it would be interesting to learn in which way deregulation of prostaglandin synthesis is involved in the development of tumors and whether other comparable defects of cellular metabolism are implicated. This is the point of departure of our own studies. We found that the temporary activation of prostaglandin formation, which is typical of injured or chemically irritated skin, does not come to a standstill in benign and malignant tumors but continues apace. This appears to back up the repeatedly expressed suspicion that tumors behave like poorly healing wounds.

Prostaglandin overproduction is due to the deregulation of enzymes involved in the process (prostaglandin synthases) and thus could be ultimately due to a genetic defect. There are two types of prostaglandin synthases (PGHS), PGHS-1 and PGHS-2. PGHS-1 is permanently produced in all tissues, whereas PGHS-2 is only formed temporarily following exposure of the cells to harmful stimuli, but also to endogenous substances, such as mediators of inflammation, growth factors and hormones. In our skin model, we also observed that PGHS-1 was present in comparable amounts both in normal and inflamed skin as well as in tumors, whereas PGHS-2 was not detected in healthy tissues. This enzyme, however, is produced in large amounts if a tumor promoter is applied to the skin. However, if applied repeatedly, the skin adapts to the condition by quickly degrading newly synthesized PGHS-2, even though the cell division rate remains high. The situation was totally different in tumors: they had lost

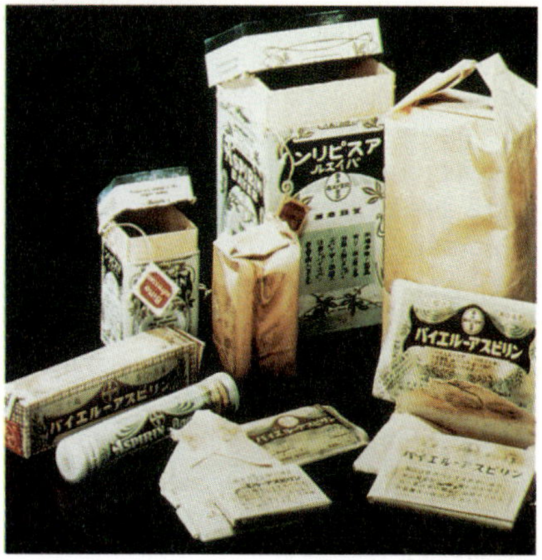

Fig. 28
Japanese aspirin boxes (ca. 1930)

their ability to adapt and accumulated large amounts of PGHS-2. This defect seems to be a typical characteristic of the tumor and does not merely result from enhanced cell division. This strengthens the suspicion that excessive prostaglandin synthesis might be an important prerequisite of tumor growth. In our opinion, the key to an understanding of the tumor-inhibitory action of NSAIDs will have to be looked for here. We are presently examining whether a similar excessive production of PGHS-2 also occurs in intestinal tumors in humans. It is critically important to know, of course, by which mechanisms prostaglandin synthases intervene in tumor development, how deregulation of PGHS-2 formation occurs, and whether the defect is repairable. Extensive and long-term research efforts will be necessary to answer this question.

Nevertheless, these studies have already provided new important insights into the cancer-preventive action of nonsteroidal anti-inflammatory drugs. Drugs of this class inhibit the activity of prostaglandin synthases but not their availability. Since cells try to counteract inhibition of an enzyme by producing more, NSAIDs must be taken on a permanent basis – controlled clinical studies have established that intestinal tumors recurred when NSAID intake was interrupted (in the animal model the inhibitory action may be overcome by the supply of prostaglandins). Permanent intake of NSAIDs, however, is risky due to the side-effects already mentioned. Again, our model studies point the way towards a solution to the problem. Even though the different physiologic functions of the two prostaglandin synthases are by no means understood, it has been shown that these enzymes respond differently to the different NSAIDs. Attempts are currently under way to develop new, more selective inhibitory substances. Preliminary studies demonstrate that specific inhibitors of PGHS-2 exhibit markedly fewer side-effects, for instance in the gastro-intestinal tract, than aspirin or other conventional NSAIDs. If the observations gained from the animal model are correct, it is precisely this enzyme which is most closely related to tumorgenesis.

At the moment, we are expanding our studies to cover skin cancer induced by ultraviolet rays. As we all know, ozone depletion means we are increasingly exposed to UV rays, and prevention of skin cancer may become a crucial medical issue in years to come. It was recently established by other authors that the especially carcinogenic UV-B rays provoke PGHS-2 production in skin cells. It is therefore possible that this enzyme also plays an important role in skin cancer in humans. Time will tell whether the same applies to other types of tumor.

Is chemoprevention using NSAIDs effective, necessary and justified? A full answer to this question cannot yet be given. There is little doubt that prostaglandins play a decisive role in intestinal tumors, even though their mode of action requires further elucidation. It is certain that NSAID have both a preventive as well as a curative effect in intestinal cancer. Preventive therapy seems to be particularly indicated in at-risk groups, such as polyposis patients, and even more so if a further reduction in side-effects is achieved. In view of the side-effects though, the idea of general cancer prevention by NSAID – following the motto "an aspirin a day" – must be treated with caution until more information is available, except with regard to high-risk patients. Other preventive measures based on nutrition, as for instance reducing the intake of fat in favor of vegetables and fruits, are certainly more promising and carry less of a risk than the uncontrolled permanent ingestion of a drug. However, the results obtained so far on the anti-cancer action of aspirin and relative substances are too important and promising to be ignored any longer.

Dr. Gerhard Fürstenberger
Prof. Dr. Friedrich Marks
Division of Biochemistry of Tissue-Specific Regulation

Participating scientists

Dr. Karin Müller-Decker
Dipl.-Biol. Kirsten Scholz

Selected puplications

Fürstenberger, G., Marks, F.: The role of eicosanoids in normal hyperplastic and neoplastic growth. In: Eicosanoids and the Skin. Ed.: Ruzicka, T., CRC Press Boca Raton, USA pp. 107–124 (1990)

Fürstenberger, G.: Role of eicosanoids in mammalian skin epidermis. Cell Biol. Rev. 24, 1–111 (1990)

Müller-Decker, K., Scholz, K., Marks, F., Fürstenberger, G.: Differential expression of prostaglandin H-synthase enzymes during multistage carcinogenesis in mouse skin. Mol. Carcinogenesis 12, 31–41 (1995)

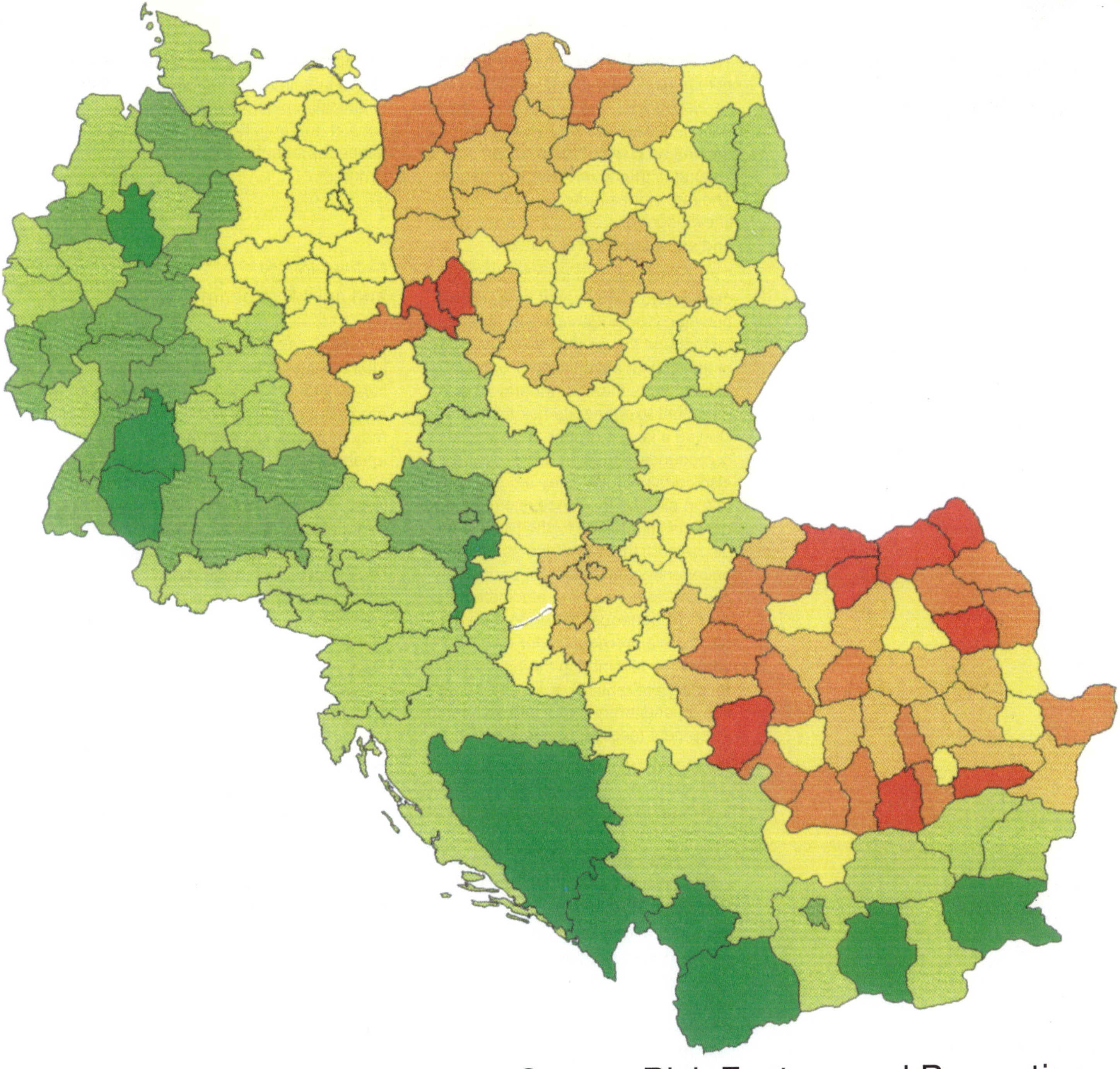

Cancer Risk Factors and Prevention

4

Cancer Risk Factors and Prevention

The Research Program regards as its primary tasks the identification of cancer risk factors, the quantitative registration of their cancer-causing potential, and the analysis of the mechanisms leading to the development of cancer. The aim of these efforts is to gain knowledge relevant for the prevention and early detection of cancer.

Carcinogenesis is a long lasting process due to complicated interactions between carcinogenic environmental factors and the genetic predisposition of the individuals afflicted. For most cancer types there is general agreement that exogeneous risk factors including a large number of chemical compounds, radiation and probably also certain viruses play the decisive role in eliciting the process of carcinogenesis. In addition to the genetic predisposition, there are also some other endogeneous risk factors, particularly certain hormones. The elucidation of such exogeneous and endogeneous factors is a prerequisite for cancer prevention by eliminating the risk factors (primary prevention) or for early detection of, and intervention into, cancer development (secondary prevention).

Direct information on environmental effects on the incidence of cancer derives from a large number of epidemiological observations showing differences in the occurrence of various forms of cancer with regard to place, time, and person (or person group).

Animal experiments (and with some restrictions also suitable tests for genetic alterations, i.e., mutagenicity test in cell cultures of certain tissues) offer an additional basis for the exploration of carcinogenic environmental factors and for the checking of findings obtained in humans. Data on the occurrence of chemical agents whose carcinogenicity is detected in animal studies also often lead to specific epidemiological investigations in humans. Both disciplines are hence represented in this Research Program.

Epidemiology and animal experiments

Chemical risk factors which, as such, or after metabolic transformation cause cancer in man or in laboratory animals are called carcinogens. Their effect may be proved by appropriate epidemiologic or animal experimental studies. Epidemiologic and experimental studies must comply with a series of methodological criteria in order to allow clear inferences with regard to the causal role of the corresponding factors in carcinogenesis. On the basis of such approaches, carcinogenic substances of the most diverse structure have been discovered up to now.

In addition to a large number of chemical compounds, physical factors like ultraviolet radiation of sunlight, x-rays or radioactive rays due to nuclear reactor accidents, as well as biological factors (viruses) have been identified as cancer risk factors. Whereas these categories of risk factors have mostly been studied in detail in experimental research, epidemiological investigations often comprise the entire diversity of potential factors.

Chemical cancer risk factors may be either widespread in the environment (ubiquitous) or delimited geographically or restricted to one location and hence associated with an exposure which can be specifically determined (occupational groups, nutritional habits). Appraisals on carcinogenicity may apply to single chemical substances as well as to groups of substances or to complex mixtures such as occur in the occupational environment or as a consequence of lifestyle (e.g. smoking or dietary habits).

The question of whether a substance has to be regarded as cancer-causing for humans is examined and decided by international expert groups under the auspices of the International Agency for Research on Cancer, an institution of the World Health Organization. So far, 50 substances or substance groups have been identified as clearly carcinogenic for humans. These include, to name just a few examples, the constituents of tar and soot (e.g., polycyclic aromatic hydrocarbons), tobacco smoke, benzene, asbestos, etc.

Besides the identification of isolated factors or groups of substances, additive or synergistic actions are also of very great importance, since they probably occur much more frequently than single effects. This holds true not only for the interaction of diverse chemical carcinogens, but also for possible synergistic effects of chemical substances with radiation or viruses. Thus, in the Deutsches Krebsforschungszentrum interactions between hepatitis viruses and the toxic fungus product aflatoxin B_1 are being intensively investigated in an experimental model of human hepatocarcinogenesis.

The occurrence and formation of suspected carcinogens in the environment are determined by means of analytical methods. In this way it is possible to appraise the exposure of a population group to such factors. Together with the investigation of nutritional habits, this can provide important information for prevention and early diagnosis. This research (e.g., the identification of nitrosamines and their analysis) is also being performed by the Deutsches Krebsforschungszentrum. Systematic animal experimental investigations with, in some cases, very elaborate methods (e.g., inhalation) are concerned both with relationships between chemical structures and carcinogenic action and with dose-effect relationships. Such data are necessary preconditions for appraisals of risks attributable to environmental carcinogens.

Co-carcinogens, which itensify the action of carcinogenic factors, can be identified by means of experiments and be isolated by biochemical methods in such a way that the structural units enable inferences with regard to the cancer-promoting action. New procedures for a quantitative assessment and evaluation of the cancer risk based on cocarcinogenic substances are being developed.

Epidemiological studies on the role of viruses in carcinogenesis are being made with respect to the incidence of papilloma virus infection in various groups of persons and their exposition to additional, particularly chemical cancer risk factors.

The follow-up investigation of the late fate of about 5000 persons in whom the radioactive x-ray contrast medium Thortrast containing thorium had been used for diagnostic reasons from 1935 to 1948 is the subject of an epidemiological study of the Deutsches Krebsforschungszentrum. In particular, this study serves to obtain more precise knowledge on the dose-effect relationship in the action of ionizing radiation on humans. The subject of this study is a comparison of the incidence of cancer cases in the exposed group of patients with that of a nonexposed control group. The persons still alive are regularly being followed up.

Other epidemiological investigations are concerned with the cancer risk of persons who were exposed to radiation for occupational reasons and for whom detailed dose measurements relating to individuals are available. These may be the staff of nuclear power stations. The detailed information on doses in this group, which are in relatively low range, should in turn provide valuable information on the dose-effect relationship of ionizing radiation. An international cohort sudy is concerned with this topic.

Besides special epidemiological studies on carcinogenesis, suitably analyzed descriptive data on the occurrence of cancer (new cases, mortalities) in western Germany and in international comparison provide an important basis for the development of specific problems and for the evaluation of cancer development in general (cancer atlases).

Molecular and cellular biomarkers

Epidemiological studies to investigate the causes of cancer and possibilities of cancer prevention will increasingly depend on laboratory-supported measurements and biomarkers in order to improve the appraisal of exposition on the level of the target tissues, to guarantee a better quantitative assessment of the cancer risk which is often influenced by genetic factors, and to understand cellular and molecular mechanisms which might be used for cancer prevention.

The research areas established at the Deutsches Krebsforschungszentrum have been contributing essential work to elucidate the metabolism of chemical carcinogens, to clarify the interaction of the metabolic products of the carcinogens with cellular macromolecules, particularly with DNA (e.g., DNA-adducts, DNA-repair), and for the detection of early changes in the function and form (phenotype) of the target cells.

The significance of DNA-repair for carcinogenesis in man is being investigated in patients with a genetically fixed repair deficiency, who run a high risk of developing skin cancer from exposure to ultraviolet rays of sunlight (Xeroderma pigmentosum). Specific cellular alterations appearing in different tissues in early stages of carcinogenesis, such as preneoplastic lesions of liver, kidney or pancreas, have generally been accepted as intermediate endpoints for the assessment of the carcinogenic risk by chemical compounds in so-called "medium term bioassays" in laboratory animals. The possibility to use such lesions for the early detection of cancer development in man is being investigated. Further studies of phenotypic cellular changes during carcinogenesis aim at an improvement of secondary cancer prevention by early diagnosis and intervention in the developmental process.

An essential supplementation and extension of these research approaches is expected from the activities of the Division of Toxicology and Cancer Risk Factors, which was newly established in 1993, and will focus its efforts on the development and application of biomarkers in molecular epidemiology and intervention studies.

The development of highly sensitive measurement methods by which lesions of DNA caused by carcinogens (actual reached sensitivity approx 1 modification per 10^{10} nucleotides) can be detected in exposed persons, makes it possible to explore more exactly the burden of carcinogenic agents. Thus, unknown sources of a carcinogenic exposition may be detected including those carcinogenic agents which were formed in the organism itself, and person groups with a higher cancer risk may be defined in a better way. For example, the potential endogeneous formation of N-nitroso-compounds as a possible risk factor for esophageal carcinogenesis (e.g., in Kashmir, India) is investigated. In addition, the genetic consequences of the carcinogen-DNA-adduct formation which in animal and in human cells often lead to characteristic mutation spectra, so-called genetic fingerprints, are investigated. Primarily, genetic alterations in human tumor cells are analyzed, which are caused by the effect of carcinogenic agents on growth-regulating genes, e.g. the p53-gene. From these fingerprints possible conclusions may be drawn on the type of the carcinogenic factors.

The role of chronic inflammation (mostly due to dusts, bacteria, parasites or viruses) in carcinogenesis, which contribute to a third of all cancer incidences worldwide, is being investigated on the molecular level. Nitrogen oxides and oxigen radicals arising in infected and inflamed tissues and overexpression of drug metabolizing enzymes may contribute to the process of carcinogenesis and lead to DNA lesions. In addition to human tumors of the head-neck region in tobacco-consuming persons, such alterations will be analyzed in an experimental model of the interaction between hepadna viruses and aflatoxin B_1 in hepatocellular carcinogenesis.

In order to clarify the mechanism of action of genotoxic substances and complex chemical mixtures, mutations and other DNA lesions, cytotoxicity and cell proliferation markers are investigated. For the evaluation of a resulting risk for humans, comparative in vitro investigations are made with freshly isolated primary cells from different organs of laboratory animals and from cells of human biopsies. The in vitro results are tested by corresponding in vivo experiments in rodents, which include mutation analyses in transgenic animals.

In the future, the interdisciplinary research area of molecular epidemiology will be extended by strengthening the cooperation between scientists of the different divisions in the Center and clinical cooperations and closer contacts with other institutions all over the world, in order to advance our understanding of cancer causes and cancer prevention.

Coordinator of the Research Program:
Prof. Dr. Jürgen Wahrendorf

Divisions and their heads:

Cellular Pathology:
Prof. Dr. Peter Bannasch

Toxicology and Cancer Risk Factors:
Prof. Dr. Helmut Bartsch

Molecular Toxicology:
Prof. Dr. Manfred Wießler

Mechanism of Tumorigenesis:
Prof. Dr. Erich Hecker

Interaction of Carcinogens and Biological Macromolecules:
Prof. Dr. Dr. Heinz W. Thielmann

Epidemiology:
Prof. Dr. Jürgen Wahrendorf

4.1 Tracing Fingerprints of Cancer-Causing Agents in Human Tumor Genes

by Monica Hollstein

Normal cells grow in an orderly, predictable way, while tumor cell growth is unrestrained and chaotic. Which of the many changes in the genetic material of the tumor cell are responsible for this new behavior? Important tasks in cancer research are to identify the genetic alterations that are crucial in carcinogenesis, to describe the nature of these changes in DNA, and to understand how they arose. Such knowledge is of more than theoretical interest, since cancer prevention programs and therapeutic strategies will be based on this information.

Research in the early decades of cancer genetics revealed major structural alterations in cancer cells such as tumor-specific chromosomal rearrangements. While it may seem logical that these substantial DNA sequence changes could elicit severe biological consequences, the more recent discoveries with techniques in molecular biology such as polymerase chain reaction (PCR) amplification and sequencing of DNA may have come as a surprise to some: tiny modifications of specific DNA sequences can also have drastic effects on health. Several inherited diseases, as well as a familial syndrome that predisposes to cancer (the Li-Fraumeni syndrome) have been traced to substitution of one single given base pair among the 3×10^9 base pairs of DNA that compose the human genome. In most sporadic cancers also (the majority of human cancers are sporadic) at least one step in the disease process is a point mutation, a single DNA base pair substitution for example, in a cancer-control gene. The p53 tumor suppressor gene in particular is a major target for these minute but devastating changes in DNA.

Point mutations are thus causative molecular events in the development of cancer. Where do these mutations come from? How do they arise? From experimental studies in the laboratory using test organisms ranging from bacteria to human cells in culture, it is clear that many known human carcinogens can cause these subtle changes in DNA. Furthermore, mutagens and carcinogens damage the genome in characteristic ways, leading to specific kinds of base changes at specific locations, a finding that has led to the concept of a "mutagen fingerprint" on DNA. The term "fingerprint" should be interpreted cautiously, however, because mutation patterns, usually referred to as spectra, are unlikely to be as unique as a human fingerprint: chemically related mutagens can have similar spectra.

An equally important dicovery from laboratory mutation research is that mutations in DNA also arise spontaneously; they are a "normal" consequence of various biological and biochemical processes in living cells. For example, when DNA polymerases replicate DNA before cell division, mistakes inevitably occur, and should the errors escape the repair machinery, a DNA sequence change – a mutation – becomes fixed in the genome.

Mutations of the kind one sees in cancer genes of human tumors could therefore arise either spontaneously or from environmental exposures. Which source is more important, or do both contribute to the mutations that lead to cancer. Since carcinogens leave mutation fingerprints on DNA, and spontanteous cellular mutagenic process also leave characteristic tell-tale DNA sequence changes, then analysis of tumor p53 mutations could provide clues

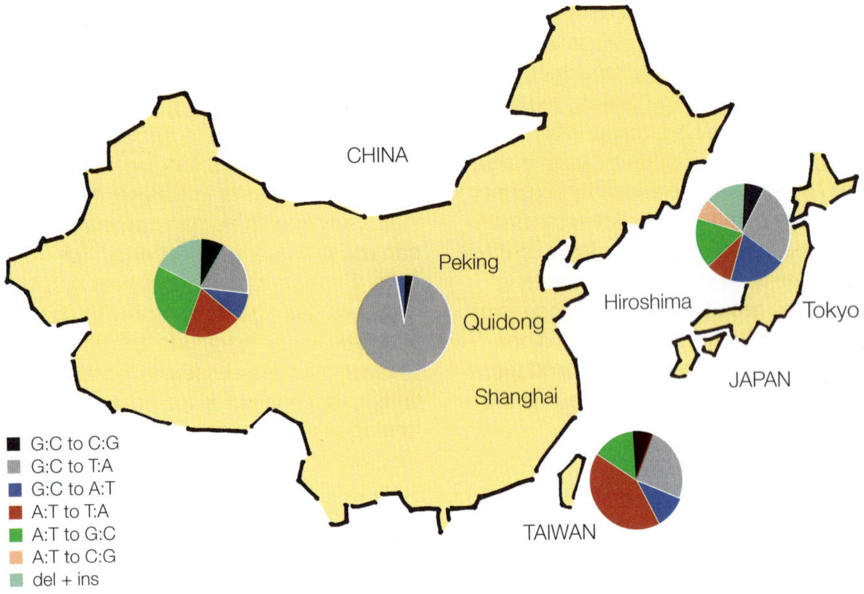

Fig. 29
In Asia the mutations associated with liver cancer vary greatly from region to region. Strikingly, a great amount of liver cell cancers in the Quidong region present the same type of mutation, G:C→T:A transversion at codon 249. A direct association has been established between this mutation and the presence of the toxic metabolic product of the fungus Aspergillus flavus contaminating the food

about the important sources of cancer gene mutation in the human setting.

To assess this approach, we have analyzed mutation spectra generated from a compilation of all the published mutations discovered in the p53 tumor suppressor gene of human cancers. About 6000 tumors have been sequenced at this location of the human genome and approximately half of these tumors harbored a single point mutation, usually the substitution of one DNA base (G A T C, the four building block bases of DNA), by another.

Several striking features of mutation spectra in the p53 tumor suppressor gene have emerged. First, the spectra vary from cancer type to cancer type, and even from risk group to risk group for a given cancer type. In lung tumors, the most common type of mutation is substitution of the base guanine to thymine (G→T), whereas colorectal tumors are likely to have an adenine at a position where guanine should be (G→A). Whether or not the mutation is G→T or G→A; the biological consequence is usually that the p53 tumor suppressor protein no longer functions properly, leading to a more "cancer-like" behavior of the cell. Whether the "G→T rich" p53 mutation pattern in lung tumors could be attributable to tobacco smoke exposure can be tested in the laboratory and in molecular epidemiology studies. Does tobacco smoke, the cause of 90% of human lung cancers, produce a G→T fingerprint on DNA ? Evidence thus far suggests that it does. Experimental work in bacteria and mammalian cells has demonstrated that a major carcinogenic component in cigarette smoke generates primarily G→T substitutions. The proportion of lung cancer p53 mutations that are G→T substitutions is higher in heavy smoker patient groups.

An undeniable concordance between the experimentally observed mutation fingerprint of a cancer agent and a p53 tumor mutation spectrum is provided by studies on skin cancers. The major risk factor for several types of skin cancers is exposure to ultraviolet rays of sunlight. Ultraviolet light has been shown in the laboratory to induce a highly unusual and characteristic type of sequence change, a tandem base substitution in which two cytosine bases (CC), side by side, are replaced with two thymine residues (CC→TT). In human skin cancers the p53 gene is frequently mutated, and typical mutations are indeed exactly those that one would expect from UV exposure: CC→TT tandem mutations. These double mutations are very rare in other human cancers; of the several hundred p53 mutations discovered in colorectal tumors, for example, not a single one was a CC→TT double substitution.

Even for a given cancer type, mutation patterns of the p53 gene can vary dramatically depending on the exposure history of the patients. The p53 mutation patterns for hepatocellular cancer (HCC) vary geographically, and the variation is linked to an environmetal carcinogen, aflatoxin, that elevates risk.

In this case, what distinguishes one spectrum from another is not only the type of base substitution but also where it occurs in the gene. In certain rural areas of China, where exposure to dietary aflatoxin is high, almost all the HCC with a p53 gene mutation are exactly alike, a G to T substitution at one unique location, codon 249. In other parts of Asia, such as urban China or Japan, many kinds of mutations in HCC are found at a variety of locations in the p53 gene. Aflatoxin causes G to T mutations in experimental systems, but laboratory studies have still not explained why the tumor mutation in rural China associated with aflatoxin exposure occurs at a unique site in the gene.

All kinds of changes in DNA sequence also occur during normal biological processes, that is, naturally. Fully one-fourth of all p53 tumor mutations belongs to a class of mutations called “base transitions at CpG dinucleotides” that can occur spontaneously by the process of deamination. This shows that some cancer-specific genetic changes arise from natural factors within the cell. In addition, some exogenous agents may increase the risk of cancer by stimulating these deleterious events.

Tumor mutation spectra are being evaluated not only for their use in the identification of environmental carcinogens, but also for the elucidation of inherently mutagenic cellular activities. p53 mutation patterns have given answers to some riddles and raised new questions about mutagenesis per se. Cancer gene mutations in tumors are a selection from an initial set of mutations following specific DNA-carcinogen interactions and DNA repair. Tests to detect non-selected mutations in normal tissue have been developed by Dr. Peter Cerutti and colleagues for calculating inital mutation loads and fingerprints. From a comparison of selected mutations (in tumors) and non-selected mutations (in normal tissue of exposed individuals) these parameters and the biological properties of various mutants in different cellular contexts can be studied.

Dr. Monica Hollstein
Division of Toxicology and Cancer Risk Factors

In collaboration with

Dr. Curtis C. Harris
Laboratory of Human Carcinogenesis, National Cancer Institute,
Bethesda, Maryland, U.S.A.

Dr. Ruggero Montesano
International Agency for Research on Cancer,
Lyon, France

Dr. Peter Cerutti
Swiss Institute for Experimental Cancer Research,
Epalinges, Lausanne, Switzerland

Dr. Kate Rice
Dr. Rainer Fuchs
European Molecular Biology Laboratory (EMBL) Datalibrary,
Heidelberg

Selected Publications

Harris, C. C., Hollstein, M.: Clinical Implications of the p53 tumor-suppressor gene. New Engl. J. Med. 329: 1318–1327 (1993)

Aguilar. F., Harris, C. C., Sun, T., Hollstein, M., Cerutti, P.: Geographic variation of p53 mutational profile in preneoplastic human liver. Science 264: 1317–1319 (1994)

Greenblatt, M. S., Bennett, W. P., Hollstein, M., Harris, C. C.: Mutations in the p53 tumor suppressor gene: clues to cancer etiology and molecular pathogenesis. Cancer Res. 54: 4855–4878 (1994)

Hollstein, M., Marion, M. J., Lehman, T., Welsh, J., Harris, C. C., Martel-Planche, G., Kusters, I., Montesano, R.: p53 mutations at A:T base pairs in angiosarcomas of vinyl chloride-exposed factory workers. Carcinogenesis 15: 1–3 (1994)

4.2 Cancer Atlases in Europe – Relevance and Results

by Nikolaus Becker

Cancer occurrence differs in term of geographical region and organs that are afflicted. Depending on factors such as lifestyle, nutrition, occupation, and natural environmental conditions, the incidence of a particular cancer may be especially high in one country while a different cancer prevails in another country. This was demonstrated impressively in one of the first „migrant studies“ in which the incidence of cancer in Japanese immigrants in the United States was investigated: their cancer risk profile shifted with the passage of time from that of their country of origin, Japan, to that of the new country, the United States. While the incidence of tumors of the bowel, lung, breast and prostate increased, the rate of esophageal or stomach tumors diminished. Such observations suggested that environmental conditions – in the widest sense – play a major role in the etiology of cancers.

In Europe, a large number of different populations inhabit a relatively small area. They live under economic and environmental conditions that are similar in some respects and very different in others; so, too, the lifestyles of the peoples. Since the beginning of the nineteen-eighties, series of national and international cancer-atlas projects have been attempting to describe the impact on cancer of the common features and differences characteristic of these populations. They preserve two goals: the first is to explain the observed mortality patterns by available knowledge on cancer risk factors. If this turns out to be not feasible, one expects, secondly, to get ideas on potential risk factors which could be investigated by future research projects. The ultimate goal of this epidemiological research project is to provide the scientific basis for effective measures for cancer prevention.

The first atlas established at a European level was the „Cancer Atlas of the European Economic Community“, published in 1992, based on mortality data for the decade 1971 to 1980 in the nine European Countries then forming the European Economic Community (Belgium, The Netherlands, Luxembourg, France, Italy, Great Britain, Ireland, Denmark, and the former West Germany). The data available for Germany covered the period 1976-1980 and had already been used to compile the German cancer atlas, published in 1984; however, in the European atlas the data were given on administrative district level rather than at a city or rural level, as in the national publication.

Figure 30 shows a map taken from this first European atlas. It displays mortality due to esophageal cancer in men: The cluster of deaths in certain regions of the north and northwest of France is particularly prominent. Those same regions also display a high incidence of tumors of the oral cavity and cancer of the larynx. By contrast, Germany had a much lower mortality from these types of tumors. When this finding became public in France at the end of the seventies, epidemiological studies were initiated to investigate the clusters. The phenomenon was found to be due to high alcohol consumption in conjunction with heavy smoking.

A joint Polish-German project to compile a Polish cancer atlas evolved into an international collaboration to produce a cancer atlas covering Central Europe. The project had been initiated as early as the mid-eighties, when the political situation was such that it was

Fig. 30
Mortality from esophageal cancer is markedly elevated in certain regions of northern and northwestern France. The map taken from the 1992 western European cancer atlas shows the mortality figures for men. The regions with the highest mortality are shown in red and those with the lowest rates in green

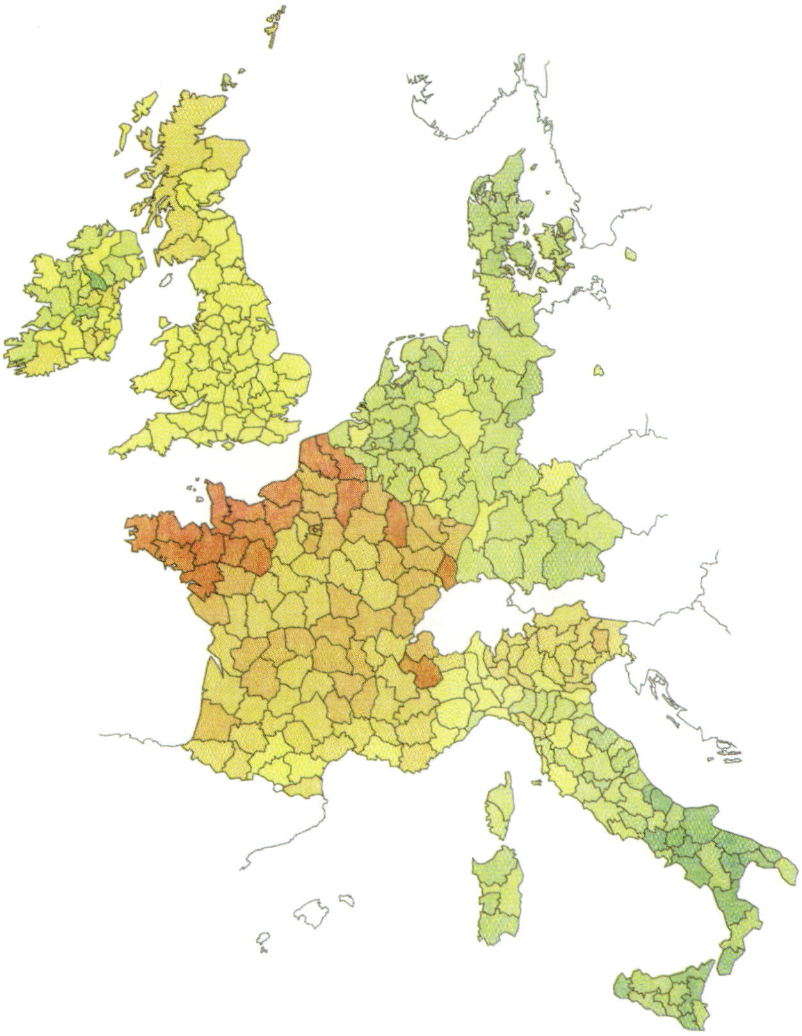

not evident whether the countries would have liked „their“ cancer mortality data to be published. This project was the first step towards illuminating the Central and Eastern European cancer scene, which until then was completely unknown. The atlas will be published in 1995 by the International Agency for Research on Cancer (IARC in Lyon, France).

Figure 31 is a map being included in the publication, showing mortality from cervical cancer in central and southeastern Europe. The highest rates are found in regions of Rumania and in parts of western Poland. While the former West Germany is one of the countries with the lowest rates, mortality in the former East Germany is somewhat higher. Whether the remarkably low rates in the former Yugoslavia are based on data of comparable quality may be called into question. A well organized early cancer screening program and willingness of women to take part in that program help prevent the occurrence of cervical cancer and death from this site. Comparison of the different countries leads to the question of whether secondary prevention of this kind is less efficient in countries or regions of countries with a high rate of cervical cancer than in other countries and might be improved. In this case, the finding of the atlas would have given rise of increased effectiveness of cancer prevention and reduction of cancer mortality in those regions.

In another cancer atlas project, initiated by the Finish cancer registry in Helsinki, epidemiological data from the Baltic countries, the bordering parts of Russia, and white Russia are being published for the first time. The work will also be published in 1995; example of maps are not yet available. In addition, data from Russia and other countries of the former Soviet Union have also become available recently, allowing work on a cancer atlas comprising the whole of Europe to be started in the future.

The examples of maps show that there is quite remarkable variation in the incidence of various types of cancers within Europe. As mentioned before, the strikingly high mortality rates found in the north of France prompted research projects at the end of the seventies which established the relationship between cancer and high alcohol consumption combined with tobacco smoking. Another approach to epidemiological research are so-called „multicenter" studies that place an arm of the study in a high-risk area and another „arm" in a low-risk area. This arrangement allows epidemiologists to verify whether and to what extent the existing risk factors are the actual cause of the reported regional differences in the incidence of cancer. An example of this procedure is the study on gastric cancer conducted at the beginning of the eighties in Bavaria and Hesse. The starting point was the map of mortality from gastric cancer in the former West Germany, published in the Cancer Atlas of the Federal Republic of Germany in 1984. The map showed a significantly increased mortality from gastric cancer in Bavaria, while parts of Hesse, relatively close to Bavaria, showed a markedly low mortality from gastric cancer. Thus, one arm of the study was located in Bavaria and the other in the neighboring region in Hesse. The study established that, independently of the region, consumption of processed meat products and smoked meat – especially that smoked using spruce wood – was associated with an increased risk of gastric cancer. Fresh fruits and vegetables were shown to have a protective effect. With regard to the considered region it turned out that the prevalence of the quoted risk factors was different and could explain at least partially the observed differences in stomach cancer mortality.

Another important aspect of cancer occurrence is the change in mortality over time. Figure 32 shows the five most frequent types of cancer most among men and women in the former West Germany. It is seen that the mortality of four of these cancers increased from 1952 to 1990. In part, the trend is still continuing. In contrast to this, the mortality of gastric cancer has declined dramatically for both sexes. Such changes over a period of time are also observed for the rarer cancer types. Cervical cancer is a revealing example in this respect. Mortality from this type of tumor increased significantly in the former West Germany up to the early seventies; since that time, however, it has been decreasing as rapidly as it had increased up to

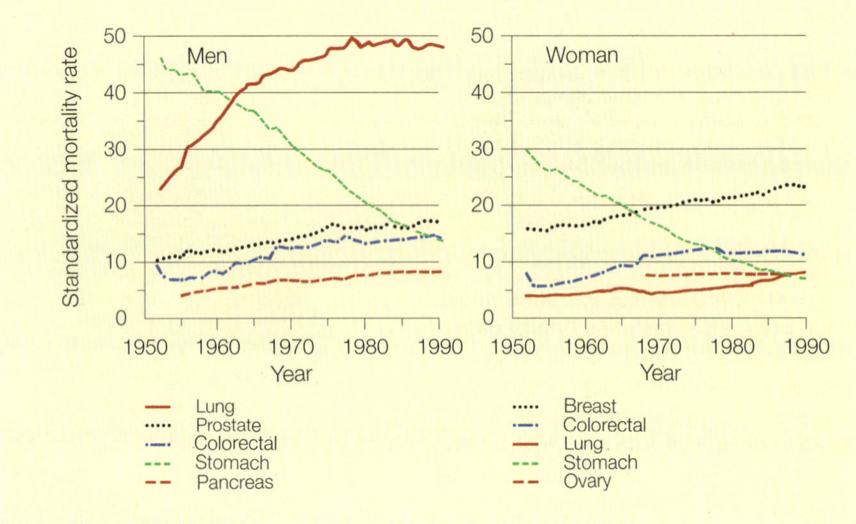

Fig. 32
The figure shows the five most common types of cancer in men and women in the former West Germany. An increase in mortality from four of them was observed from 1952 to 1993

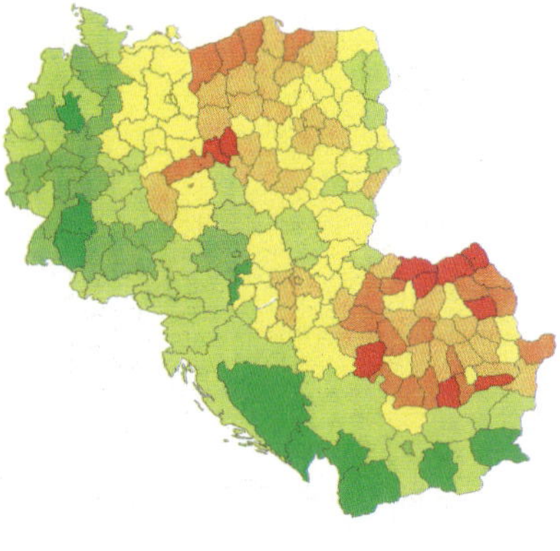

Fig. 31
This map from the central European cancer atlas shows mortality from cervical cancer in central and southeastern Europe in the 1983–1988 period. Mortality from cervical cancer was highest in certain regions of Romania and parts of western Poland

Fig. 33 a, b
Mortality trends in the former West Germany (broken line) and in the former East Germany (dotted line). Figure a shows mortality from colorectal cancer, which has been steadily decreasing since the mid-1970s in women and men. Figure b shows the impressive reduction in mortality from testicular cancer since the introduction of improved means of treatment

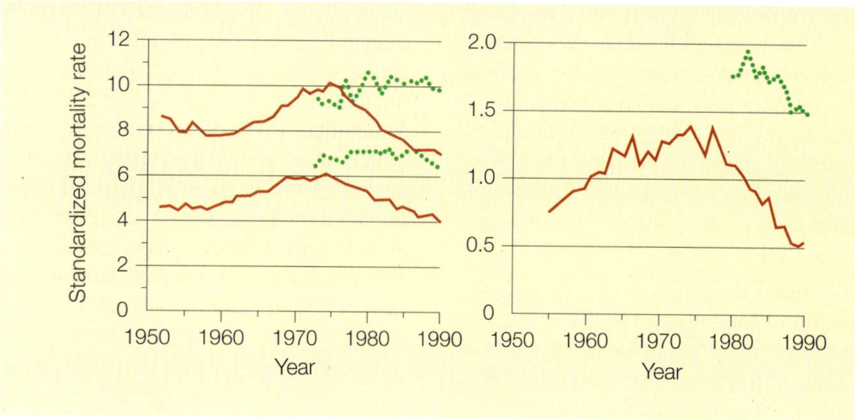

then. The turning point was marked by the introduction of early cancer screening programs for cervical and other cancers in the then West Germany. Mortality rates in the former East Germany were slightly higher than those in Western Germany. Although East Germany also experienced a rapid fall in mortality over the period for which data are available (since 1973 for some types of cancer) the initial rates here were much higher than in the West. The difference between the two parts of Germany has hardly diminished, an indication that, after reunification, efforts to improve early detection of cervical cancer should be made so as to reduce the difference between Eastern and Western Germany as soon as possible.

Some remarks should be included on the changes in mortality from the various cancers demonstrated in Figure 33a. This figure shows the death rate due to rectal tumors. The rate is seen to have increased up to the end of the seventies since then to have declined dramatically in both sexes. In contrast, data from the mid-seventies onwards from the former East Germany show an almost constant level. Dedicated epidemiological studies indicate that the decrease reported in West Germany is due only slightly, if at all, to early cancer detection measures. It is more likely that better diagnostic procedures and possibly a change in dietary habits have played a role.

A major risk factor for tumors of the gall bladder are gall stones. The decline in mortality from this type of cancer is attributable to the preventive removal of the gall bladder in gall stone carriers.

Mortality from melanomas increased markedly over the whole period, although, data are only available from 1968 onwards. Excessive sun-bathing is thought to be the main risk factor. The data from the former East Germany that are available since the eighties are interesting. They do not follow the trend towards increased rates, a fact that may be explained by the different vacationing habits in the two parts of Germany. It should be added that the increase in the incidence of melanomas started from a very low baseline level.

Testicular tumors (Fig. 33b) provide an excellent example of how the introduction of a new, efficient treatment is directly reflected in cause-of-death statistics. In 1979, a new therapy with cisplatin was approved for this type of cancer. Since then, mortality from testicular tumors has decreased dramatically.

The deaths due to kidney tumors also reflect a possible impact of improved therapy. Since the mid-eighties, the hitherto rapidly increasing mortality rate has levelled off, an effect which coincided with the introduction of a new type of treatment. However, the data available from the former East Germany show increased mortality. This might be due to the relatively slow implementation of new diagnostic procedures and therapeutic methods there.

Finally, the data basis of cancer atlases and some of the associated problems will be considered in a few sentences. Cancer atlases are usually based on official cause-of-death statistics of the participating countries. The World Health Organization (WHO) has drawn up guidelines for the documentation of cause of death and these are followed in almost all European countries. The guidelines include information on such matters as how a death certificate should be laid out and that it must be completed by a physician. The cause of death indicated is then coded according to the International Classification of Diseases (ICD). Finally, all deaths and the ascertained causes of death are reported to statistics offices, where they are stored as official cause-of-death statistics.

For the compilation of cancer atlases, epidemiologists retrieve these data from the statistics offices of the participating countries in a condensed form. The Deutsches Krebsforschungszentrum, for example, receives the number of deaths from different cancer sites, e.g. lung, stomach, separated according to sex and broken down in 5-year age groups. For groups of calendar years (for instance from 1976–1980), which cover all individual districts and cities in Germany. This means that no individual data or even personal data are used. The first cancer atlas compiled according to district was the Cancer Atlas of the Federal Republic of Germany“, published in 1984 by Springer Verlag, Heidelberg, Germany.

Detailed investigations confirm that these data achieve the necessary quality, at least with respect to the western European countries. Whether the same applies to the central and eastern European countries remains to be decided by future studies. A fundamental problem of all regional and time-based analyses of cancer on the basis of mortality data is that only fatal cancers are included. The incidence of tumors that do not usually lead to death, for instance skin cancer (melanoma excepted), and tumors in which efficient early detection or therapeutic successes lead to improved survival, is either not amenable at all to presentation by this method, or can only be presented in a distorted fashion. For instance, the rate of new cases of a cancer may rise, while the mortality rate drops due to major therapeutic advances. The discrepancy only becomes visible if statistics concerning new cases are available. Such data can be obtained from cancer registers. Countries running cancer registers, for instance the Scandinavian countries, are then able to study incidence in parallel to mortality and can thus identify diverging developments. Of all the German States, only Saarland has well-performing register. However, laws on cancer registers are being prepared on a federal and country level or have already been passed. A major argument for the rapid establishment of cancer registers all over Germany is the problem described, namely, only a uncomplete or, in some instances, distorted description of the cancer landscape is possible on the basis of a country's mortality data alone.

Dr. Nikolaus Becker
Division of Epidemiology

Selected Publications:

Becker, N., Frentzel-Beyme, R., Wagner, G.: Krebsatlas der Bundesrepublik Deutschland – Atlas of Cancer Mortality in the Federal Republic of Germany. Second Edition. Springer, Berlin Heidelberg New York Tokyo, (1984)

Zatonski, W., Becker, N.: Atlas of Cancer Mortality in Poland. Springer, Berlin Heidelberg New York (1988)

Boeing, H., Frentzel-Beyme, R., Berger, M. et al: Case-Control Study on Stomach Cancer in Germany. Int. J. Cancer 47, 858–864 (1991)

Hölzel, D., Altwein, J.E.: Hodentumoren. Deutsches Ärzteblatt 88 (47), 4123–4130 (1991)

Smans, M., Muir, C.S., Boyle, P.: Atlas of Cancer Mortality in the European Economic Community. IARC Scientific Publications No.117, Lyon (1992)

4.3 Ways to Eliminate Carcinogenic Substances in the Occupational Surrounding – the Prevention of Nitrosamine Exposure in the Rubber Industry

by Jens Seibel
and Bertold Spiegelhalder

Today, carcinogenic substances exist in the surrounding of many occupational fields. In the following contribution, we especially examine the chemical class of nitrsamines in a selected industrial area. Nitrosamines are a group of chemical substances characterized by their pronounced organ specificity and high carcinogenic potential even at very low doses.

Carcinogenic nitrosamines are found in the surroundings in which secondary amines and nitrosating agents, the basic material of nitrosamines, occur. This means that the spread of this problem extends from the metal-consuming industry, the steel industry, and the chemical industry to the leather industry and the rubber industry. In the following, we will concentrate on the initial basis and the attempts to solve these problems in the rubber and tyre industry.

Epidemiological studies, carried out in the early 1980s in Scandinavia and the USA, showed a high risk of cancer among workers in the rubber industry. A probable cause was postulated as being due to the occurrence of volatile carcinogenic nitrosamines in the production and storage process. Also, air measurements performed in the German rubber industry (1982–1984) engaging more than 85 000 workers showed nitrosamine concentrations in the range between 0.1 and 90 $\mu g/m^3$. The following nitrosamines were detected:

N-nitrosodimethylamine (NDMA), N-nirosodiethylamine (NDEA), N-nitrosodibutylamine (NDBA), N-nitrosomorpholine (NMOR), and N-nitrosopiperidine (NPIP). The reduction of nitrosamine exposure in the rubber industry is of great preventive medical interest. The high production capacity existing in all industrial countries coupled with the expansive use of rubber products in our daily life requires effective improvement.

Legalities

Personell measurements taken in more then 500 workplaces in the year 1987 revealed volatile nitrosamine concentrations up to 41 $\mu g/m^3$. Therefore, the Board for Dangerous Chemical Substances (Ausschuß für Gefahrstoffe, AGS) enacted the Technical Rule for Substances of a Critical Nature (Technische Regel für Gefahrstoffe; TRGS 552/"nitrosamines"). These rules for criti-cal substances enacted by the Minister of Labor and the Minister of Environmental Affairs, illustrate the technical and medical standard requirements. The preliminary permitted concentration of nitrosamines in the rubber industry at this time was 2.5 $\mu g/m^3$. New measurements conducted at the end of the year 1989 showed reduced nitrosamine concentrations. However, the measured values in 13.7% of the cases (rubber products, not including tire) were still higher than 2.5 $\mu g/m^3$. All nitrosamines found in the rubber industry are volatile carcinogenic substances. Since the end of 1992, permitted concentrations of these substances accord the normal values (Technische Richtkonzentrationen (TRK)-values). These values, given in the TRGS 102, lay down maximal permitted concentrations of a compound obtainable with modern methods. By the observation of these values, the health risk for workers could be reduced to as low as possible. The value nevertheless does not exclude a rest risk for those concerned.

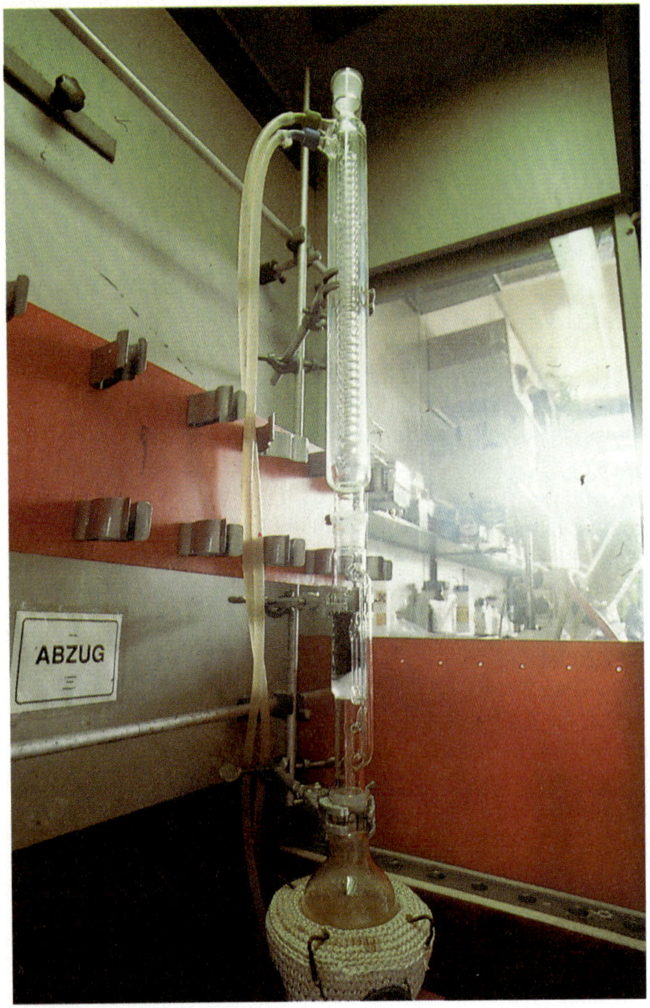

Fig. 34
Extraction of nitrosamines from rubber samples for analysis

Presently, the TRK-value amounts to 2.5 µg/m³ in the rubber industry for the curing process and in storage. In all other areas of production the permitted value is 1 µg/m³ (this value also applies for all the above-mentioned industrial areas). In the near future an amendment of the TRGS 552 will restrict the relative high value of 25 µg/m³ of the respective working areas.

Characteristics of the rubber production/causes of nitrosamine exposure

Rubber is an elastomeric material which is characterized by high elasticity as well as low brittleness at low temperatures. This characteristic feature is caused by the cross-linking of the macromolecules through a chemical reaction at high tem-peratures and pressure (vulcanization).

The high requirements needed, especially for sealing, V-belts, tubes, and tires, are reached by utilizing very complex product mixtures. Polymer is the basis of the rubber material. Additionally, rubber contains inorganic rubber additives, for example zinc oxide or carbon black, pigments, softening agents, aging protective substances, and vulcanization accelerators. These vulcanization accelerators induce the cross-linking of the polymer at moderate reaction conditions. Subsequently, the obtained product is suitable for diverse applications.

The used vulcanization accelerators predominantly contain sulphur-nitrogen compounds, wherein the structure of secondary amines is found. During the curing process the secondary amines react with oxides of nitrogen in the air, nitrite from salt-baths or with nitrosating rubber chemicals (organic nitro- and nitroso compounds) to form the carcinogenic nitrosamines. These nitrosamines correspond to the used vulcanisation accelerators. This implies that only those nitrosamines are formed which correspond to the secondary amine moiety of the accelerators.

Approaches to reduce nitrosamines exposure

The set norm values (TRK-values), given by the legislature, are supervised by the industrial inspection board and

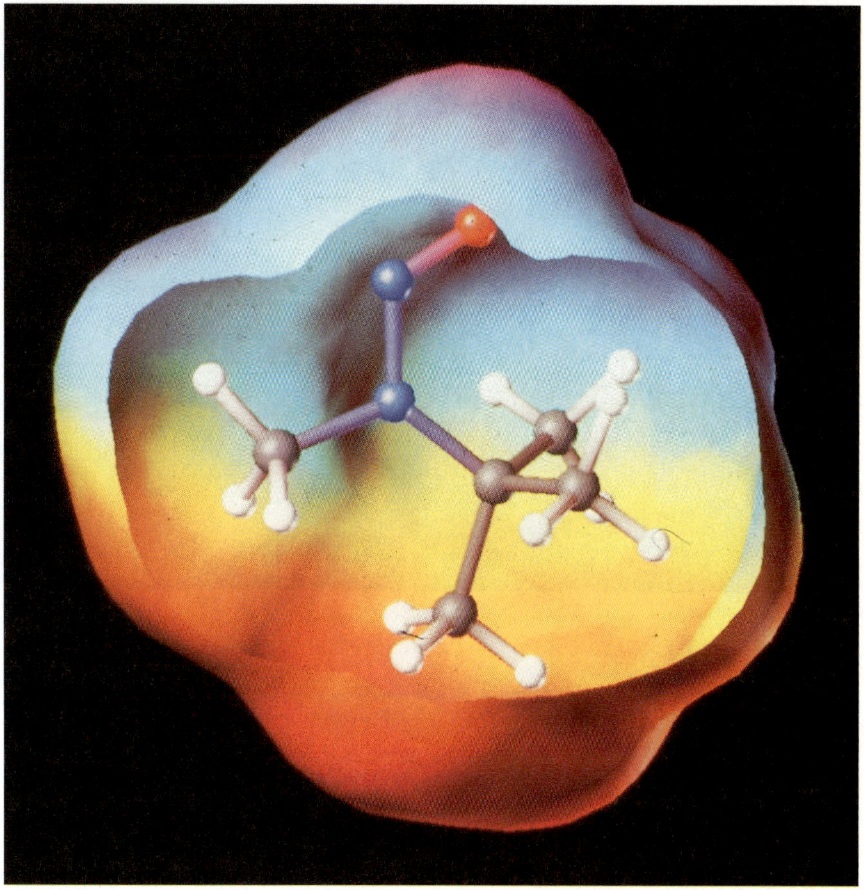

Fig. 35
A computer model (MOLCAD) of a non-carcinogenic nitrosamine, derived from a "safe amine"

the professional association. In order to meet these values, the industry undertook different measures with varying success. The different approaches to prevent the formation of carcinogenic nitrosamines are listed as follows:

The exclusion of nitrosating substances at the site of vulcanization is not realistic because this would require production under an inert-gas atmosphere. Additionally, a part of the oxides of nitrogen is absorbed on the large surface of the inorganic rubber additives.

The use of inhibitors (α-tocopherol, urea), which are able to inhibit the formation of nitosamines in the rubber mixture, is still on trial.

The best results are achieved by the use of ventilation techniques, especially in the depot of rubber material. During the curing itself, these approaches are not sufficient to reach the so-called TRK-values.

The best alternative procedure to these methods is the introduction of substitutes instead of the commonly used accelerators. These substitutes should be free of secondary amines or at least should not be able to form carcinogenic nitrosamines. The use of nitrogen-free accelerators (for example, thiophosphates, peroxides) is definitely the best way to avoid the formation of nitrosamines, but the application of nitrogen-free accelerators is, however, limited to specific rubber mixtures. In the past, the industry tried to replace the used vulcanization mixtures with new combinations of harmless accelerators. A novel development of a new vulcanization accelerator has been successful in only one of the four large groups of accelerators. The widely used sulfenamides can, in most cases, be substituted by accelerators containing primary amines instead of secondary amines. The other classes of accelerators, thiurames, dithiocarbamates and bisaminodisulfides, are still necessary for rubber to achieve good technical properties.

Concept of "safe amines"

An alternative approach to avoid the formation of carcinogenic nitrosamines has been followed by our group for several years. This work is financed by the Ministry of Research and Technology in the program "Work and Technique". Our aim is to synthesise new accelerators bases on "safe-amines". "Safe-amines" are characterized by low nitrosibility and/or formation of non-carcinogenic nitrosamines. The properties of the

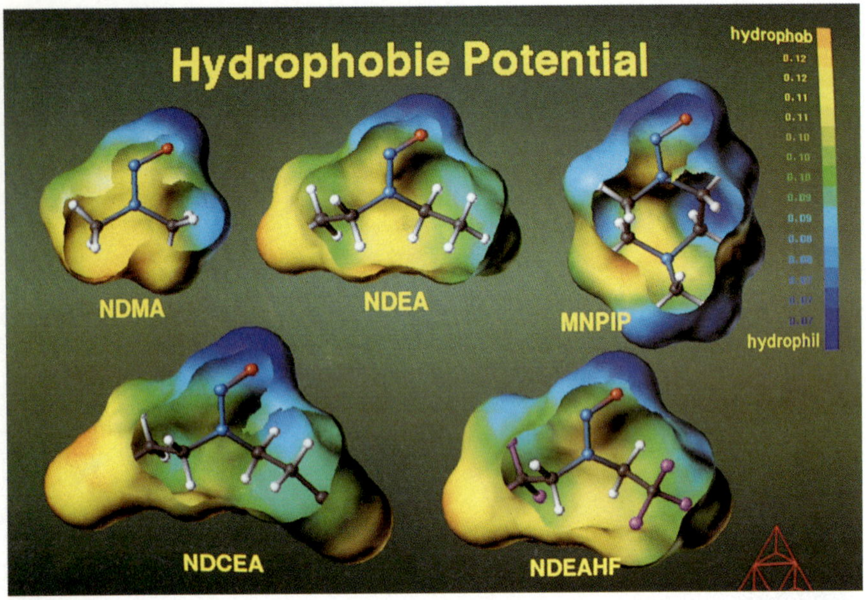

Fig. 36
A computer model of various nitrosamines: N-nitrosodimethylamine (NDMA, carcinogenic) and N-nitroso-methylpiperazine (MNPIP, derived from a "safe amine")

"safe-amines" correspond to special structural and electronic factors in the amine molecules. Therefore, substitution of "safe-amines" for the traditional amino compounds in different types of accelerators give compounds that are still active as accelerators, but unable to form carcinogenic nitrosamines.

Realisation of the "safe-amines" concept

Following the concept of "safe-amines," it is principally possible to exchange the commonly used secondary amines with "safe-amines" in all classes of accelerators (sulfenamides, dithiocarbamates, thiuramdisulfides, and bisaminodisulfides). Over 100 "safe-amines", predominantly newly synthesised, showed an important relationship between the structure of the amines and the possibility to obtain accelerators of good yields. In spite to some synthetic difficulties, the synthesis of more than 150 vulcanization accelerators was successful.

In a second step, the technological properties of the new compounds are tested by our industrial cooperation partner. The examination of the rubber, after a general prescreening, gives typical properties such as cross linking, tensile strength, elongation at break and rebound elasticity. The comparison of these data with industrial standards give first insights for the applicability of a new compound. Consequently, the applicable substance is tested in several different rubber formulations, for example, nature rubber and different synthetic rubbers. In the following step, the new accelerator will be synthesized in an amount of 50–100 kg. These quantities enable use to supply those interested firms in the rubber branch, so that the product can be tested under different conditions, especially rubber formulations. From the feedback, we can conclude the acceptance of the new product in the industry.

Accompanying this procedure, we synthesize the corresponding nitrosamines to the utilized "safe-amines". In cooperation with our partner in Hungary, we carry out the toxicological evaluations (mutagenic and carcinogenic behavior) of these nitrosamines. In all examined cases so far, it was shown that the nitrosamines derived from "safe-amines" are non-carcinogenic.

Furthermore, the rubber manufactured with the new accelerators is examined in order to evaluate the amount of formed nitrosamines.

Thirty compounds of the 150 synthesized accelerators showed very similar vulcanization characteristics to those of the industrial standard, but only some of these substances are suitable for technical production. This marked reduction is mainly due to two factors. First, the new compounds require a wide spread application and second, the production must be simple and economical. Only these factors give the guarantee for a good acceptance in the industry.

In each of the classes of dithiocarbamates and thiuramdisulfides, one compound was developed and all the predescribed test and synthesis procedures were completed. From the product development side, the marketability will not be hindered. In the case of the bisaminodisulfide, technical production will soon start. This will enable us to send the new product to several German rubber factories. Presently, several other tests of new copunds are in progress, and will lead to the availability of optimal accelerators under high specific formulation conditions on the basis of "safe-amine". In spite of some synthetic difficulties, the formed products possess very high technological value.

Our concept for harmless subsitutes for commonly used compounds is an important primary preventive measure. This method, which avoids the formation of carcinogenic nitrosamines, is favored over all attempts made to eliminate the nitrosamines after their formation. At the close of this project, it can be inferred that the accomplished work, based on the "safe-amines" concept, is one of the most successful methods to solve the nitrosamine exposure in the rubber industry.

Dr. Jens Seibel
Dr. Bertold Spiegelhalder
Division of Toxicology and Cancer Risk Factors

Participating staff

Dr. Claus-Dieter Wacker
(until February 1993)

Prof. Dr. Rudolf Preußmann
(until October 1993)

Helmut Kehl
Dr. Gerd Moeckel
Eva Schleicher
Ina Theobald

In collaboration with

Schill & Seilacher, Rubber chemicals, Hamburg

Spieß & Sohn, Chemical plant, Kleinkarlbach

Dr. Alan Pintér
National Institute of Hygiene, Budapest, Hungary

Selected publications

Preussmann, R., Spiegelhalder, B., Wacker, C.-D.: Präventionsmaßnahmen zur Verringerung der Nitrosaminexposition in der Gummiindustrie, Ergo-Med 13, 64–66 (1989)

Wacker, C.-D., Spiegelhalder, B., Preussmann, R.: New sulfenamide accelerators derived from "safe amines" for the rubber and tyre industry. In: Relevance to Human Cancer of N-Nitroso Compounds, Tobacco Smoke and Mycotoxins. Eds.: O'Neill, I., Chen, J., Bartsch, H., IARC Scientific Publications, Lyon, No. 105, 592–595 (1991)

Wacker, C.-D., Kehl, H., Theobald, I., Schleicher, E., Preussmann, R., Spiegelhalder, B.: Vorkommen von Nitrosaminen in der Gummiindustrie: Prävention durch "Safe Amine"-Beschleuniger. In: Krebsrisiken am Arbeitsplatz. Hrsg.: Horst, A., Norpoth, K., Verkoyen, C., Springer-Verlag, Berlin, 247–262 (1992)

Spielgelhalder, B., Wacker, C.-D.: Prevention of nitrosamine exposure in the rubber industry. In: Nitrosamines and N-Nitroso Compounds. Ed.: Loeppky, R.N., ACS Books, Washington, 42–51 (1993)

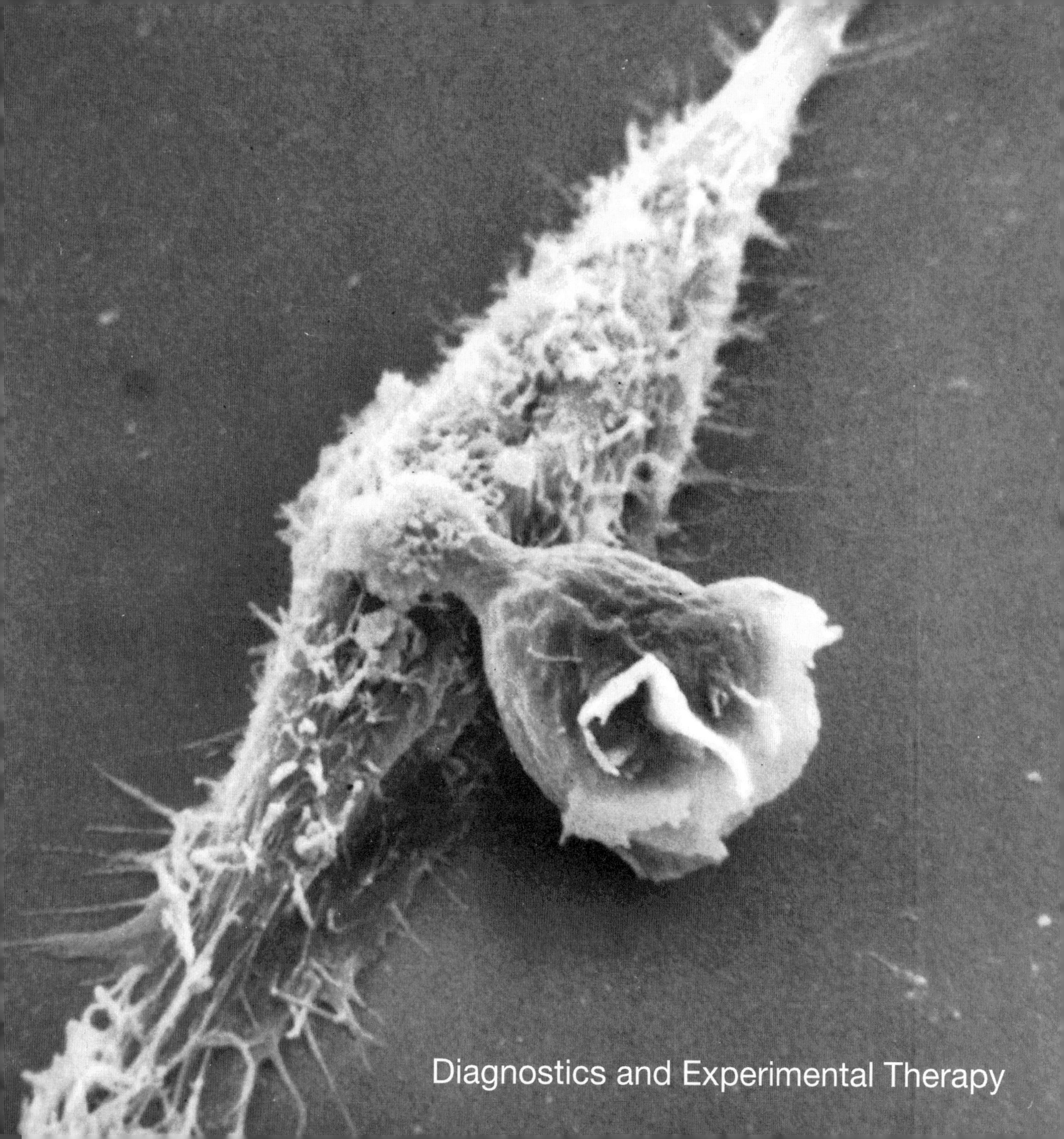

Diagnostics and Experimental Therapy

5

Diagnostics and Experimental Therapy

It is the Research Program's goal to make new molecular-biological developments in the areas of cell biology, virology, and immunology accessible for cancer diagnosis and therapy.

The Division of Histodiagnostics and Pathomorphological Documentation is responsible for all the centralized histopathological examinations within the Deutsches Krebsforschungszentrum. Its research activities include the expansion of computerized image analysis aimed at quantitatively describing the nucleus' morphology, on the basis of which the structural and cellular heterogeneity of tumors may be characterized. For this purpose, the Division utilizes a most advanced image processing system.

Closely related to these morphological evaluations are investigations in which transgenic mice serve as model systems for diseases in humans and the elaboration of a catalog of experimental tumors. A tumor bank made up of animal and human tumor models cryopreserved in liquid nitrogen has been in existence for twenty years and can be accessed by scientists of the Deutsches Krebsforschungszentrum and other research institutions at any time. The tumor bank also houses duplicates of all cell systems stored elsewhere. At present there are approximately 70,000 samples deposited. The functions of the tumor bank were recently expanded by the establishment of an embryonic bank. Murine embryos at the earliest stages of development (2-, 4- or 8-cell stage) are cryopreserved in order to allow easy access as required without having to continuously breed the particular strains. This is particularly important for the maintenance of transgenic murine strains.

The research done by the Division of Cell Growth and Division mainly focuses on the examination of molecular processes during cell division using biochemical, histochemical and cytochemical techniques, as well as on in-situ hybridization.

The malignant transformation of cells is usually accompanied by alterations in the structure and number of chromosomes. Defects in the distribution of chromosomes become visible during or after cell division, when the mitotic spindle separates the chromosomes into chromatides. In this process the centromere, visible as a constriction in the chromosome, plays an important role. The process is controlled by specific proteins.

The Division of Perinatal Toxicology deals with cancer chemotherapy. One focus is the development of strategies to overcome therapy resistance in ovarian tumors. The researchers are particularly interested in the role which intracellular enzymes play in the development of resistance and the importance of selective inhibitors of these enzymes. These studies are based on animal experiments and on the examination of human ovarian carcinomas. A further objective is the investigation of the mechanism of action of new metal complex compounds. In cooperation with the Neurosurgical Clinic of the University of Heidelberg, this Division is also involved in the development of new carrier systems which, after surgical implantation, slowly release medications.

Antitumor and antivirus mechanisms are the focus of work of the Division of Molecular Biology of DNA Tumor Viruses. It concentrates on intracellular signal transmission systems which regulate the growth of tumor cells, and which may also be used by viruses for proliferation. Presently, a new class of intracellular signal transmission inhibitors is being studied. Further research includes the investigation of the effects of biomodulators in combination with chemical substances that both enhance the desired effect of body effector substances and simultaneously reduce their adverse side effects.

The Division of Applied Immunology analyzes the activation processes of human T-lymphocytes, which are responsible for tumor control and defense. One focus of research is the analysis of receptor-mediated intracellular signal tr3ansmission processes which control genes that are relevant for differentiation and growth.

Cytoplasmic enzyme systems are characterized molecularly in order to develop new growth-inhibiting and immunomodulatory substances. Another focus of work is the clarification of the cell-to-cell-interaction. The processes taking place there are of major importance in the defense against tumor cells. Tumor cells alter their interaction structures and thus behave abnormally, thus allowing them to escape detection by defense cells. Endogenous biomodulators (cytokines) are tested with regard to their effect on the expression of interaction structures and adhesion molecules. Monoclonal antibodies against functional determinants of these molecules are produced and they serve to establish new diagnostic reagents which may be used for investigating the tumor cell's phenotype. Current clinical activities in the Division focus on improving the control of transplant rejection (a reciprocal model of tumor defense), as well as on the improvement of vaccination strategies against viral infections favoring tumor growth.

In 1993 the Division of Tumor Progression and Immune Defense was founded. It originated from the project group Immune Regulation and Tolerance, the main focus of which was the evaluation of mechanisms of peripheral tolerance, and the elaboration of new approaches to interrupting tolerance and eliciting an immune response to malignant cells. Based on the observation that in a lymphogenic metastatic tumor model of the rat variants of a lymphocyte receptor (CD44) proved to be essential for the metastatic process, the original topic was expanded to include work on the following topics: role of CD44 in the lymphogenic metastatic process, role of CD44 in lymphocyte maturation and activation, and the diagnostic and therapeutic implications of CD44 expression in oncology and hematology.

Since splice variants of CD44 are also expressed in some human tumors and probably play an important role in the metastatic process, attempts are being made to exploit CD44v expression for diagnostic purposes. The therapeutic potential role of CD44v in oncology remains to be seen.

The objective of the working group Recombinant antibodies is to develop new techniques for obtaining recombinant antibodies from bacteria for the diagnosis and treatment of cancer. These antibodies can be specifically altered and linked to other proteins, peptides, and toxins. Small „mini-antibodies“ are for instance capable of binding tumor cells to cells of the immune system and thus of eliciting an immune response to these tumor cells. Another advantage is that human antibodies can be produced in bacteria that are associated with less treatment-related side-effects than those produced in animal cells. To be able to isolate antibodies of any desired specificity from bacteria, the group has developed techniques and vectors permitting the imitation of the basic principles of human antibody immune response in bacteria. Antibody libraries are produced from the gene repertoire of human lymphocytes and by gene synthesis applying random sequences for antigen-binding regions. To obtain the desired antibodies from such libraries, the antibodies were fused with proteins situated on the surface of phage particles or bacteria, permitting the selection via immobilized antigens of specific antibodies carrying their own genes, „piggy-back“ fashion.

The overall concept of the Research Program also includes new Clinical Cooperation Units, which will be divisions of the Deutsches Krebsforschungszentrum that closely cooperate with the Hospitals of the University of Heidelberg. This is to ensure that new clinical strategies in cancer diagnosis and therapy can be introduced quickly and efficiently into the treatment of patients. Presently, the first clinical cooperation units are being established in the Medical Clinic V and in the University Pediatric Clinic. In view of the new dynamic developments in the field of hemato-oncology, it is planned that the new units will first focus their work on research in this area. A clinically oriented research group working on approaches of somatic gene therapy was established in cooperation with the Surgical Department of Heidelberg University Hospital.

Coordinator of the Research Project:
Prof. Dr. Stefan C. Meuer

Divisions and their heads:

Histodiagnostics and Pathomorphological Documentation
Prof. Dr. Dymitr Komitowski

Perinatal Toxicology
Prof. Dr. W. Jens Zeller

Cell Growth and Division
Prof. Dr. Neidhard Paweletz

Applied Immunology
Prof. Dr. Stefan C. Meuer

Tumor Progression
and Immune Defense
Prof. Dr. Margot Zöller

Experimental Therapy
Prof. Dr. Thomas Boehm

Clinical Cooperation Unit
Molecular Oncology/Pediatry
Priv.-Doz. Dr. Klaus-Michael Debatin

Clinical Cooperation Unit
Molecular Hematology/Oncology
Priv.-Doz. Dr. Rainer Haas

5.1 Immune Defense and Cancer

by Stefan C. Meuer

A scientifically proven and clinically established form of immunotherapy against cancer remains to be discovered. This is as clear as it is disappointing at first glance. After all, tumor immunology has long been one of the more promising approaches in the fight against cancer.

There is no doubt that immunologists have contributed considerably to the diagnostics of cancer, for instance, by developing monoclonal antibodies that indicate the degree of proliferation and differentiation of malignant cells. Such information has become indispensable for the physician with respect to treatment and the course a cancer takes, and evaluation of the prognosis of tumor patients.

Why has it not been possible so far to use the body's own defense mechanisms as a therapeutic weapon in the fight against cancer? The question of whether monoclonal antibodies against tumor cells, immune mediators such as interleukin-2, tumor necrosis factor, and interferons, or killer cells activated outside the organism are effective against cancer has been the topic of a large number of clinical studies. However, a beneficial effect on the course of cancer has been demonstrated in only a few of the patients treated. In addition, treatment was associated with severe side effects. This is mainly due to the fact that, while the substances used are usually effective at one particular site in the organism, the only way of administration has been systemic so far, thereby eliciting vigorous defense reactions throughout the whole organism.

For this reason, new, focused forms of treatment specifically directed against the tumor have to be developed. The key to more specific treatment modalities lies in an understanding of the interactions between defense system and cancer cells. Essential new insights into this complex topic have been gained recently. This and the considerably expanded range of methods may provide grounds for cautious optimism.

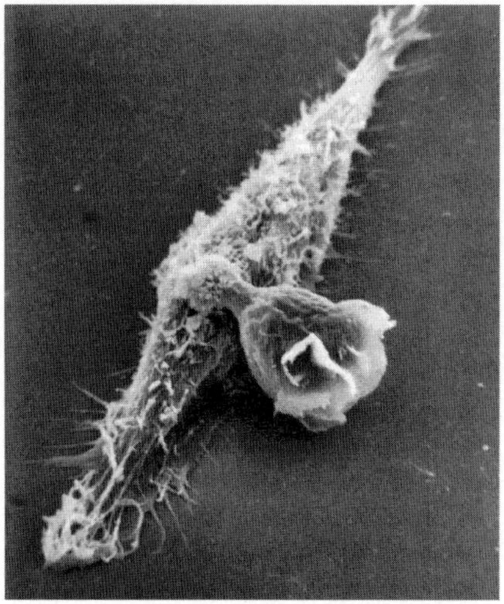

Fig. 37
A club-shaped stimulated lymphocyte attacks a considerably larger cancer cell

The immune system consists of a variety of cell types which, at least under experimental laboratory conditions, are capable of destroying cancer cells. Much of the hope placed in the immune system's role in cancer therapy is based on its precise specificity, i.e., its propensity for activation solely against cancer cells, leaving normal cells untouched: the immune system is capable of distinguishing clearly between "nonself" and "self". This is how it protects us from microbial pathogens and rejects foreign tissue; it is not, however, usually directed against the body's own cells.

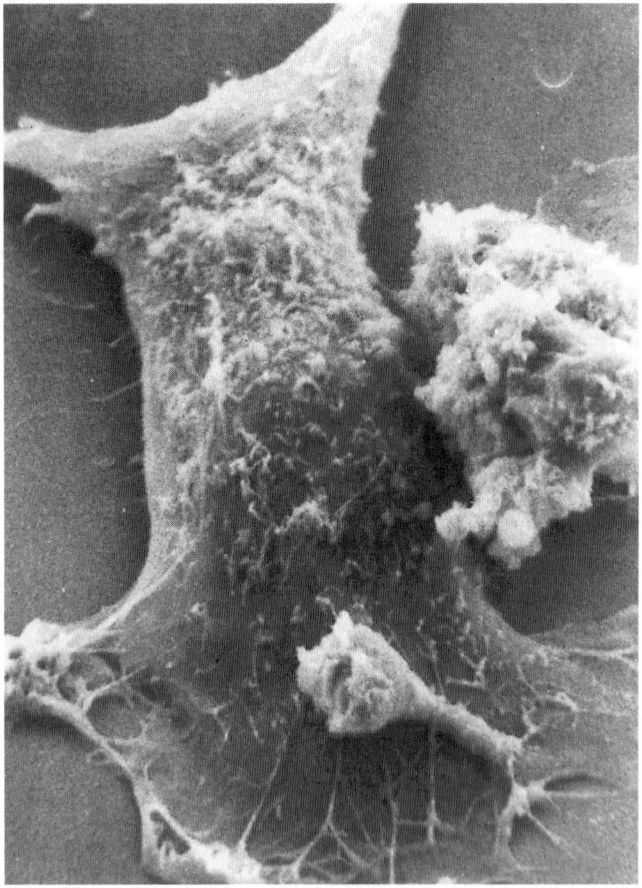

Fig. 38
A cancer cell (above right) is dying already, leaving nothing but debris. The lymphocyte (center) moves on to attack another cell

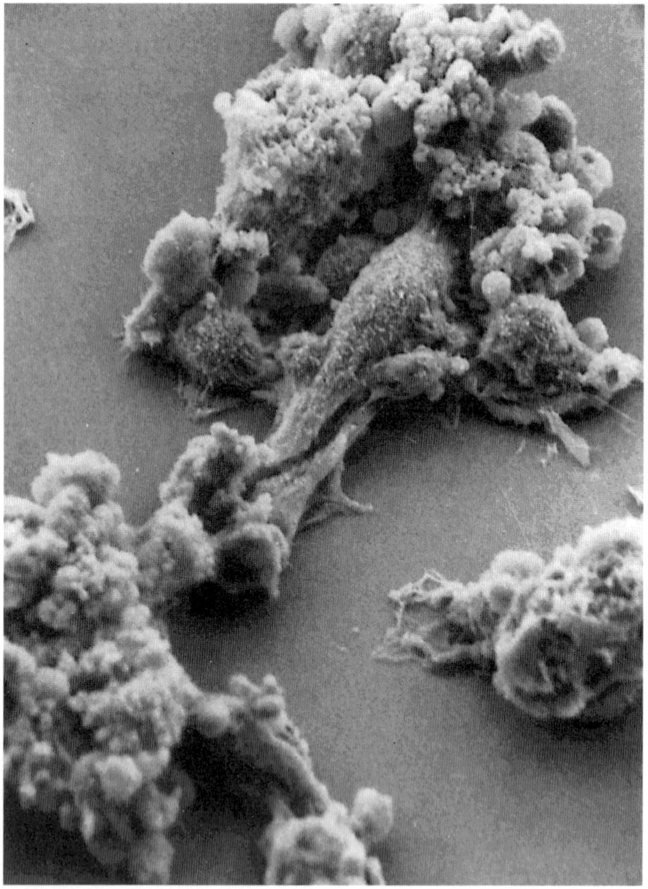

Fig. 39
The lymphocyte attack was successful, resulting in the disintegration and death of the cancer cell

Is the immune system capable of distinguishing "malignant" from "benign" cells? This question has long been contentiously discussed, but for about 2 years now, we have known that the answer is an unequivocal "yes," for it has been possible to elucidate the underlying molecular mechanisms of recognition and differentiation. Scientists at the Deutsches Krebsforschungszentrum contributed to this important advance. Two articles in the present edition of "Current Cancer Research" are dedicated to a detailed presentation of the results obtained (Hans-Georg Rammensee: "How the Immune System Controls the Inside of Cells"; and Günter Hämmerling/Bernd Arnold: "Immune Tolerance and Cancer"), offering key insights in the design of new rational strategies for immunotherapies.

The cells of our body present their products to the immune system on the cell surface. These products are protein molecules in the form of short peptide fragments which combine with the Class I HLA antigens present on all nucleated cells of the organism. Proteins are products of cellular genes. Since tumor cells contain abnormally modified genes (mutations, chromosomal translocations, etc.) they also produce abnormal protein molecules. The immune system may identify the fragments of these proteins as abnormal, i.e., "foreign," and should provoke defense reactions against tumor cells. The hunt for, and identification of "tumor peptides" is currently in full swing, and sophisticated physico-chemical techniques, such as mass spectrometry, are of invaluable help. However, it will also be necessary to elucidate how peptide fragments are formed from cellular proteins and how they are transported to the cell surface – a prerequisite for being recognized by the immune system. Scientists at the Deutsches Krebsforschungszentrum are contributing with internationally outstanding work to the elucidation of these central questions. Soon, it will be known whether and how these important transportation processes are disturbed in tumor cells and how they might be influenced. A knowledge of tumor-specific peptides could be used for the synthetic production of such molecules. Subsequently, they would be loaded onto antigen-presenting cells taken from the blood of the cancer patient and be used specifically as a "vaccine against cancer".

The process of recognition on its own does not provoke an immune response – this is also a new insight gained in recent years. Recognition is only the first signal in the activation of defense cells. The Division of Applied Immunology is devoting much effort to work on what are called accessory/secondary signals which, in conjunction with the first "switch-on" signal, are necessary to activate lymphocytes, for instance for the formation of defense substances indispensable for directly or indirectly attacking tumor cells (by switching on other effector cells). The following facts have become evident:

a) lymphocytes are stimulated into defensive action only if the first and second signals are transmitted to the immune system in close temporal and spatial proximity;

b) if the second signal is missing after the first one, the immune system is switched off, and specific tolerance occurs.

In fact, tumor cells indeed seem to take advantage of this tolerance-inducing mechanism, thereby evading an attack by the immune system despite their foreignness. We have known this ever since the time receptors for accessory signals of the immune system were identified and since finding out about their corresponding ligands, which must be present on tumor cells to induce secondary signals by binding to receptors. The density of ligand molecules on tumor cells can be exactly measured using specific monoclonal antibodies. Studies on malignantly transformed cells demonstrate that these cells do not, or not sufficiently, possess the crucial ligands – which confirms the assumption expressed above. In addition, it has since become evident that the absence of such ligand molecules is associated with a very poor prognosis of certain cancers, whereas the presence of at least a small number of such molecules stimulating the immune system is associated with a much better prognosis with respect to the course of the disease.

These findings mark a watershed in immunotherapy. Due to advances in gene technology it has become possible, via gene transfer, to insert molecules into tumor cells which they do not normally produce themselves. A project group specially concerned with this question was founded last year in cooperation with the Surgical Department of Heidelberg University Hospital. It is their task to find out which molecules must be inserted in tumor cells in order to provoke a defense reaction and break the body's tolerance towards cancer.

The new strategies for immunotherapy discussed are not causal in their approach. They do not target the "sick" genes causing cancer. However, since many and diverse gene modifications occur in tumor cells and since it is not yet known which of these are responsible for malignancy (which would then be targeted to receive specific "gene therapy"), immunologic techniques can provide a way of destroying tumor cells due to their "foreignness" without having to have a detailed knowledge of the relevant modifications of individual genes. In this manner, the strategies discussed could contribute to the treatment of cancer. For instance, enhancement of the immune system's surveillance function, which certainly exists and by which early cancers are detected and destroyed, would provide a means to avoid or delay relapses.

Prof. Dr. Stefan C. Meuer
Division of Applied Immunology

5.2 Computer-Assisted Techniques for the Description of the Cytoskeletal Structure in Modern Cancer Diagnostics

by Dymitr Komitowski, Svetlana Karnaoukhova, and Ralf Bracht

Modern techniques used to visualize specific cellular structures have demonstrated that the morphological organization of the cytoplasm of tumor cells correlates with the origin and degree of differentiation of the tumors. Features of this organization permit a more distinct differentiation between histologically and clinically diverse tumors and thus has diagnostic implications. The detection of different classes of fibrillar proteins which form a complex skeleton in the cytoplasm, the cytoskeleton, is of special interest in this respect. The cytoskeleton is responsible for a number of cell functions: it gives the cell its ability to maintain its characteristic shape, to move, and to communicate with other cells.

In diagnostics, it is above all the intensity of expression of cytoskeleton proteins that needs to be considered. The structural properties and the architectural characteristics are usually not taken into consideration, due to the limited ability of the human eye to make out architectural elements of complex networks, to compare their patterns, and to classify them. A number of observations indicate that external factors are also capable of changing the cytoskeletal structure, including viral infections that impair the biological properties of cells. It is still unclear to what extent such changes are predictive of a malignant transformation of cells.

In order to elucidate this question we applied automatic computer-assisted image analysis techniques in studying the cytoskeleton. Four methodical approaches were applied:

- immunohistochemical presentation of the cytoskeletal structure using antibodies against characteristic cytokeratin fibers of epidermal cells;
- confocal laser scanning microscopy for three-dimensional presentation of the cytoskeletal structure;
- registration of a great number of subvisual parameters describing the three-dimensional cytoskeletal architecture;
- classification of the identified structural patterns using neural networks.

The cytoskeletal structures must be visualized with confocal laser scanning microscopy. Immunohistochemical techniques can be used to label the structures with fluorescent dyes which emit a typical fluorescent color when stimulated by laser. The microscope emits this light to every point in the visual field so as to generate a three-dimensional scanning image of the cell.

The technique of presenting the three-dimensional organization of the cytoskeleton by quantitative image analysis can be divided into three steps: reduction of the huge amount of data, extraction of structural parameters, and identification of characteristic patterns.

In reducing the data it is important that only the information on the cytoskeletal structure is maintained, thus eliminating for instance differences in thickness and the fluorescence intensity of individual fibers. The images present the cytoskeletal structure as a network of uniform fibers stained with the same dye. The image is referred to as „binary image“ since it contains only two elements: the cytoskeleton network and the background.

A great number of parameters are used to describe the structure, including parameters which define the length and thickness of fibers, and how they are bound together. In addition complex

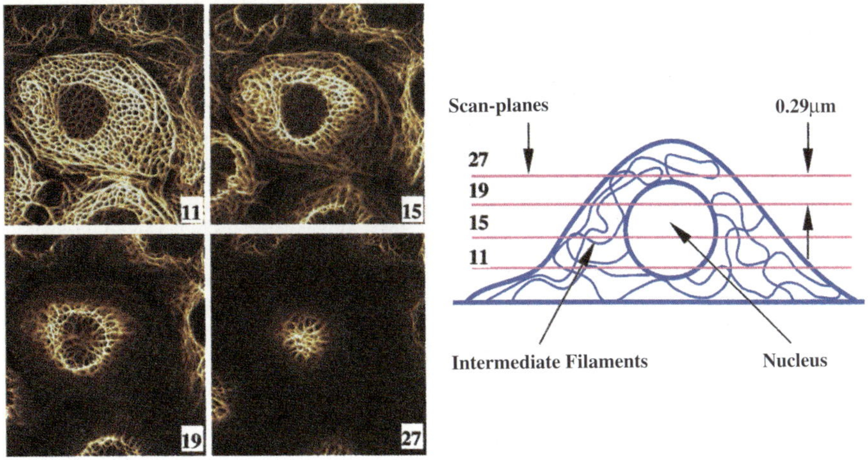

Fig. 40
Three-dimensional image of a cytoskeleton seen with a confocal laser scanning microscope. The four projections show different optical sections of a hepatic cell. The imaging technique is presented on the right. The distance between the sections is about a three ten-thousandth parts of a millimeter. This allows precise presentation of the spatial structure of the cytoskeleton

structural parameters including fractal dimension and Fourier coefficients are calculated and used to characterize the architecture. Fractal dimension describes the complexity of the structures: the higher the dimension, the higher the density of the cytoskeleton. Periodic repetition of specific fiber arrangements is determined using Fourier coefficients. In order to achieve adequate characterization of the cytoskeletal structure 400 different parameters were applied in our studies.

The huge amounts of data generated in image analysis pose considerable problems when it comes to identifying cytoskeleton patterns associated with defined biological properties. For this purpose we use modern classification methods such as neural networks are used.

In a first step the values from all cytoskeleton parameters of each individual cell are integrated as vectors of a multidimensional space. Similar cytoskeletal structures form circumscribed clouds. The task consists now in differentiating between the clouds, the sensible solution being neural networks. Advantages of the method include the detection and description of connections between individual parameters defining the cytoskeleton that would not be recognized with other techniques of data analysis.

A neural network consists of several input and output units, known as nodes. These nodes are crosslinked by a great number of connections. A particular in-

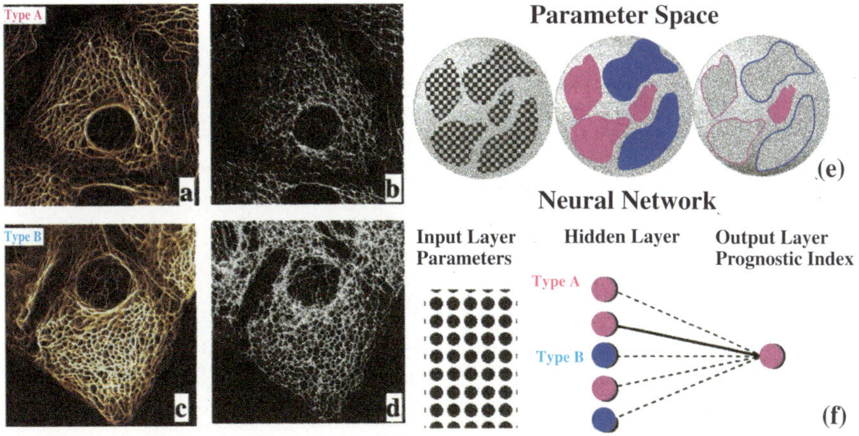

Fig. 41
The cytoskeleton is analyzed in four steps. A three-dimensional image of cell types A and B is taken by confocal laser scanning microscopy (left). The imaging data are reduced to the major cytoskeletal parameters (right), in which each cell corresponds to a region in a multiparametric space. During the learning process similar cells are grouped into "clouds" (e). The parameters are fed into the neural network (input node), which classifies the clouds in particular cell types (f) in multiple computational steps (hidden node). Different cells can thus be classified by means of neural network. Because of their characteristic cytoskeleton organization they gravitate towards particular clouds in the multiparametric space

formational content, such as measured values, can be assigned to each node. The informational content, described as the state of the node, is fed forward to the next node via an interconnecting network. The state of the input nodes is defined by the measured values that were already determined for each network. The output nodes provide data describing the different cytoskeleton patterns. The connections within the network are established during the so-called learning process.

Our studies demonstrate that computer-assisted image analysis of the cellular organization permits the identification of still unknown associations between morphological and biological properties of cells when many and diverse parameters, combined with modern evaluation and classification techniques of great amounts of data, are taken into account by the use of neural networks.

This is the basis for defining morphological properties that correlate with differences in the clinical manifestation and response to therapy of tumors of the same kind, opening up the possibility of improving the accuracy of the individual prognosis and allowing treatment decisions.

Prof. Dr. Dymitr Komitowski
Dr. Svetlana Karnaoukhova
Dr. Ralf Bracht
Division of Histology and Pathomorphological Documentation

In cooperation with

Prof. Dr. Josef Bille
Institute of Applied Physics,
University of Heidelberg

Selected Publications

Komitowski, D., Bracht, R.: Computergestützte Analyse von mikroskopischen Bildern – subjektive Entscheidungswege zur objektiven Befunderhebung. Bioscope I, 8–16 (1993)

Karnaoukhova, S., Komitowski, D., Bille, J.: Quantitative Beschreibung und Klassifizierung von 3-dimensionalen Bildern des Zytoskeletts. In: Mustererkennung '93. Ed.: Deutsche Arbeitsgemeinschaft Mustererkennung, Springer Verlag, Heidelberg, 222–227 (1993)

Karnaoukhova, S., Bille, J., Komitowski, D.: Quantitative changes in a three-dimensional cytoskeletal structure analysed with neural network. In: Proceedings of the International Conference on Confocal and Near-Field Microscopy '94, Munich (1994)

5.3 The Driving Force Behind Metastasis – the Surface Molecule CD44v

by Margot Zöller

Most primary tumors can be treated curatively. The high mortality rate in cancer patients is due to the ability of tumor cells to form secondary growths (metastases). Despite intensive research carried out in the field, the properties a tumor cell must possess in order to metastasize are still largely unknown, as is the sequence of events leading to the growth of metastatic cells in the target organ. This lack of understanding is due to the complexity of the metastatic process: the tumor cell must separate from the tumor tissue, migrate through the adjacent tissue, enter the lymph or blood vessels, invade other tissues via the lymph or blood stream, and finally leave the vessels, embed itself into foreign tissue and grow. For these processes the cell must acquire not only one but a whole series of new properties. A cell may acquire new properties during cell division by random changes in the genome. Since tumor cells have a high division rate, it is thus feasible that they acquire the properties required for the metastatic process over time. However, since this process is accidental and would be different in each tumor, it is almost impossible to establish a generally valid concept of the metastatic cascade. However, there is an alternative to this Darwinian theory of the metastatic process: if there are cells in the body which use a similar program – migrating in the tissue and blood, embedding themselves in other organs in order to multiply – to fulfill their physiologic function, then tumor cells might be able to “steal” this program and thereby acquire the ability to form secondary growths in a single step.

Tumor cells do indeed seem to use this trick. Metastases from pancreatic cancer in rats express a surface molecule, CD44v, that is also found in white blood cells (lymphocytes) under certain conditions. White blood cells are quiescent for most of their lives. During this period of inactivity they carry CD44s (s = standard) on their surface. They only become active in response to a threat to the organism, whereupon they migrate through the tissue and multiply. During this process the molecules on their surface change and express CD44v (v = variant) – just like the metastatic rat tumor cells. Does this happen by chance, or does CD44v play a role in the activation of lymphocytes and the metastatic process?

CD44v is essential to metastasis in the rat because: 1) whereas locally growing rat tumors do not carry the molecule, all rat tumors metastasizing via the lymph vessels do express CD44v; 2) when the genetic material of CD44v is introduced in nonmetastatic rat tumors, these tumors acquire the ability to metastasize; 3) in rats it is possible to block CD44v by the administration of antibodies and thus to considerably delay the metastatic process. Rat lymphocytes also require CD44v. If the molecule is blocked by an antibody they are not able to multiply sufficiently to prevent infection or combat a foreign substance.

These findings obtained from animal experiments are of primary importance for medical research. The first thing it is important to establish is whether the expression of CD44v is necessary and sufficient to cause human tumors to metastasize. The second set of problems that needs to be answered relates to the function of the molecule. If we can find out why and how expression of CD44v helps lymphocytes in their activation and enables tumor cells to metastasize, this might help us to work out therapeutic strategies to prevent the formation of secondary growths. Studies investigating these two questions have not yet been concluded. However, there is evidence that CD44v may play a role in the metastasis of human tumors. In elucidating the function of this molecule in metastasis it has proven useful to investigate, first of all, its role in the physiologic processes, since the same mechanism appears to underlie the metastasis of tumor cells.

CD44v: A "Marker of Metastasis" only in the Rat?

The finding that the expression of a single molecule is sufficient to initiate the metastatic spreading of locally growing tumors in the rat was so alarming that screening programs for human tumor material were initiated worldwide in order to establish whether expression of CD44v also correlates with the metastasis of human tumors.

Based on the findings obtained so far, it can be assumed that CD44v is not expressed in all human tumors that form secondaries, unlike in the rat. According to findings already published, intestinal tumors frequently express CD44v even before metastasis, during the precancerous and in-situ cancer stage. The situation is similar with stomach cancer, in which two different variants of CD44 are expressed depending on the histologic type of the tumor. CD44v is also expressed in breast cancer and appears to be a crucial prognostic marker since patient survival time strictly correlates with the expression of the genome portion exon v6. However, expression of CD44v in tumors of the skin and mucosa of the buccal cavity and the pharynx has no diagnostic implications since the expression of split variants of CD44 in these tissues is physiologic in humans. Malignant melanoma is an exception. Unlike the adjacent skin, the primary tumor in malignant melanoma does not express any variant forms of CD44. However, expression of a certain type of CD44v is seen in almost all metastases from this type of skin cancer. Further proof that CD44v is essential to the metastasis of malignant melanoma – as reported in the rat – is provided by the study of a series of human melanoma lines in nude mice in which the only cell lines to metastasize were those expressing the same exon observed in metastases. Renal cancers seem to behave in a similar way: CD44v is only found in primary renal tumors which have already formed secondaries, while in-situ cancers are negative for the molecule. Finally, it should be mentioned that expression of CD44v is reported in some but not all malignant diseases of the hematopoietic system (Table 1).

Insights into which human tumors express CD44v can be directly exploited for diagnostic purposes. Immune scintigraphy has been an established clinical procedure for many years. Some of the technical limitations of the procedure were eliminated recently by refinement of the system. For example, the use of bispecific monoclonal antibodies binding both to the tumor and to a radionuclide permits the application of higher amounts of radioactivity required for tumor detection. These so-called "bispecific" antibodies have the disadvantage of reduced binding capacity to the tumor. To compensate for this, bispecific antibodies with three binding sites, so-called F(ab')3 fragments, can be produced. In any of the human tumors shown to require CD44v for the metastatic process, or in which CD44v is at least expressed in all metastases, there are legitimate grounds for hoping that the search for metastases will be successful at a very early stage.

Whether and how the expression of CD44v can be harnessed for therapeutic use will essentially depend on the success of attempts to define the molecule's mode of action. The findings we have obtained so far permit the establishment of a working hypothesis which may help to throw some light on the matter.

Table 1: Hematological Malignancies: Expression of CD44v

Disorder	Number of Patients	Expression of CD44v (% of Patients)
Iron-deficiency anemia	7	0
Polycythemia vera	9	75
Non-Hodgkin Lymphoma	35	54
Chronic-lymphatic Leukemia	11	48
Chronic-myeloid Leukemia	7	58

Function of CD44v: Physiology and Pathology

CD44 is an adhesion molecule. What is/are the function(s) of the variants of this molecule? Since CD44v is expressed on metastatic tumor cells and temporarily on lymphocytes, it is important to establish which cellular biological phenomena are common to both metastatic tumor cells and lymphocytes. The basic elements of the lymphocyte activation cascade do indeed correspond to the principles underlying lymphogenic metastasis: migration from the periphery to the draining lymph nodes, embedment, adhesion to defined antigen presenting cells, expansion, emigration with the efferent lymph. Only then do the two processes go their separate ways. While the activated lymphocyte returns to the periphery, to the site of tissue injury, the tumor cell re-embeds itself into the next lymph node.

Given the parallelism of the lymphocyte activation process and lymphogenic metastasis it is hardly surprising that the "metastases antigen" CD44v is also found on lymphocytes. While CD44v is not expressed on quiescent lymphocytes it is however found on antigen presenting cells, T cells, and B cells following antigenic stimulation. Just as in the metastatic process, lymphocyte activation can be prevented by a CD44v (v6) specific antibody.

A look at the different steps in tumor progression and lymphocyte activation shows that the process starts with the separation of tumor cells from the primary tumor tissue. There is no evidence so far that CD44v is involved in this process. For migration through the tissue into the draining lymph vessel it is possible that both tumor cells and lymphocytes use the molecule's constant regions: it is known that CD44 binds to hyaluronic acid and that cells use this extremely long molecule as a

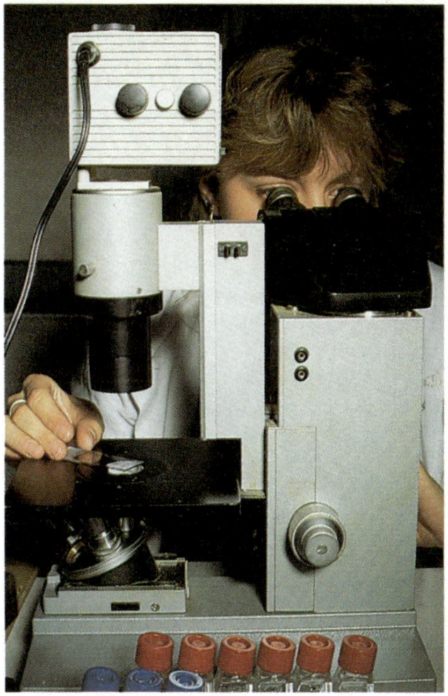

Fig. 43
CD44 antibody staining shows up the variant CD44. Light microscopy can thus be used to show whether a tumor expresses aberrant forms of CD44

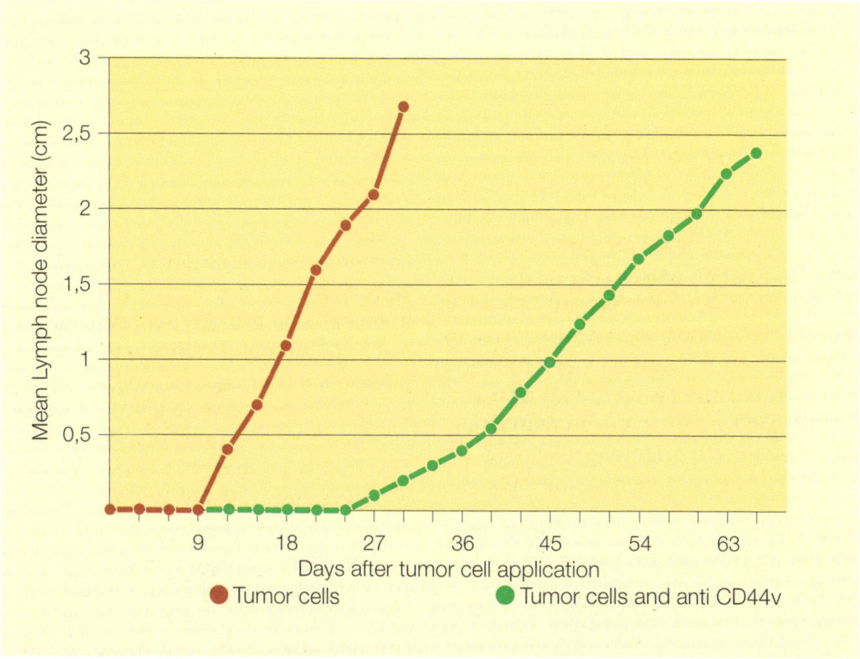

Fig. 42
The significance of variants of the CD44 surface molecule was detected in pancreatic cancers of the rat. Only variants of this molecule enable tumors to form secondaries. An antibody against mutated CD44 delays the growth of secondary tumors, as shown here

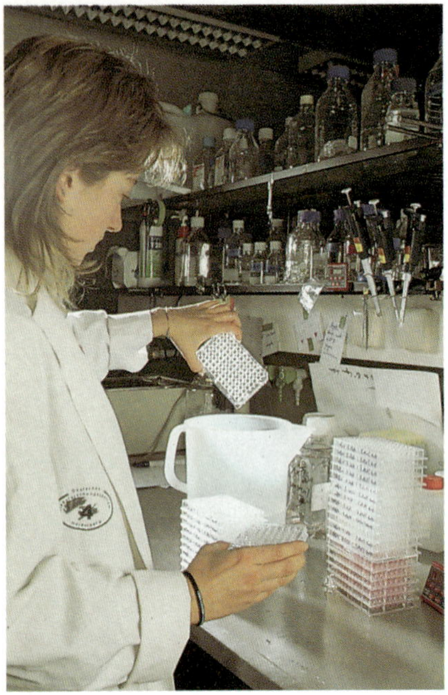

Fig. 44
Mice are immunized with variant CD44 to stimulate the production of monoclonal antibodies. The antibodies thus obtained are then tested for efficacy in the microtiter plates shown here. If the antibodies bind to the variant CD44 against which they are directed, the plates change color

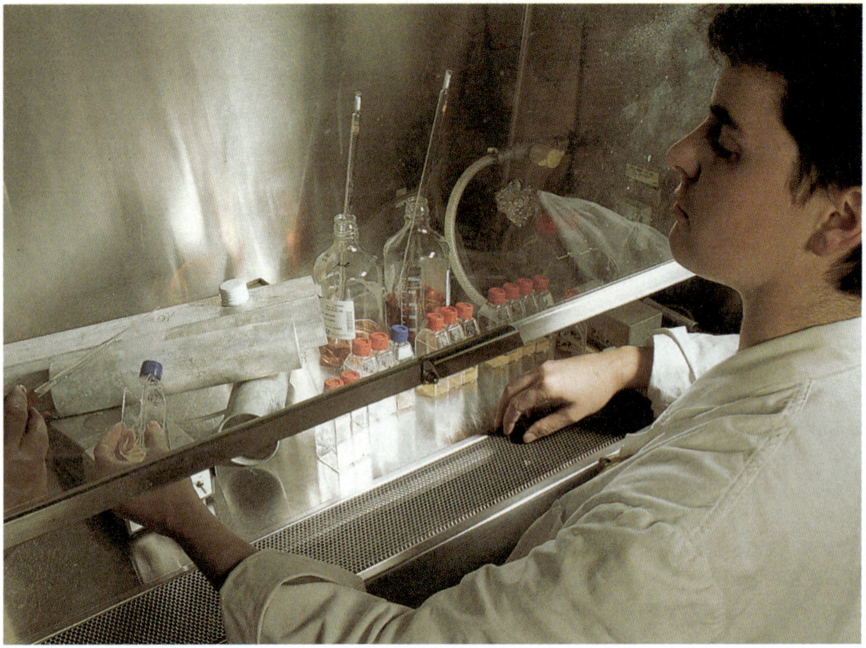

Fig. 45
Cancer cells isolated from rat pancreatic cancer can be kept indefinitely in storage bottles. Sterile conditions are necessary to protect the cell cultures from infection by fungi and bacteria. All work, including the "feeding" of the tumor cells with a special nutritive solution (shown here), is therefore done on a sterile bench

guide during migration. Interestingly, the expression of CD44s is upregulated very quickly during lymphocyte activation, well before the expression of CD44v. Transportation with the lymph is passive to a large extent and possibly does not require expression of specific transport molecules either in metastatic tumor cells or in lymphocytes. In any case CD44v appears not to be involved in this process since immigration of tumor cells and lymphocytes into draining lymph nodes is not inhibited by anti CD44v. By contrast, expansion both of tumor cell populations and of lymphocytes in the draining lymph nodes is considerably impaired by anti CD44v.

Lymphocytes bind in the draining lymph node to antigen presenting cells that produce cytokines in a specific way, allowing lymphocytes to mature and expand. In vitro studies have demonstrated firstly that metastasizing tumor cells bind to these antigen presenting cells via CD44v since anti CD44v inhibits the binding and secondly that anti CD44v inhibits the expansion of lymphocytes in the presence of these antigen presenting cells. If these cells are removed and substituted by adding the corresponding growth factors, lymphocytes also multiply in the presence of anti CD44v.

These findings suggest that growth signals are transmitted to the lymphocyte and/or the metastasizing tumor cell when CD44v binds to a ligand on antigen presenting cells. It is still unknown to which structure on the antigen presenting cells CD44v binds, nor is it known whether the signals are only transmitted to the antigen presenting cell or whether the signals are then passed on from the antigen presenting cell to the tumor cell and/or the lymphocyte via CD44v. Available findings indicate, however, that CD44v is required, at least initially, as a bystander molecule on lymphocytes and as a "marker of metastasis" on tumor cells for activation of the target cell. The provision of growth factors for CD44v by a target cell may explain why a single molecule is equally necessary for such divergent processes as lymphocyte activation and lymphatic metastasis. The observation that tumors of different histologic types can fall back on a uniform principle of action is consistent with this working hypothesis.

Can CD44v be considered as central to the activation of a cellular biological program in lymphogenic metastasis and in the induction of an immune response? We assume that both cases represent only one of several possibilities. Apart from other genetic programs that may lead to the same goal, it should be possible to manipulate this central molecule and thus decode the principle of action underlying metastasis and the establishment of the multiple steps leading to an immune response.

Prof. Dr. Margot Zöller
Division of Tumor Progression
and Immune Defense

Participating Scientists

Dr. Robert Arch
Dr. Sophia Khaldoyanidi
Simone Seiter
Karin Wirth

In collaboration with

Prof. Dr. Peter Herrlich
Prof. Dr. Helmut Ponta
Institute of Genetics,
Nuclear Research Center Karlsruhe

Dr. Günter Adolf
Bender / Boehringer, Ingelheim/Vienna

Dr. Jochen Schumacher
Division of Radiochemistry and
Radiopharmacology,
Deutsches Krebsforschungszentrum,
Heidelberg

Priv.-Doz. Dr. Wolfgang Tilgen
Skin Clinic,
University Clinic of Heidelberg

Dr. Dr. Joachim Zöller
Department of Maxillofacial Surgery
and Dentistry,
University Clinic of Heidelberg

Dr. Franz-Xaver Bosch
Ear, Nose and Throat Clinic,
University Clinic of Heidelberg

Dr. Martin Achtnich
Faculty of Clinical Medicine Mannheim
of Heidelberg University, Municipal
Clinics Mannheim,
Medical Clinic –
Chair of Internal Medicine III,
Mannheim

Selected publications

Günthert, U., Hofmann, M., Rudy, W., Reber, S., Zöller, M., Haußmann, I., Matzku, S., Wenzel, A., Ponta, H., Herrlich, P,: A new variant of glycoprotein CD44 confers metastatic potential to rat carcinoma cells. Cell, 65, 13–24 (1991)

Arch, R., Wirth, K., Hofmann, M., Ponta, H., Matzku, S., Herrlich, P., Zöller, M.: Participation of a metastasis-inducing splice variant of CD44 in normal immune response. Science, 257, 682–685 (1992)

Seiter, S., Arch, R., Komitowski, D., Hofmann, M., Ponta, H., Herrlich, P., Matzku, S., Zöller, M.: Prevention of tumor metastasis formation by anti-variant CD44. J. Exp. Med., 177, 443–455 (1993)

Wirth, K., Seiter, S., Hofman, M., Herrlich, P., Matzku, S., Zöller, M.: Expression of CD44 isoforms including domain III in newborn and adult rats. Eur. J. Cancer, 291, 1172–1177 (1993)

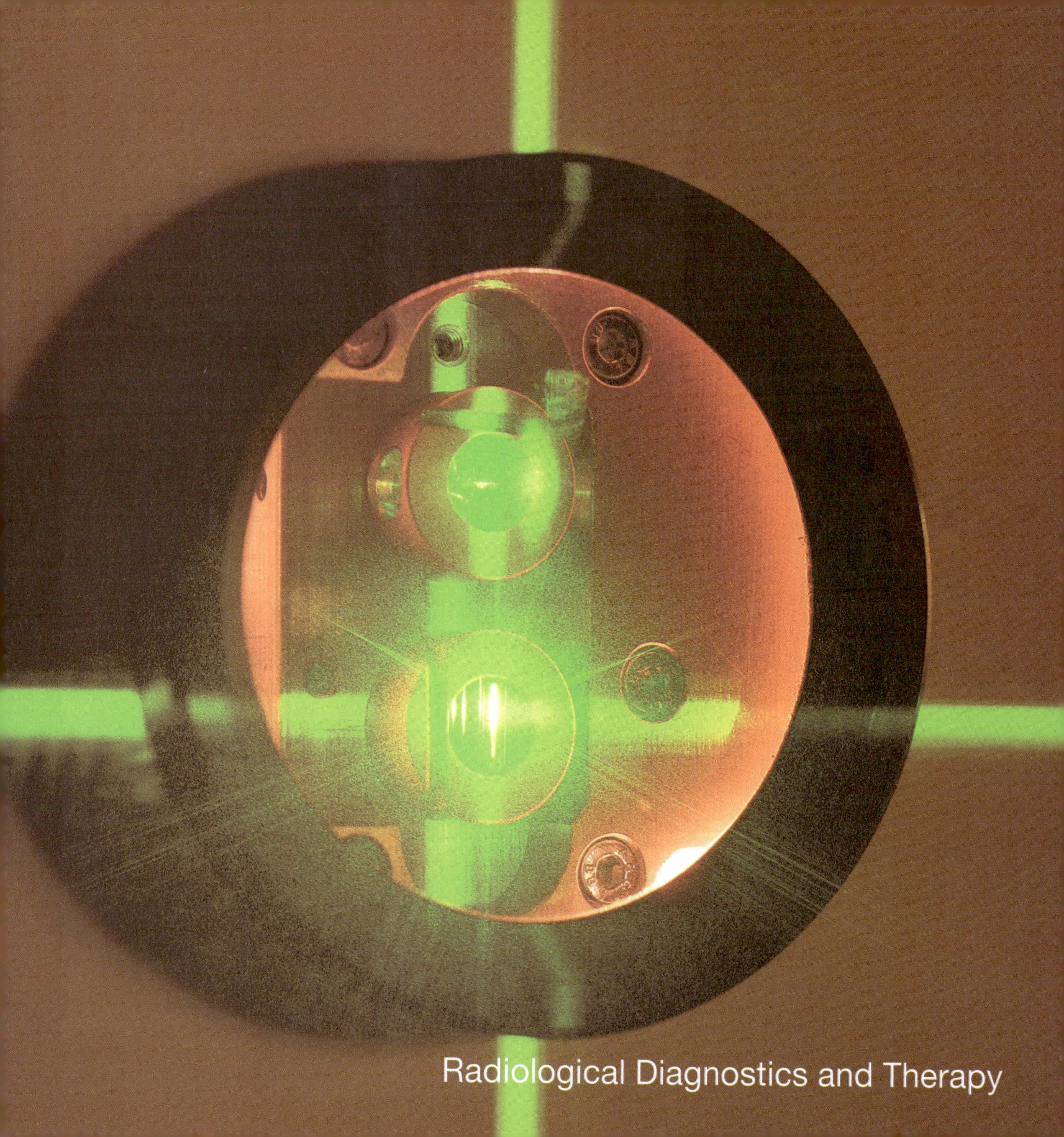

Radiological Diagnostics and Therapy

6

Radiological Diagnostics and Therapy

Radiology is one of the most important specializations in medicine for the detection, treatment, and follow-up of cancer diseases. Today, radiology not only encompasses conventional radiological methods of diagnosis and therapy, but also advanced techniques that make use of non-ionizing forms of radiation.

Research in Radiological Diagnostics

In the fight against cancer, diagnostics is of strategic importance. Failures in diagnosis can hardly be compensated by therapy.

Tumor diagnostics basically has the following tasks:

1. Detection of the tumor in the earliest possible stage;
2. Determination of its size, localization, relationship to organs, and spread ("staging");
3. Characterization of the tumor tissue through morphological, physiological, and biochemical parameters;
4. Control of the course of therapy, and
5. Diagnostic postoperative care.

The decisive first step in treating the individual cancer disease is the earliest possible detection of the tumor. Diagnostic procedures should put little strain on the patient so that they can be used as soon as suspicion arises. In general, the tumor develops without symptoms for several years before it is detected. At the time it is detected or when symptoms become evident, it has usually grown to a size of more than 1 centimeter. This means that, even in the case of an early detection, several million tumor cells have already grown.

After tumor detection, the next important diagnostical step is the determination of the tumor stage (staging). Staging is the basis for both the planning of the therapy and the evaluation of its success. Each tumor type requires the use of specific examination methods to determine its size, its spatial relationship to other structures, and its spread within the organism. Here, computed tomography has proven to be of great value. Computed tomography also is the basis for calculating advanced radiotherapy plans. Another goal of diagnostics is to find out the tumor's individual characteristics and its "internals". This is done by evaluating the tumor's histological properties in the microscope and, if necessary, in the electron microscope (grading). Recent approaches aim at detecting and quantifying physiological and biochemical parameters such as blood circulation and metabolism within the tumor, in the healthy surrounding tissue, and in metastases. This data provides important information for therapy planning and for the evaluation of the success of the therapy.

Modern diagnostic methods that make it possible to exactly monitor the effect of a therapy considerably help to optimize the treatment. The tumor's response to therapy can now be detected more precisely and earlier than it could have been 20 years ago. In the case of poor response, the treatment plan can thus be altered at an earlier stage of the therapy. After successful removal or apocatastasis of the tumor, the patient has to be continuously monitored in order to detect local relapses or metastases as early as possible. In follow-up examinations, of course, non-invasive methods that do not strain the patient are preferred over invasive techniques.

Various diagnostic methods are available for the detection and evaluation of the cancer disease:

1. Biochemical and immunologic examinations of body fluids (blood, urine, discharges, etc.);
2. Detection of tumor tissue with imaging techniques:
   a) radiodiagnostics
   b) endoscopy
   c) ultrasound diagnostics
   d) computed tomography
   e) magnetic resonance tomography
   f) scintigraphy, including immunoscintigraphy
   g) positron emission tomography;
3. Detection of individual tumor cells (cytodiagnostics) in the sputum, in smear, or in puncture fluid;
4. Pathological detection of tumor cell clusters through sampling of suspicious tissue.

Imaging techniques make it possible to detect tumors and metastases that are larger than 1 to 2 centimeters. Due to physical and biophysical limitations, however, it cannot be expected to enhance the resolution in the near future. Instead, the development in diagnostics is aimed at better specifying the characteristics of the detected foci.

In the recent past, diagnostic research focused on improving the evaluation of the tumor's size, its structure, and its functional performance on the basis of newly developed, advanced radiological methods. Such examinations have now become possible with magnetic resonance tomography and positron emission tomography.

Magnetic resonance tomography (MRT) images a specified portion of the body slice-by-slice; the slice images can then be evaluated by the physician. For the examination, the patient is placed in a strong magnetic field. Certain atomic nuclei, which have an intrinsic angular momentum (spin), behave like small magnets and align with the external magnetic field. They may be excited by radio waves whose frequency corresponds to the nuclei's precession frequency. The excited nuclei emit high-frequency signals that give information on the state of the tissue they are located in. However, these signals have to be decoded with the help of modern data processing methods. The use of even stronger magnetic fields makes it possible to also investigate specific metabolic processes occurring in the tissue (magnetic resonance spectroscopy).

Parallel to and supplementing MRT, the tumor tissue is also examined with positron emission tomography (PET). PET renders slice images of the distribution of radiolabeled organic substances within the body. A radiolabeled molecule, in which one of its atoms is replaced with a radioactive atom of the same kind, has the same biological properties as the corresponding unlabeled molecule. A fact of great importance for the analysis of metabolic processes is that radiolabelling makes it possible to measure quantitatively.

Positron emission tomography and magnetic resonance tomography make it possible to non-invasively measure important metabolic parameters (perfusion, metabolisms of glucose, phosphorus, and proteins, catabolism) of cancer drugs in the tumor. By comparing the treatment data with the data collected prior to and at the beginning of the treatment, the physician can draw conclusions about the success of the therapy or optimize the treatment protocol.

Therefore, both techniques are used in the search for tumors, in tumor staging, for monitoring the course of therapy and, most importantly, for the characterization of tumor tissue in the living organism.

Radiological Therapy Research

The term "cancer" does not mean one specific disease but is a comprehensive term for a multitude of different tumor types. Thus, it cannot be expected that all malignant tumors can be influenced or cured with one and the same therapy. One basic difficulty for some therapeutic techniques comes from the fact that the tumor cell has developed from a normal cell. Consequently, much lesser differences to normal cells can be exploited for therapy than, for example, in the case of bacteria.

There are various approaches to cancer therapy: surgical removal of the tumor tissue, radiotherapy, hyperthermia, hormone therapy, chemotherapy, and immunotherapy. Surgery and radiotherapy are local tumor treatments. They cannot be used, however, if the tumor has infiltrated vital organs, as a consequence of which radical removal or destruction of the tumor is no longer possible without damaging the healthy tissue. Preliminary results show that radiotherapy of various tumors can be effectively supplemented by local hyperthermia.

Chemotherapy is used for several types of solid tumors after they have metastasized. Chemotherapy has shown important results in the treatment of malignant diseases of the hematopoietic tissue (leukemia). Positive effects on primarily malignant tumors of the lymph nodes can be achieved through radiotherapy and/or chemotherapy, depending on the tumor's stage. In general, hormone therapy is limited to tumors whose cells carry hormone receptors.

In the field of radiotherapy, the activities of the Deutsches Krebsforschungszentrum aim at the complete elimination of the tumor while optimally sparing the neighboring healthy tissue. This objective can be realized by improving radiotherapy planning, in particular, by using computerized tomography and electronic data processing.

A particularly powerful radiotherapeutic technique being developed at the Deutsches Krebsforschungszentrum is photon conformation therapy. In conformation therapy, the tumor is irradiated from various directions, and an adjustable multi-leaf collimator adjusts the shape of the irradiating beam to that of the tumor for each direction of irradiation. Thus, the dose is concentrated and homogeneously distributed within the tumor, while the neighboring tissues are protected.

Another technique used for precision radiotherapy, stereotactic convergent beam irradiation, has been developed for the treatment of small tumors in the brain or in the region of the head and neck. The patient's head is immobilized, and the tumor is irradiated from various directions with highly collimated photon beams. Again, the dose is concentrated within the tumor and the neighboring healthy tissue is spared. This technique is used for single-high-dose irradiations of tumors, metastases and vessel deformations in the brain.

Another research project focuses on interstitial stereotactic brain tumor therapy. A special puncturing device allows the surgeon to precisely introduce a needle into the brain and advance it to a specified target point. The needle then serves to inject liquid or solid radioactive substances into the tumor. This makes it possible to irradiate the tumor from within while sparing the surrounding tissue. This technique also allows the surgeon to inject chemotherapeutic agents or to introduce special antennas, with the aid of which the tumor volume can be locally heated. The combined application of radiation, heat, and cytostatics may improve the success of the therapy.

Radiobiological factors limit the effect of photons and electrons in the treatment of highly differentiated and slowly growing tumors, as well as in the treatment of large tumors with central necroses. The use of high-energy neutrons may improve these results. Researchers of the Deutsches Krebsforschungszentrum have developed an angle-weighted isocentric radiation technique with fast neutrons. This method, too, produces a high dose concentration within the target volume and helps to protect the surrounding tissue. It is being used in the treatment of sialomas, soft-tissue sarcomas, and recurrences of rectal tumors.

Presently, a combined therapy of irradiation and hyperthermia is being tested for the treatment of tumors of the esophagus, the bile duct, the cervix, and the rectum. Controlled local hyperthermia can be produced with special antenna systems.

For many years, pulsed high-energy ultrasound has been used to destroy nephroliths. Experimental studies have shown that a modified form of this technique, in combination with radiation, heat, and chemical substances, is suitable for the local treatment of tumors. Clinical trials are planned to follow these preliminary experiments.

Another promising concept which is being further developed and applied at the Deutsches Krebsforschungszentrum is photodynamic therapy. A photo-sensitizer is introduced into the tumor via the circulating blood, and the tumor is irradiated with suitable laser light. The resulting chemical processes destroy the tumor from within. Researchers of the Deutsches Krebsforschungszentrum have succeeded in developing photosensitive substances with considerably higher accumulation rates in the tumor than has been achieved with previous substances. This method may improve the treatment of superficial tumors.

Clinical studies on all of the mentioned techniques are being carried out in close cooperation with the clinics of the Tumor Center Heidelberg/Mannheim and the Department of Stereotactic Neurosurgery of the University of Cologne.

Coordinator of the Research Program:
Prof. Dr. Walter J. Lorenz

Divisions and their heads:

Oncological Diagnostics and Therapy:
Prof. Dr. Gerhard van Kaick

Biophysics and Medical Radiation Physics:
Prof. Dr. Walter Lorenz

Radiochemistry and Radiopharmacology:
Dr. Wolfgang Maier-Borst

Medical Physics:
Prof. Dr. Wolfgang Schlegel

6.1 Improvement in Breast Cancer Diagnostics

by Michael V. Knopp
and Stefan Delorme

Breast cancer is the most common malignant tumor in women. Epidemiological studies have shown that the incidence of this cancer is still rising. Nevertheless a remarkable increase in survival rates of affected women has been achieved in recent decades due to early diagnosis and constantly improving

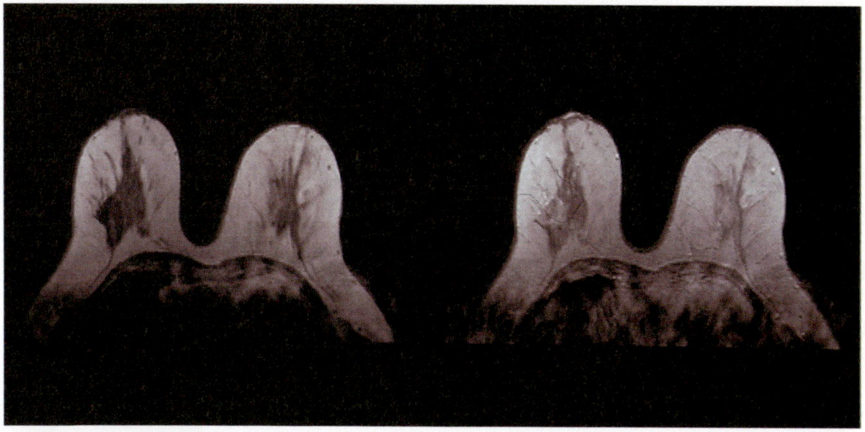

Fig. 46a

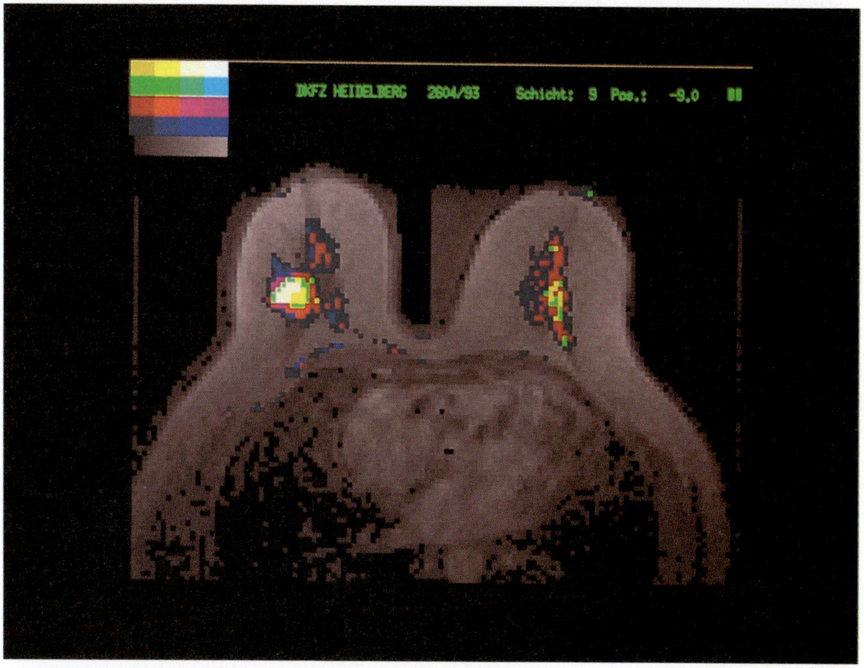

Fig. 46b

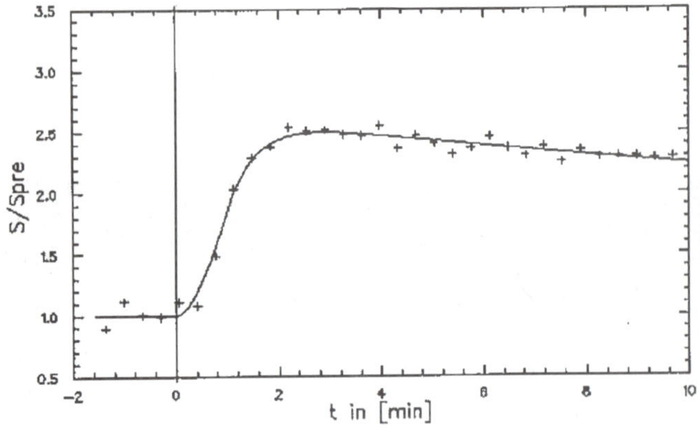

Fig. 46c

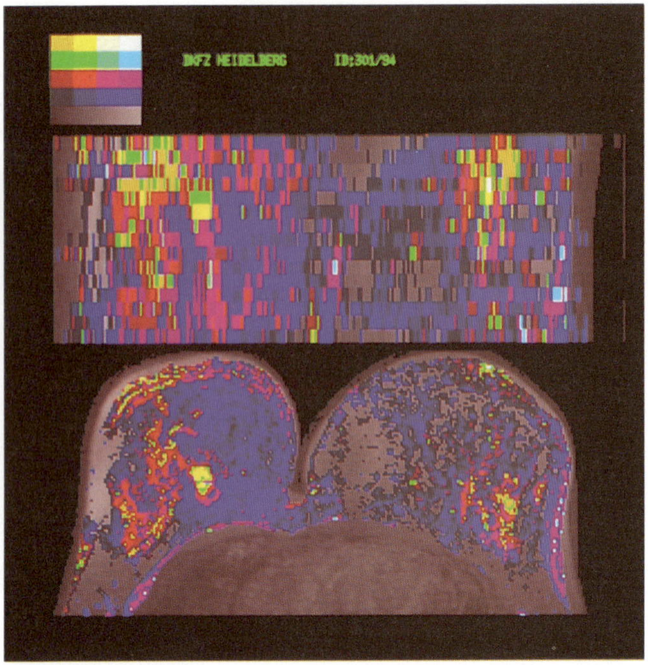

Fig. 46d

treatment. Advances in imaging diagnostics and better patient awareness have both contributed to early and improved tumor detection. X-ray mammography is the most important imaging technique. Continuous technical innovation has led to better quality images with minimum exposure to radiation. Large-scale international studies have demonstrated that the survival rates can be increased by regular mammographic screening in women 50 years of age and older. The technique is highly sensitive in the detection of suspicious regions; however, the findings are difficult to interpret from the x-ray image. For this reason, ultrasound scanning is used in conjunction with mammography for better evaluation of whether a suspicious finding is benign or malignant. Ultrasound scanning is highly reliable for instance in detecting cysts, i.e., harmless fluid pools, and in interpreting them correctly. However, the method is often not suitable to clearly determine whether dense lumps are benign. Therefore tissue samples taken by needle and punch biopsies are of primary importance for verification of the diagnosis. The tissue samples taken are conclusively classified by histopathology. However, tissue sampling is an invasive procedure and only makes sense if the ratio of the number of positive findings to the total number of tissue sampling procedures performed is justifiable.

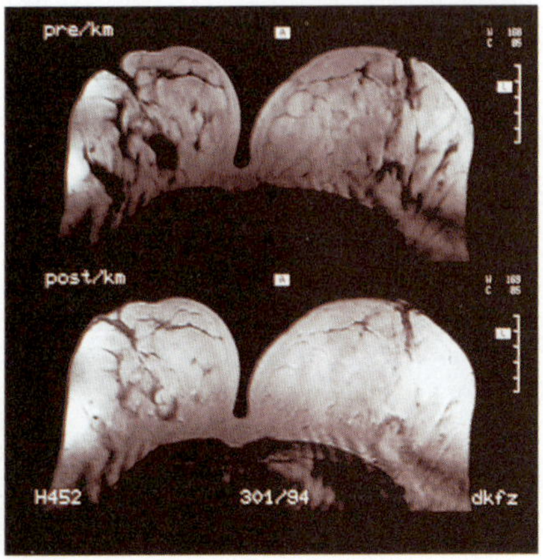

Fig. 46e

Magnetic Resonance Imaging (MRI)

For all the diagnostic options described above, there is still considerable room for improvement. Another diagnostic technique with high sensitivity and specificity is required to enhance those already described. This is currently the objective in applying and further developing magnetic resonance mammography (MRM). This tomographic imaging technique can detect changes in blood circulation in a tumor and can be represented in an image following administration of a paramagnetic contrast medium. The good sensitivity of the method has been demonstrated in clinical studies. However, a problem of this technique is that benign lesions such as fibroadenomas, mastopathic changes, and inflammatory regions also take up contrast medium, resulting in a significantly decreased specificity at first. The use of special temporal high-resolution dynamic imaging techniques has demonstrated that benign and malignant lumps take up contrast medium differently. The differences in enhancement can only be described by way of a mathematical calculation. Figure 46 shows the images from a patient suffering from breast cancer (a-c), and from a patient with a benign fibroadenoma (d-g). The signal-time curves of the two patients differ significantly although both tumors take up contrast medium. This indicates that the dynamic time-dependent high-resolution imaging technique is clearly superior to time-independent studies. The disadvantage is that more than 480 images are acquired within twelve minutes with the technique, making a visual analysis virtually impossible for the physician. Therefore, a color-coded parametric image is computed per section, summarizing the characteristics of contrast medium enhancement. By summarizing these parametric images as maximum intensity projections (MIP) in the sagittal, coronal, transverse plane one can reduce the total information contained in more than 480 sections to three color-coded images. These images allow the physician to identify conspicuous regions

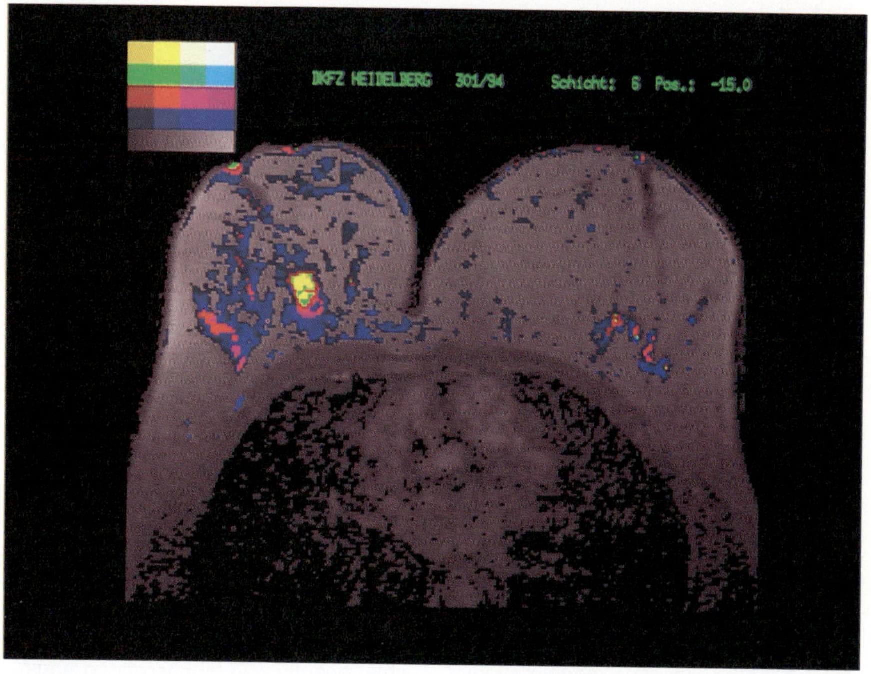

Abb. 46f

and to regard them in a cinematographic display and clarify them by further evaluation. In order to achieve an optimal morphologic representation in addition to the possibility of functional assessment, spatial high-resolution 3-D-FLASH imaging is performed prior to and following administration of contrast medium. In a collaborative clinical study we have already performed over 300 of these examinations, revealing that the sensitivity and specificity of this imaging technique for correct classification of focal changes are very high.

The technique is also suitable for early identification of functional changes occurring during chemotherapy, and is currently being applied in a clinical study in order to establish early and reliable criteria for assessment during so-called neoadjuvant chemotherapy with subsequent breast-conserving surgery.

Doppler Ultrasound-Scanning

Doppler ultrasound-scanning is based on the phenomenon that the perceived frequency of an acoustic wave changes when the source is moving towards or away from the receiver. This phenomenon is commonly experienced when the noise of a car becomes deeper as the vehicle passes by and is referred to as the „Doppler phenomenon“. When an ultrasound wave is transmitted into a medium in motion, such as blood, the superposition of the transmitted and the reflected waves results in a sound

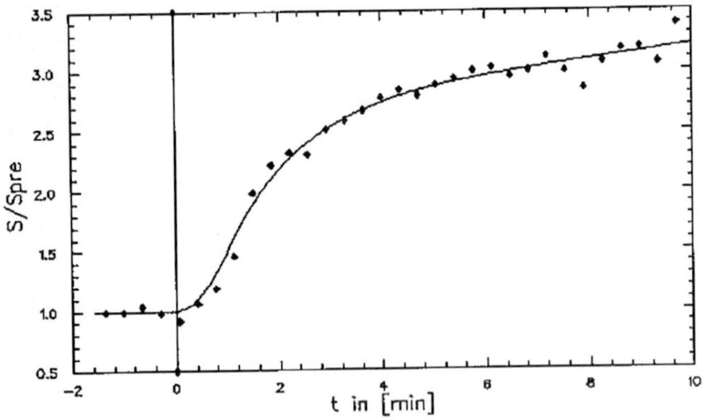

Fig. 46g

(„Doppler signal“) whose frequency is equal to the difference between the frequencies of the transmitted and the reflected waves and is dependent on the velocity of the reflecting medium (flow velocity if blood vessels are examined). The combination with conventional („B-mode“) ultrasound imaging permits to determine the location where the Doppler signal is acquired. „Spectral Doppler“ expresses the detected blood flow velocities in a single location as a velocity-time diagram. With „color Doppler imaging“, an entire image section is mapped for Doppler signals. The detected flow velocities are color coded and superimposed on the black and white B-mode image in real time. Where blood flow is detected, the black and white image points (picture elements, „pixels“) are replaced by isolated or confluent color spots, enabling not only a clear delineation of the perfused vessel lumen but also an assessment of the dynamic properties of the local blood flow. This method has advanced to a state-of-the-art modality in vascular imaging and has partly replaced X-ray angiography with intravascular application of contrast medium. Satisfactory imaging of very small vessels, such as those in tumors, has only become possible recently with highly refined equipment, and is only applicable in rather superficial lesions such as in breast tumors or lymph nodes. According to histopathological studies, the majority of breast carcinomas have more blood vessels per volume (higher „vascularity“) than benign lesions (such as fibroadenomas) or normal breast tissue. The degree of vascularity in the tumor appears to be positively correlated to the risk of distant metastases. If Doppler sonography is capable of reliably quantifying tumor vascularity, it may be a helpful non-invasive adjunct to predict whether a tumor is cancer or not, as well as to identify patients at high risk of distant metastases. Due to the tedious character of the Doppler examination, it is not suitable for early cancer detection.

Quantification of the Doppler information is a major challenge. Since spectral Doppler evaluates blood flow in a single small sample volume only, it will not help to assess vascular density. It facilitates the measuring of physical blood flow velocity with a certain reliability, but only in a single vessel and thereby with questionable validity. Color Doppler imaging gives at least an impression of vessel density (restricted to detectable vessels) and carries some limited information on flow velocities encoded by color. However, an exact quantification of the findings is difficult.

A first approach is to count detectable vessels in the color Doppler image and to measure blood flow velocities with spectral Doppler in a few standardised locations. A study based on this method showed that the density of detectable vessels as well as the measured flow velocities are exceedingly variant in breast carcinomas. Ten percent of the examined tumors were void of any detectable Doppler signal.

In a second approach, we applied a computer-assisted image analysis routine to statistically evaluate the color Doppler image. The image is frame-grabbed from the video output and stored on a personal computer. In a dedicated evaluation routine, the examiner recalls a set of stored images and delineates the tumor by a region of interest (ROI) in order to define the cross-section area as well as to exclude vessels outside the tumor from evaluation. Thereupon, the system calculates the percentage of color pixels inside the ROI and the first order statistics of color hues (color values), to express the vessel density and the flow velocities. This method permitted a differentiation of benign and malignant le-

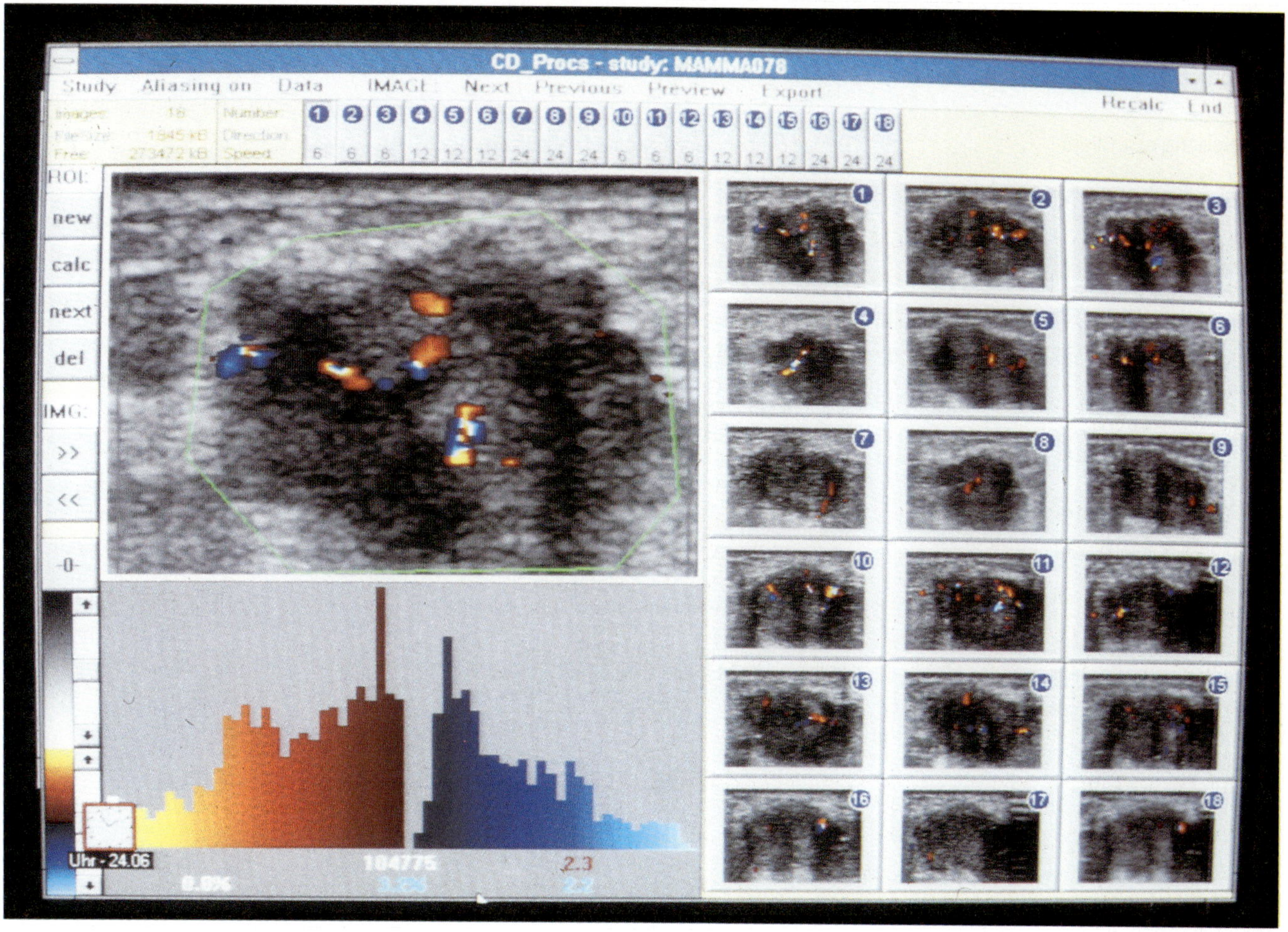

Fig. 47
Screen from the evaluation program of a color Doppler examination. All the images stored from a given examination are shown on the right half of the screen in miniature. The physician can then select the images for viewing in consecutive order on the left-hand side of the screen in their original size. Once the tumor has been outlined (green line) the computer calculates the area quotient of the colored dots and the mean color value. A malignant tumor is often better perfused and therefore has more "color" than a benign one

sions with a sensitivity of 92% and a specificity of 78%.

Although the role of Doppler sonography in the diagnosis of breast cancer has not yet been determined sufficiently to justify its routine use, it appears that a high degree of detectable vascularity in a suspicious nodule suggests malignancy. However, Doppler sonography does not make it possible to rule out cancer since up to 10% of carcinomas lack any detectable signal, and with sensitive equipment, there may be some detectable flow in benign lesions also. Its application for prognostic implications requires quantitative methods as described above. Results on this issue are pending until our patients have been followed long enough for preliminary estimation of their outcome.

Dr. Michael V. Knopp
Dr. Stefan Delorme
Division of Oncological Diagnostics and Therapy

Participating scientists

Beatrix Albert
Dr. Malte Bahner
Dr. Thomas Heß
Dr. Sabine Huber
Traudel Polzer
Prof. Dr. Gerhard van Kaick
Division of Oncological Diagnostics and Therapy

Dr. Gunnar Brix
Dipl.-Phys. Ulf Hoffmann
Dr. Dr. Ivan Zuna
Prof. Dr. Walter J. Lorenz
Division of Biophysics and Medical Radiation Physics

In cooperation with

Dr. Hans Junkermann
Prof. Dr. Dietrich von Fournier
Division of Gynecological and Obstetrical Radiology,
University of Heidelberg

Prof. Dr. Dr. Gunther Bastert
Gynecological Hospital of University of Heidelberg

Prof. Dr. Herwart F. Otto
Dr. Peter Sinn
Pathological Institute of the University of Heidelberg

Selected Publications

Delorme, S.: Dopplersonographie des Mammakarzinoms. Radiologe 33, 287–291 (1993)

Delorme, S., Anton, H.W., Knopp, M.V. et al.: Breast cancer: assessment of vascularity by color Doppler. Eur. Radiol. 3, 253–257 (1993)

Knopp. M. V., Heß, T., Bachert, P., Ende, G., Junkermann, H., Hesterkamp, T., van Kaick, G.: Magnetresonanzspektroskopie des Mammakarzinoms. Radiologe 33, 300–307 (1993)

Heß, T., Knopp, M. V., Hoffmann, U., Brix, G., Junkermann, H., Zuna, I., von Fournier, D., van Kaick, G.: Pharmakokinetische Analyse der Gd-DTPA-Anreicherung in der MRT beim Mammakarzinom. RöFo 6, 518–523 (1994)

Huber, S., Delorme, S., Knopp, M.V. et al.: Breast tumors: computer-assisted quantitative assessment with color Doppler US. Radiology 192, 797–801 (1994)

Knopp, M. V., Brix, G., Junkermann, H., Sinn, H. P.: MR-Mammography with Pharmakokinetic Mapping for Monotoring of Breast Cancer Treatment During Neoadjuvant Therapy. Ju: Magnetic Resonance Imaging, Ed.: Peter L. Davis. Saunders, Philadelphia (1994)

6.2 Positron Emission Tomography (PET) in Tumor Diagnosis and Therapy Management

by Antonia Dimitrakopoulou-Strauss

The diagnosis and choice of a suitable chemotherapeutic protocol poses basic problems in the treatment of tumors.

After a tumor has been found, the treating physician has to decide which type of chemotherapy seems most promising. A great variety of agents which suppress cell division, referred to as antineoplastics or cytotoxic drugs, are available for chemotherapeutic use. The therapeutic efficacy of a cytostatic agent differs not only from patient to patient but also from tumor to tumor. Even different metastases in the same patient frequently respond differently to therapy. Procedures for an early assessment of a patient's response to an administered cytotoxic drug are particularly important in cancer therapy for selecting an optimal therapy for the patient and for avoiding unnecessary side-effects due to switching drugs. Today the therapeutic efficacy of a drug is mainly evaluated by imaging techniques such as computed tomography (CT), magnetic resonance imaging (MRI), and ultrasound scanning (ultrasonography), which provide morphologic information such as tumor size, position, and shape. A change in tumor volume and an increase or decrease in tumor size are indicators of the therapeutic efficacy. Such changes in the tumor, however, are only detectable several days after the onset of chemotherapy.

Positron emission tomography (PET), an imaging technique used in nuclear medicine, provides further information about what goes on inside a tumor such as tissue perfusion and metabolic activity. The information is a measure of tumor viability and is assessed non-invasively by PET scanning without exposing the patient to undue risk. The metabolic activity in the tumor, for example, responds very rapidly to therapy and precedes changes in tumor morphology. Very early in therapy, conclusions about the therapeutic efficacy can be drawn from metabolic changes. It is possible to identify patients whose tumors do not respond to therapy soon after the onset of therapy, allowing the medication to be stopped or modified, and avoiding the administration of drugs ineffective in a given patient and associated with a high risk of side-effects. The information also allows prognoses to be made on the therapeutic efficacy prior to chemotherapy, making it easier for the physician to choose an adequate therapy for the patient.

PET provides information on the following:

- tissue perfusion of the tumor,
- metabolism of tumors,
- accumulation and kinetics of cytotoxic drugs, and
- determination of resistance against cytotoxic drugs (multi-drug resistance).

Before a patient undergoes PET scanning he or she is given an injection of radioactively labeled substances, known as radiopharmaceuticals, which indicate specific biochemical processes in the tumor. With PET, the difference between their accumulation in normal and tumor tissues can be monitored and assessed quantitatively and very precisely. Conclusions can be drawn from cross-sectional computational images of the involved region about the concentration of the radioactive drug in a particular tissue and thus about the degree of metabolic activity in the tumor.

In addition to primary diagnostics of a tumor, basic problems in clinical oncology are: the determination of the tumor stage (staging), the diagnosis of recur-

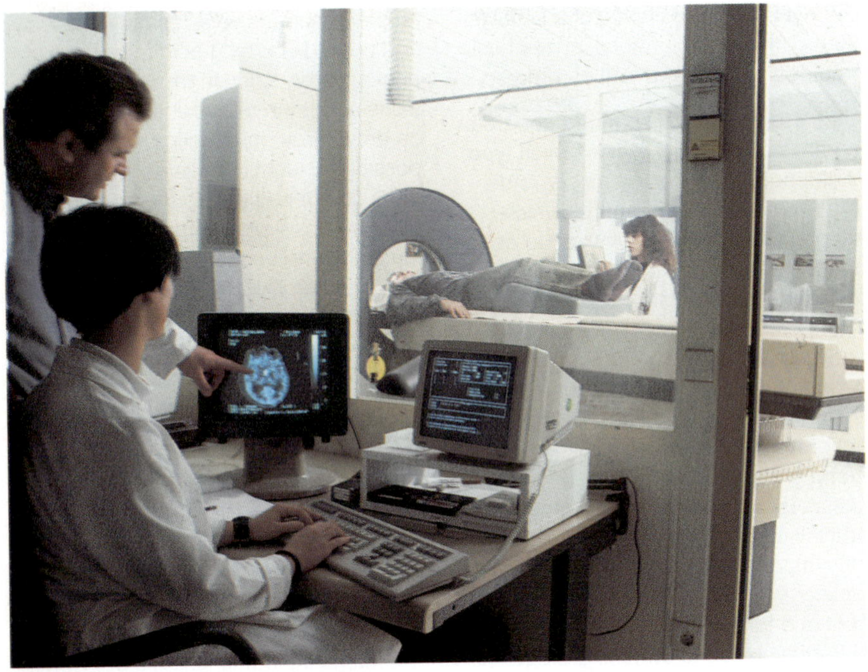

Fig. 48
Positron emission tomography (PET) provides detailed information on the processes in a tumor. The cross-sectional computer images can indicate the degree of metabolic activity in a tumor and thus provide important information on the likely efficacy of chemotherapy

rent disease, the detection of therapy-related changes, and the monitoring of tumor response. This is where PET scanning can be applied.

PET scanning for perfusion and metabolic studies in the diagnostics of recurrent disease

While CT and MRI scanning are successfully applied in the primary diagnostics of tumors, the usefulness of these techniques is limited to patients who have already undergone treatment. For instance, a new CT finding does not always permit an accurate differentiation between recurrent tumor and surgical scarring. One of the main problems in treating malignant disease, beside the detection of changes related to therapy and the evaluation of tumor viability, is the detection of tumor recurrence. Morphologic procedures are often inappropriate. The application of PET scanning with actively metabolized substances considerably improves diagnostics since an enhanced metabolic activity compared to healthy tissue is usually an indication of viable tumor tissue, thus permitting an early decision on a suitable therapeutic method.

We applied PET in patients with colorectal tumors, melanomas, and lymphomas in order to measure the metabolic activity of the tumors. We used fluorine-18-labeled deoxyglucose (FDG), a glucose analogon which is a marker of glucose metabolism in tumors. The activity concentrations measured with PET was put in relation to the patient's weight and the injected dosage, and expressed as what is known as the Standardized Uptake Value (SUV).

The Standardized Uptake Value is a measure of tumor viability: the higher it is, the more viable the tumor tissue is. Untreated tumors showed a markedly increased metabolic activity (SUV above 2) compared to normal tissue. A somewhat lower metabolic activity (SUV above 1.5) was measured in histologically confirmed recurrent tumors compared to healthy tissue. Involved lymph nodes in patients with lymphomas and melanomas showed markedly increased activity concentrations. The highest values were measured in melanoma patients. Bone metastases were also found to have an increased metabolic activity. Primary diagnostics of recurrent disease by means of PET scanning and the radioactive substance FDG was successful in 95 percent of patients. However, problems existed in individual cases where inflammatory processes were present. The sites of inflammation also proved to be metabolically very active, showing FDG uptake values in the range of those observed in tumors. In these cases further clinical and morphologic examinations are required for PET data evaluation.

PET scanning in chemotherapy

Several criteria can be applied to evaluate therapeutic efficacy including, for instance, various laboratory values, the

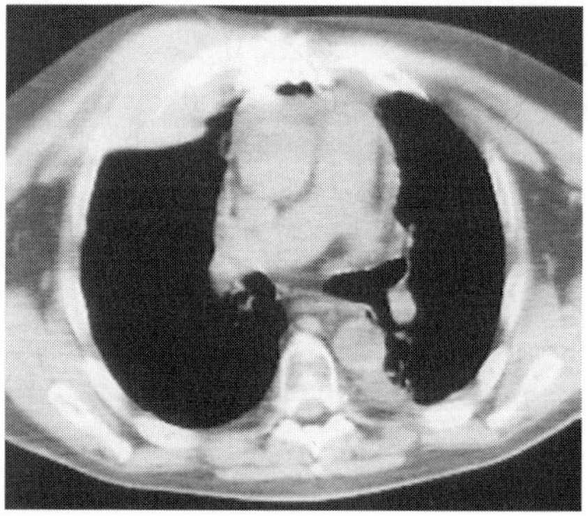

Fig. 49
These computed tomography scans of a patient with non-Hodgkin's lymphoma show changes in the chest wall, breastbone and diaphragm. It is impossible to tell whether the changes are benign or malignant

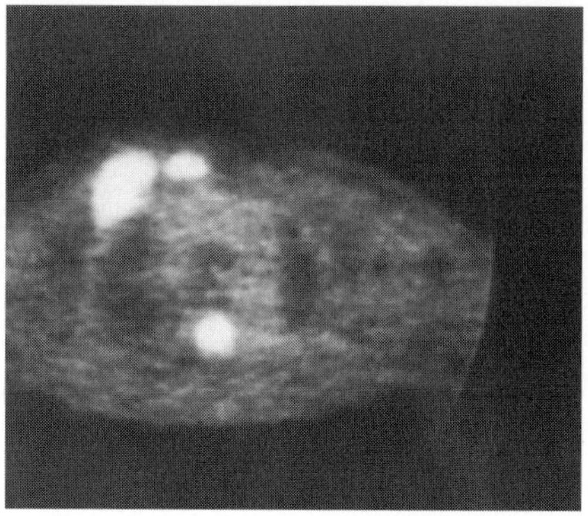

Fig. 50
Positron emission tomography in the same patient. Injection of radiolabeled fluorodeoxyglucose showed up vital tumor tissue in three places – two (chest wall, breastbone) of which were visible in the computed tomogram and one of which was not (spine)

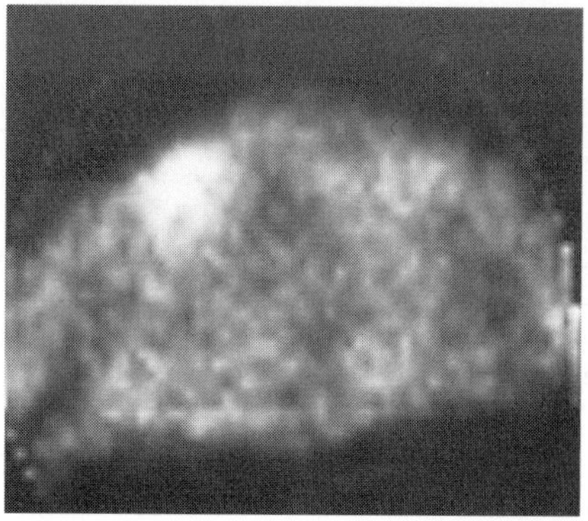

Fig. 51
Single photon emission computed tomography (SPECT) allows the observer to assess the response to anticancer drugs. The tumor in the chest wall appears to be sensitive to chemotherapy while the other two tumors seem to be resistant

clinical presentation of the patient, and information on tumor morphology as provided by ultrasound, computed tomography, and magnetic resonance imaging. These modern imaging techniques permit high spatial resolution and thus the assessment of tumor volume, position, and infiltration in adjacent tissues. Since morphologic changes following initiation of therapy are frequently detected only very late, more sensitive parameters are required that provide information on tumor metabolism or the behavior of drugs earlier in the process.

We applied positron emission tomography to investigate new parameters that permit early determination of therapeutic efficacy. Examinations of tumor metabolism, measurements of the metabolism of a cytotoxic drug in the tumor tissue, and determination of resistance against anticancer drugs, so-called multi-drug resistance (MDR), permit a timely evaluation of the selected form of therapy. Assessment of each parameter requires the application of a very specific radioactive substance. F-18-deoxyglucose (FDG) and C-11-aminoisobutyric acid (AIB) are primarily used in studies on metabolism while studies on the uptake and metabolism of a cytotoxic agent require labeling of the agent used in therapy. To date, studies with labeled fluorouracil (FU) have been performed that may provide a model for the application of other cytotoxic drugs. New radioactive drugs not yet available for PET examinations are required for the determination of MDR.

For the planning and monitoring of chemotherapy with PET three strategies requiring the application of differently labeled radioactive substances are feasible:

- Metabolic examinations before, during, and after chemotherapy, permitting the assessment of therapeutic response on the basis of change in metabolism and the identification of patients who do not respond to therapy.
- PET examinations with labeled cytostatic drugs. These examinations provide information about the behavior of a drug in the target area, in normal tissue, and in the vascular system.
- PET examinations and examinations with related single-photon emission tomography (SPECT) for determination of MDR in order to evaluate the therapeutic efficacy of combined chemotherapy.

PET follow-up studies demonstrated that a decrease in FDG uptake correlated with clinical response to therapy, while an increase in FDG uptake was indicative of increasing metabolic activity of the tumor and thus tumor growth.

In some of our patients we observed a continuous increase in FDG metabolism using PET, even 1 day after onset of therapy. In these cases it was possible to forecast that the patients would not respond to chemotherapy. Further monitoring of the course of the disease using imaging techniques and observation of the patient's clinical state confirmed our diagnosis.

Application of FDG for evaluation of therapeutic efficacy

PET examinations with FDG for the monitoring of therapy allow early identification of patients who will not respond to therapy.

Furthermore, we performed PET FDG examinations after a test dose of a cytostatic agent to assess different parameters providing information on therapeutic efficacy. These so called profile measurements provide information on the following parameters:

- Tumor metabolism before therapy

A baseline PET measurement prior to chemotherapy provides information on the baseline metabolism of the tumor, a measure of tumor viability prior to therapy.

- Short-term metabolic changes

PET examinations immediately after the end of therapy demonstrate the initial response to therapy. An FDG decrease in the tumor cells means that a number of the tumor cells have already died within this short period of time due to the uptake and the effects of the antineoplastic.

- Time to maximum therapeutic effect

Further PET examinations in the course of the next days were performed to determine the time of the minimum metabolic activity (this is called maximum therapeutic effect). We were able to confirm our finding by CT scanning several days later.

We performed several PET monitoring sessions using FDG in patients with Hodgkin's disease and non-Hodgkin lymphoma who had undergone treatment. A decrease in the FDG uptake was shown to correlate with a clinical response to therapy while an increase in the FDG uptake and thus metabolic activity resulted in tumor growth.

If repeated PET monitoring examinations are performed it is difficult to interpret the course of therapy since a cyclic behavior of therapy is demonstrated, with an increase in metabolic activity during the therapy-free interval and a decrease immediately after the end of chemotherapy. This suggests that in this case some cells are resistant against the antineoplastic and cause new tumor growth. The other nonresistant cells are destroyed during chemotherapy, resulting in a short-term drop in the tumor's metabolic activity.

We are presently developing a method designed to facilitate interpretation of such therapy courses. Preliminary evaluations in 15 patients were successful.

Application of labeled cytostatic agents for evaluation of therapeutic efficacy

PET examinations with labeled cytostatic agents allow the direct measurement of the kinetics of the drugs in the tumor, and thus the evaluation of the prospective response to therapy. Examinations with a cytostatic agent require very complex drug labeling. To date, there is only one drug that can be radioactively labeled with a positron emitter and thus be used for routine PET scanning: fluorouracil (FU). This cytotoxic drug is mainly used to treat patients with colorectal tumors. We applied labeled FU and performed sequential PET scanning over two hours. Early imaging with PET approximately 20 minutes after starting FU infusion gives information on the transport of the drug into the tumor cell. Late PET scanning two hours following infusion shows the therapeutically active part of the drug („trapped FU"). This value is used as a measure for therapy evaluation.

Different metastases even in the same patient showed a different FU uptake and thus varied in their response to therapy. Our findings demonstrated that a high uptake of the cytostatic drug in the tumor was principally associated with metastatic regression while low concentrations of the antineoplastic were not capable of preventing tumor growth during chemotherapy. Our data demonstrate that PET with F-18-FU makes it possible to assess the probable therapeutic response even prior to chemotherapy.

We also studied the perfusion of tumor tissue using PET and 0-15 labeled water and found out that an increase in tumor perfusion alone is no guarantee of chemotherapeutic success. On the contrary, it is only a prerequisite of therapeutic efficacy since good perfusion allows a larger amount of the antineoplastic to get into the tumor by way of the bloodstream. The data of our studies demonstrated that even a ten-fold increase in perfusion resulted in only a five percent increase in FU uptake in the tumor. Further prerequisites are an adequate transport of the cytostatic agent into the cell and the trapping of the cytostatic agent in the tumor cell.

Examinations to determine multi-drug resistance (MDR)

Multi-drug resistance is a major limitation to the efficacy of chemotherapy, whereby cytotoxic drugs are eliminated from the tumor, thus preventing the therapeutic agent from taking effect. Experimental studies show P-glycoprotein, a membrane protein, to be the responsible agent. It is expressed by the so-called mdr-1-gene and is responsible for the elimination of a number of substances from the cell. Studies performed by the Boston working group under Piwnica-Worms demonstrated that not only cytotoxic drugs, but also a radioactive drug used in nuclear medicine, Tc-99m-sestamibi, can be eliminated from tumor cells by P-glycoprotein.

To determine the MDR of tumors we examined patients with recurrent lymphoma using single photon emission tomography (SPECT) and determined the degree of Tc-99m-sestamibi uptake. Preliminary results indicate that a high uptake of this substance in the tumor correlates with a low P-glycoprotein expression. Elimination of the administered cytotoxic drug by the tumor will therefore also be slight, chemotherapy will be effective, and regression of the tumor will be seen. This shows that the patient can only be expected to respond to therapy if Tc-99m-sestamibi is taken up in sufficient quantities. Presently a drug analog of this specific radioactive drug is being developed that will be available for use in PET examinations.

Dr. Antonia Dimitrakopoulou-Strauss
Division of Oncological Diagnostics and Therapy

Editorial assistance

Dipl.-Biol. Karin Henke

In cooperation with

Dr. Franz Oberdorfer
Division of Radiology and Radiopharmacology,
Deutsches Krebsforschungszentrum

Dr. Gunnar Brix
Division of Biophysics and Medical Radiation Physics,
Deutsches Krebsforschungszentrum

Dr. Hartmut Goldschmidt
Medical University Hospital and Outpatient Hospital, Heidelberg

Dr. Thomas Möhler
Medical University Hospital and Outpatient Hospital, Heidelberg

Priv.-Doz. Dr. Wolfgang Tilgen
University Hospital for Skin Diseases, Heidelberg

Prof. Dr. Wolfgang Queißer
Medical Hospital - Chair for Internal Medicine III, Municipal Hospital Center, Mannheim

Ausgewählte Publikationen

Strauss, L.G., Clorius, J.H., Schlag, P., Lehner, B., Kimmig, B., Engenhart, R., Marin-Grez, M., Helus, F., Oberdorfer, F., Schmidlin, P., van Kaick, G.: Recurrence of colorectal tumors: PET evaluation. Radiology 170, 329–332 (1989)

Strauss, L.G., Dimitrakopoulou, A., Haberkorn, U., Knopp, M., Helus, F., Lorenz, W.J.: Einsatz der Positronenemissionstomographie (PET) zur onkologischen Diagnostik. Zentralblatt Radiologie 141, 255–256 (1990)

Strauss, L.G., Conti, P.S.: The applications of PET in clinical oncology. J. Nucl. Med. 32, 623–648 (1991)

Dimitrakopoulou, A., Strauss, L.G., Clorius, J.H., Ostertag, H., Schlag, P., Heim, M., Oberdorfer, F., Helus, F., Haberkorn, U., van Kaick, G.: Studies with Positron Emission Tomography after systemic administration of Fluorine-18-Uracil in patients with liver metastases from colorectal carcinoma. J. Nucl. Med. 34, 1075–1081 (1993)

Piwnica-Worms, D., Chiu M.L., Budding, M., Kronauge, J.F., Kramer, R.A., Croop, J.M.: Functional imaging of multidrug-resistant P-Glycoprotein with an organotechnetium complex. Cancer Res. 53, 977–984 (1993)

6.3 Radiosurgical Treatment of Patients with Brain Metastases

by Rita Engenhart and Jürgen Debus

Brain metastases are one of the hardest kinds of secondary growths to treat. They occur in 20 to 30 percent of all cancer patients. Although virtually any tumor can metastasize to the brain, brain metastases arise most commonly from lung or breast cancer, usually when the primary tumor is out of therapeutic control and proliferating. Brain metastases occur most frequently within two years after detection of the primary tumor. In 25% of the cases brain metastases present the first symptoms of a tumor undetected up to that time. Common manifestations of brain metastases are headaches, neurologic symptoms, convulsive seizures, and mental changes.

If untreated, brain metastases are fatal within a few weeks. Due to advances in neurosurgery and radiotherapy in recent years, it is now possible to considerably improve the quality of life and prolong the survival of many patients.

Rapid, precise diagnosis and starting therapy on time are crucial for the successful management of brain metastases. Depending on the patient's condition at the outset, one of the following three modes of treatment is generally applied:

- surgical removal of the secondary growth,
- fractionated whole brain irradiation in which the total dose is delivered in fractions over several days, and
- radiosurgical single-session treatment in which the patients receive the total radiation dose in a single session.

Surgical removal of a brain metastasis is the preferred therapy for patients with a favorable prognosis. These patients include those suffering from one or two isolated metastases in the brain tissue and whose general physical condition is good, i.e., the primary tumor is considered to be cured, metastases in other organs are absent, and the patient is under 60 years of age. These positive prognostic factors are found in 20 to 30 percent of all patients suffering from brain metastases. If in addition the metastasis is located at a favorable site it may be removed surgically without damaging adjacent healthy brain tissue. Patients suspected to have further brain metastases are given adjuvant fractionated whole brain irradiation following surgery. In patients with such a favorable prognosis, survival can be prolonged by many months, on average one to two years. Most importantly, the patient's quality of life is improved considerably. The 25% of patients still surviving five years after treatment can generally be considered cured.

Surgery is not an option in patients with an unfavorable prognosis. This group includes patients with more than two brain metastases; patients with additional metastases in other organs from an uncontrolled primary tumor; and patients in poor health. These patients are usually given fractionated whole brain irradiation therapy in which cumulative radiation doses totaling 40 Gy are administered over four weeks. In order to boost the therapeutic effect, some patients additionally receive so-called „boost irradiation“ in which a part of the tumor is again irradiated and the dose in this region „saturated“. Due to the poor initial prognosis in these patients, radiotherapy alone is less successful than surgery alone. Survival is prolonged by three to six months on average, and in every tenth patient by as much as two years.

Today, radiosurgery is applied in the treatment of inoperable metastases and metastases unresponsive to conventional radiotherapy. Twenty to forty percent of patients presenting with favorable prognostic factors cannot undergo surgery because the brain metastases are located at such an unfavorable site that the risk of irreversible neurologic injury is too high.

Some patients have brain metastases that originate from primary tumors with a low degree of sensitivity to radiation, such as melanomas, non-small-cell lung cancer, and cancer of the kidney and the intestines. In these cases, conventional whole brain irradiation alone has only limited therapeutic success. Although metastases insensitive to irradiation may regress during therapy the patient usually suffers a relapse after a few months. Administration of higher doses is not possible since healthy brain tissue would be injured, resulting in atrophy (wasting and loss of tissue), poor oxygen supply to the brain tissue, or necrosis (death of brain tissue).

In such cases radiosurgical irradiation may be the answer. Radiosurgery is a generic term for radiation techniques that deliver high-concentration and high-precision radiation to the target volume in the brain. The radiation effect is limited to a small target area in the brain, sharply demarcated from adjacent healthy tissue, and ranging in size from a few millimeters to a few centimeters. A larger dose is built up in the target area than in the adjacent healthy tissue. This ensures that healthy tissue is largely spared.

Brain metastases are well-suited for radiosurgical irradiation because they are generally spherical in shape and do not infiltrate normal tissue. They can be clearly distinguished and demarcated from healthy brain tissue using imaging techniques such as computed tomography (CT) and magnetic resonance imaging (MRI). Brain metastases are usually not more than three centimeters in diameter at the time of detection.

In cooperation with the Radiological and Neurosurgical Departments of Heidelberg University Hospital, we have been investigating the therapeutic efficacy of this specific radiation technique on brain metastases for several years and we have successfully applied the technique to inoperable and radioresistant brain metastases. Since 1986 we have radiosurgically treated 158 patients with inoperable and apparently radioresistant brain metastases at the the linear accelerator at the Deutsches Krebsforschungszentrum. The cumulative dose administered in single-session irradiation ranged from 15 to 20 Gy. During linear accelerator radiotherapy the source of radiation is rotated around the patient's head. In addition, the patient treatment couch can be moved in the horizontal plane and adjusted to different positions, thus permitting application of radiotherapy from multiple directions so that overcrossing of the individual beams of radiation, and hence administration of the cumulative dose, only occurs in the target volume.

Much higher radiation doses can be applied in radiosurgical irradiation than in fractionated radiotherapy. Since the effect is similar to that of surgical removal of the brain tissue affected by the tumor, this form of radiotherapy is referred to as radiosurgery, in analogy to the term „neurosurgery". Special stereotactic fixation options ensure complete immobilization of the patient's skull, exact location of the tumor in CT or MRI, and precise positioning of the patient under the source of radiation. High precision in radiation is achieved using this technique.

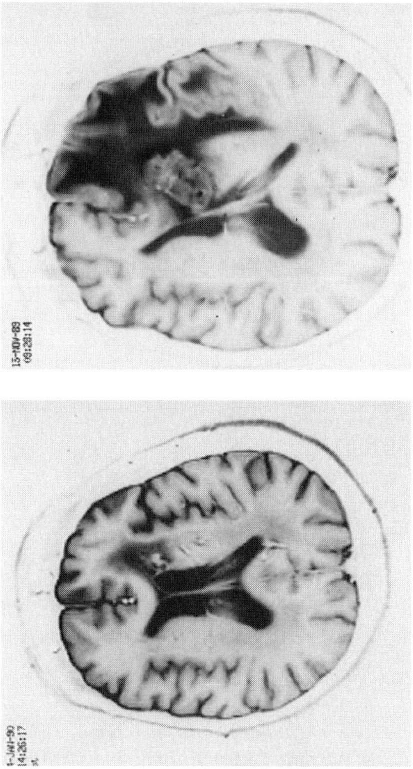

Fig. 52 a, b
Magnetic resonance tomography scans of a patient's brain. Image a shows a brain metastasis surrounded by an area of cerebral edema. The patient is paralyzed on one side. The image was taken before radiosurgical therapy. Two months later (b): Complete regression of the metastasis and edema after radiation. The patient is no longer paralyzed

We have applied radiosurgery both for primary treatment of brain metastases

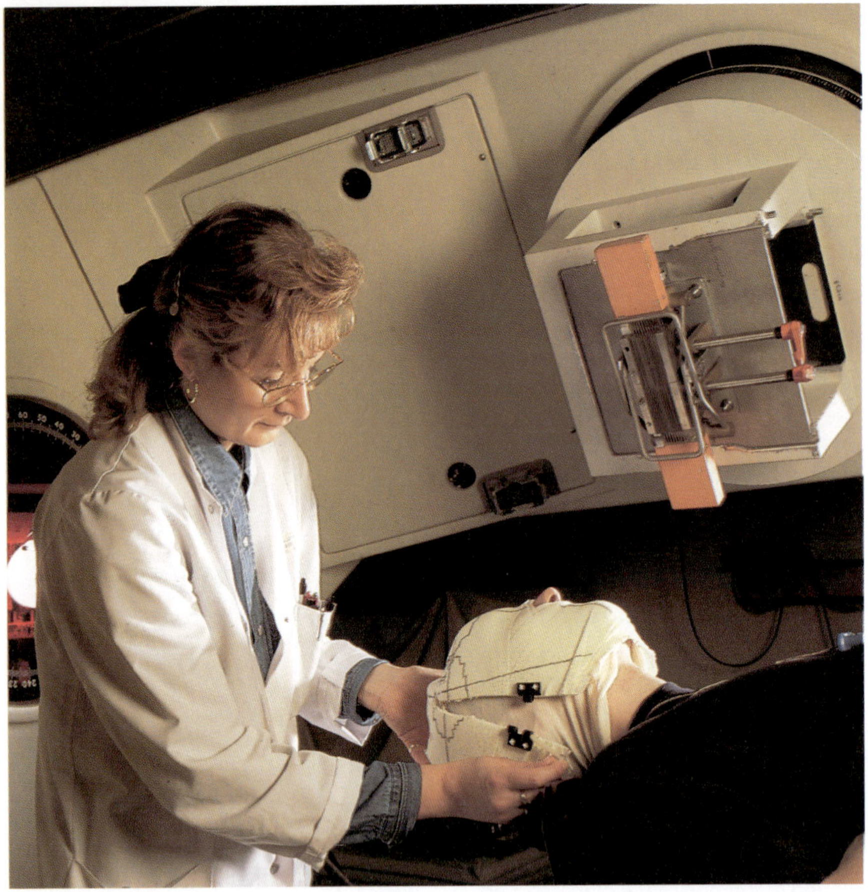

Fig. 53a
The precise position of the patient is adjusted by a laser system

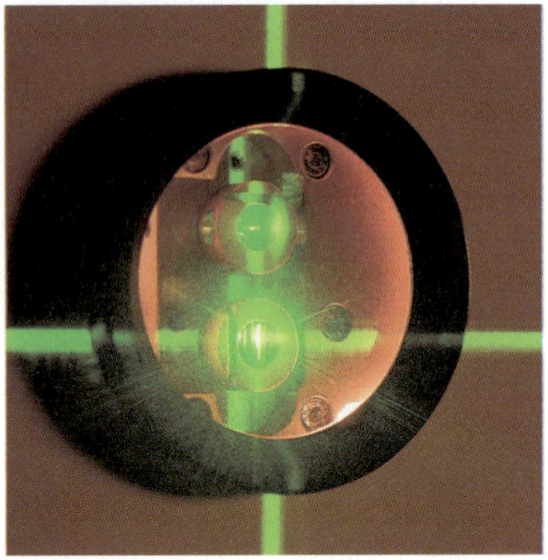

Fig. 53b
A patient is being prepared for radiation. The precision mask means that the patient can be positioned accurately down to the last millimeter. The tumor is located precisely by magnetic resonance tomography. The direction of the radiation beam and the dose of radiation to be directed at the tumor are then calculated. Great care is taken to target the tumor effectively and avoid damaging healthy tissue

and as boost therapy along with fractionated whole brain irradiation. Some of the patients we treated had suffered a relapse and once again developed brain metastases following surgery or fractionated whole brain irradiation.

In the treatment of these patients we were interested in the following questions:

- Does radiosurgical irradiation permit the destruction of radioresistant metastases without irreversibly damaging the surrounding healthy tissue?
- If yes, does this noninvasive technique present an alternative to surgery?
- Is radiosurgery successful in the treatment of patients who suffer a relapse following fractionated radiotherapy?

Our patients underwent neurologic examination and CT scanning or magnetic resonance imaging six weeks after radiotherapy and subsequently every three months. We succeeded in controlling the tumor locally, stopping growth of the brain metastases in 93 percent of the patients by radiosurgical irradiation. In just over one third of this patient group the metastasis decreased by more than half, and in 20 percent it was no longer detectable by imaging techniques. Eighty-two percent of all radiosurgically treated patients experienced considerable improvement of their disease-related neurologic symptoms within a few weeks.

All in all, radiosurgery was well tolerated by the patients. Side-effects, such as brain necroses or edema, were more rarely observed than following surgery.

Patient survival was prolonged by one and a half years on average, depending on the initial prognosis. In 10 percent of our patients, radiosurgical therapy was performed five years ago or even longer. It is safe to assume that some of these long-term survivors are completely cured. Hence, our studies demonstrate that with respect to survival and the quality of life, radiosurgery alone was as effective as surgery alone or a combination of surgery and fractionated brain irradiation.

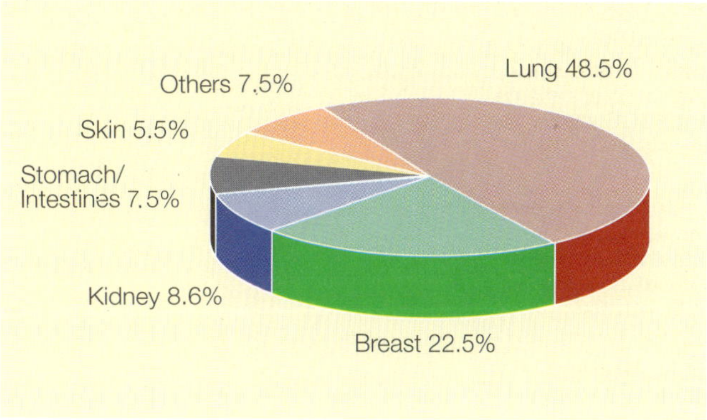

Fig. 54
Schematic representation of primary tumor distribution in patients with brain metastases. The incidence of brain metastases is highest in lung and breast cancer patients

In summary, radiosurgery is a highly effective technique for the treatment of solitary brain metastases and rapidly restores neurologic normality, significantly improving the quality of life. Radiosurgery can also be recommended if there are two, or at the most three metastases originating from radioresistant primary tumors since the technique does not appear to cause irreversible injury to adjacent brain tissue.

The question as to whether radiosurgery is an alternative to surgery can be answered with an unequivocal yes, on the basis of our results from patients with a favorable prognosis. Radiosurgery even has some advantages over surgical resection: it is noninvasive and therefore accompanied by less strain for the patient. After the radiation session lasting twenty to thirty minutes, the patient is required to stay in hospital for only one day. In addition, the therapy is less expensive than surgery although it is just as effective. Since radiosurgery is such a „gentle" and efficient technique, it should also be considered in cases where surgery is possible but difficult to perform. In some patients, however, in whom the pressure of the tumor on the brain must be relieved as a matter of urgency, surgery should still be the preferred therapy.

Furthermore, radiosurgery enlarges the indication spectrum of radiotherapy to include patients with recurrent disease who usually no longer respond to further fractionated brain irradiation. We have administered radiosurgical therapy to such patients with excellent results. Conversely, fractionated whole brain irradiation can also be performed following radiosurgical irradiation if the tumor continues to grow or the patient suffers a relapse.

Despite these positive results there are still a number of open questions. For instance, we intend to investigate whether prophylactic whole brain irradiation as an adjunct to each course of radiosurgery would improve the outcome of therapy. This strategy is aimed at fighting any metastase precursors, known as micrometastases, which may be present but are too small to be detected with currently available imaging techniques.

To elucidate this question, a joint European study involving several European research centers and sponsored by the European Union will be performed.

Priv.-Doz. Dr. Rita Engenhart
Division of Oncological Diagnostics and Therapy

Dr. Dr. Jürgen Debus
Division of Biophysics and Medical Radiation Physics

Participating scientists

Dr. Karl-Heinz Höver
Dipl.-Ing. Bernhard Rhein
Priv.-Doz. Dr. Lothar Schad
Division of Biophysics and Medical Radiation Physics

Prof. Dr. Wolfgang Schlegel
Division of Medical Physics

Prof. Dr. Gerhard van Kaick
Division of Oncological Diagnostics and Therapy

Editorial assistance

Dipl.-Biol. Karin Henke

In cooperation with

Prof. Dr. Dr. Michael Wannenmacher
Radiological University Hospital, Heidelberg

Prof. Dr. Stefan Kunze
Neurosurgical University Hospital, Heidelberg

Selected publications

Diener-West, M., Dobbins, T. W., Phillips, T. L., Nelson, D. F.: Identification of an optimal subgroup for treatment evaluation of patients with brain metastasis using RTOG study 7916. Int. J. Radiat. Oncol Biol. Phys. 16, 669–673 (1989)

Engenhart, R., Wowra, B., Kimmig, B., Hoever, K. H., Kunze, S., Wannenmacher, M.: Stereotaktische Konvergenzbestrahlung: Aktuelle Perspektiven auf der Grundlage klinischer Ergebnisse. Strahlenther. Onkol. 168, 245–259 (1992)

Engenhart, R., Kimmig, B. N., Hoever, K. H., Wowra, B., Romahn, J., Lorenz, W. J., van Kaick, G.: Long-Term Follow-Up for Brain Metastases Treated by Percutanous Stereotactic Single High-Dose Irradiation. Cancer 71, 1353–1361 (1993)

6.4 Ultrasound in the Treatment of Tumors

by Jürgen Debus and Peter Huber

The vast majority of cancers remains undetected until the patient has symptoms, by which time the tumors have usually grown to a considerable size. The first step in treatment is therefore to initiate local therapy, i.e., directed at the tumor itself. Local therapy usually involves surgical removal and radiotherapy, backed up by adjunctive chemotherapy. Presently, it is possible to cure about 70% of cancer patients whose disease is detected in the early stages. More than half of the other 30% of patients die of an uncontrollable in situ cancer, accounting for roughly 100 000 people annually in Germany alone. There are therefore many of patients who stand to benefit from any new technique which leads to improvements in the field of local therapy in the treatment of tumors. The search for new therapeutic forms has led to discussions about the possibility of applying ultrasound in the treatment of tumors.

Ultrasound is widely used in almost all medical specialities, mainly for diagnostic purposes. The technique has the advantage over conventional diagnostic procedures such as x-ray, of being quicker, fairly low-cost, and of not exposing the body to ionizing radiation. The great advantage of ultrasound for therapeutic purposes lies in its excellent focusability combined with a high penetration depth, allowing for high energy densities in deep tissue layers and sparing the intermediate tissues at the same time.

Ultrasound is also ideal for the palliative treatment of cancer patients due to its ease of use in combination with its minimally invasive properties. Palliative treatment is the term used to describe an approach to care that is primarily directed at improving the patient's comfort and quality of life (pain management, reduction in tumor size, and so on) rather than curing the patient. Radiotherapy using electromagnetic waves or atomic particles has already been valuable in this respect. However, radiation therapy is not always applicable near certain organs such as the kidneys and the liver which are intolerant of major doses of radiation. Ultrasound treatment promises to alleviate symptoms in these patients.

Basically, our research is intended to investigate the mechanisms of interaction between ultrasound and tissues and how effective tumor treatments may be derived from them. Research into these interaction mechanisms is important to gain reliable information on possible harmful effects of clinical ultrasound use. The question of side-effects has been the topic of controversial discussions ever since (in conventional ultrasound scanning) high-intensity Doppler techniques started to be more widely used than lower-intensity ultrasound B scanning.

From the point of view of physics, ultrasound is a mechanical oscillation, similar to ocean waves and audible sound waves, but occurring at frequencies inaudible to the human ear. The biological effects of ultrasound are due to both heat and mechanical processes. Both effects usually occur in combination. However, by changing physical parameters, such as duration or intensity of ultrasound pulses, a domination of either heat or the mechanical action is achieved. The mechanical action has important therapeutic implications since it may occur as a thresholding phenomena, i.e., it is conceivable that its genesis and hence also its effect

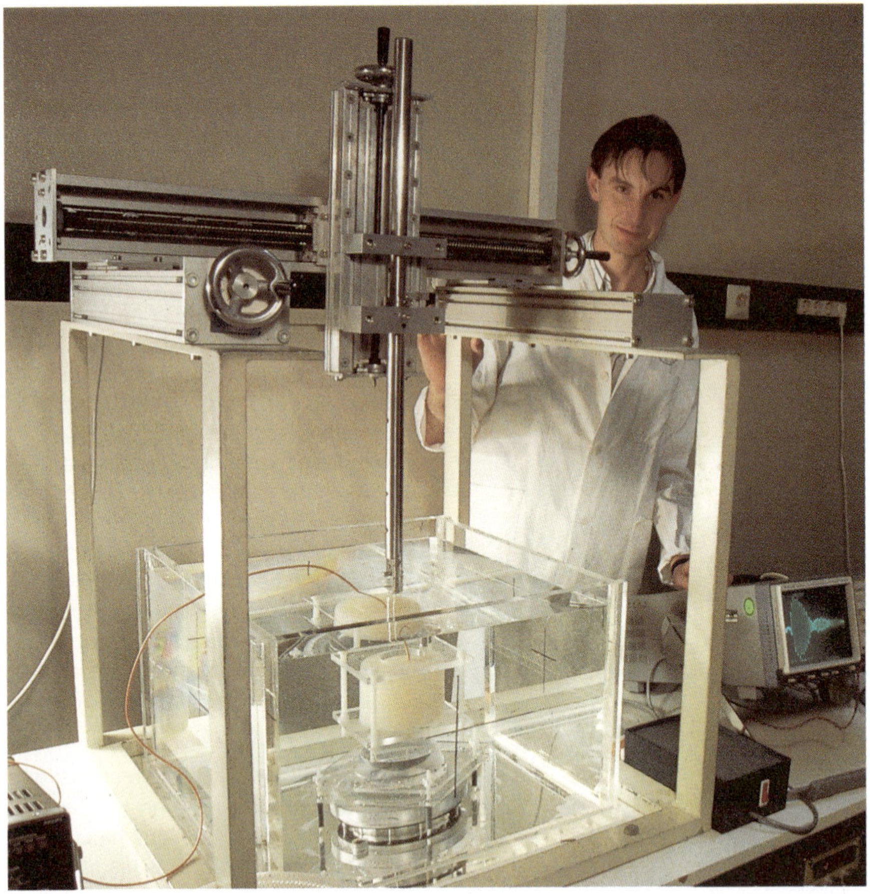

Fig. 55
A newly developed ultrasound device for the experimental treatment of tumors in the rat. Treatment considerably slowed down tumor growth in animal models

may be controlled so as to achieve a local effect in a circumscribed zone, the so-called target volume. The formation of what are called cavitations is an example of such a mechanism. Cavitations are tiny, hollowed-out spaces which may occur when applying sufficiently strong low pressure to a medium over a short time. The cavity collapses upon removing low pressure. Implosion of the cavity may be so violent as to destroy adjacent biological structures.

The experimental device

Part of our work conducted so far has been to develop and build an ultrasonic device that offers the great variability required for the implementation of basic experiments. An electromagnetic sound-source, a device similar to a huge loudspeaker in operation, is used to generate ultrasonic pulses and an acoustic lens is used for focusing. A high-voltage capacitor charged up to 21 kilovolts supplies the device with the electrical energy required for the generation of sound pulses. The characteristic sound pulse in the focus shows a steeply rising high-pressure proportion and a flat low-pressure proportion. Other sound-sources with an enormous range of potential sound pulses have recently been developed. At first, the sound-sources were precisely characterized using measurement techniques. Peak pressures of up to 600 bar were measured, the duration of the sound pulse being as brief as only a few millionths of a second.

Cavitations

A major result of physico-technical characterization of ultrasonic effects was the detection of cavitations in the ultrasonic fields. These cavitations last a mere thousandth of a second. However, we succeeded in taking photographs of these effects using ultrashort flashes light. Numerous studies were conducted on the kinetics of these cavitations, demonstrating that the effect is dependent on the other sound-field parameters. We further succeeded in demonstrating that radicals may be produced due to these cavitations in a similar way as in the application of ionizing radiation. These biologically and chemically highly reactive groups of atoms play a central role in the tumor-destructive effect of radiotherapy. This is however not only of great interest with regard to the potential use of ultrasound for therapeutic purposes, but also shows the importance of safety limits in diagnostic ultrasound use, as it is essential to prevent damage to healthy tissues by radicals.

The development of new techniques for determining cavitation activity in vivo was based on these measurements. A small glass fiber, 0.05 millimeter in diameter, is placed in the tissue. Using laser light, it is then possible both to measure pressure and to demonstrate cavitation itself. A major finding was the similarity between the dynamics of the cavitation in tissue and in water. The results obtained so far in water have therefore been useful as a basis for roughly judging cavitation dynamics in tissue and hence the associated biological effect. Furthermore, it was possible to directly quantify the energy involved in a single cavitation event by assessing the size of the cavitation. Total cavitation intensity was shown to increase disproportionately as the repeat frequency of ultrasonic pulses increased. These quantifications of energetic deposition in the tissue are especially important for a dose-response relationship, which is the essential basis of radiotherapy using ionizing radiation.

The effect of ultrasound on tumor tissue was investigated in animal experiments on the basis of the examination of morphological changes in tissue sections and functional parameters, such as blood flow to the tumor. However, the most important task was to elucidate to what extent tumor growth is suppressed or even stopped by ultrasound treatment.

Histological changes following ultrasound therapy

We obtained the following results from a model of cancer of the prostate in the rat:

Treatment of tumors in rats with 1000 ultrasonic pulses applied at 1-second intervals resulted in death of the tumor cells within 72 hours of ultrasound treatment of a localizable, circumscribed area, as confirmed by classical staining techniques and evaluation of immunohistochemical staining following integration of a proliferation marker (bromide deoxyribonucleotide, BrdUrd). Tiny hemorrhages, and sometimes smaller hematomas, occurred at the sound entry and exit sites, and they disappeared in the course of several days.

Tumor growth delay

The growth profile of tumors approximately 1 square centimeter large was examined following treatment with 1000 ultrasonic pulses constantly focused on the center of the tumors during a single session. The following results were obtained:

Therapy with high-energy ultrasound alone produced a highly significant growth delay (significance level $p<0.05$) of one tumor volume doubling time, i.e. 5 days, compared to untreated control animals. This means that the application of ultrasound dramatically suppresses the growth of certain tumors – at least in animal experiments.

Reduction of blood flow to the tumor

We know from a magnetic resonance imaging study in the same animal model that blood flow to the tumor is dramatically reduced following ultrasound treatment. This effect is reversible; blood flow is gradually restored within 24 hours of ultrasound treatment. In some tumors no signal increase of the contrast medium applied as a signal amplifier was demonstrable 8 hours following ultrasound treatment. In contrast to this, blood flow was not altered in the neighboring muscle which was used as reference tissue. This suggests that blood vessels in tumors are especially sensitive to ultrasound therapy. This in turn sets the stage for an already established supplementary therapeutic approach, namely the application of heat. Ultrasound treatment considerably reduces the blood's capability of carrying away heat, which is consequently maintained in the tumor for a longer time after hyperthermic treatment.

Combined therapy with local tumor hyperthermia

Starting from the presently held concept that the main therapeutic application of ultrasound would be as an adjunct in combined therapy, we investigated both the effect of combination therapy as well as that of local overheating of tumor tissue. We wanted to discover to what extent pretreatment with ultrasound might additionally enhance sensitivity of tumor tissue to local hyperthermia applied over 30 min at a temperature of 43.5° C, or even have other than purely additive effects. We found out that local tumor hyperthermia on its own does not significantly affect tumor growth of the chosen prostate carcinoma in the rat. Combined therapy of ultrasound plus hyperthermia however was able to slow down tumor growth significantly by two volume-doubling times compared to the untreated control group, and by one volume-doubling time compared to the group treated only with ultrasound. This suggests that the effect is more than additive. We expected increased thermosensitivity of the tumor tissue due to ultrasound since we knew from the above mentioned magnetic resonance imaging study that the blood vessels in the tumor are especially sensitive to ultrasound treatment. The more than additive effect is probably due to the increased heat retention at the site and the interruption of oxygen supply to the tumor tissue caused by restriction of the blood flow, thereby increasing the sensitivity to hyperthermia.

These studies on the effect of high-energy ultrasound on tumors represent a new therapeutic concept for the treatment of soft-tissue tumors, although the ideal therapeutic application of high-energy ultrasound remains to be found. We know today that each of the following mechanisms is capable of destroying tumor tissue: mechanical force of pressure, tear and shear forces, cavitation, and ultrasound-induced hyperthermia. Ultrasound has not yet found its place in the treatment of tumors, and its role will remain uncertain as long as the discussion as to its optimal effect continues.

Conclusions

These preliminary results give us reason to hope that, due to its easy in-depth focusability, high-energy ultrasound will be applicable as a supplementary therapeutic technique in sonically accessible tumors, i.e., all regions of the body which can be visualized in ultrasound diagnostics, such as the liver, the urogenital tract, and the neck. The changes we observed in our biological studies are clearly a function of physical parameters. The exactitude of the physical parameters we use permits us to achieve defined biological effects in a potential therapeutic application. Ultrasound treatment of tumors may be performed in addition to therapy, so as to control the outcome. Our study group is therefore investigating the potential of noninvasive magnetic resonance imaging and ultrasonic diagnostic techniques which record biological and physical parameters in the target area.

Having obtained these encouraging preliminary results, we will examine whether the results can be extrapolated to other forms of tumors. We shall also try to further explore the question of whether ultrasound enhances the effect of other regionally applied local therapeutic modalities, such as ionizing radiation, or is a useful adjunct to local or systemic chemotherapy.

Dr. Dr. Jürgen Debus
Dr. Peter Huber
Division of Biophysics
and Medical Radiation Physics

Participating scientists

Dr. Peter Peschke
Prof. Dr. Eric W. Hahn
Dr. Gunnar Brix

In cooperation with:

Siemens AG,
Unternehmensbereich Medizin

Prof. Dr. Franz M.J. Debryune
Department of Urology,
University Hospital Nijmegen,
Netherlands

Prof. Dr. Peter Antich
Department of Radiology,
University of Texas, Dallas, U.S.A.

Selected Publications:

Debus, J., Peschke, P., Hahn, E.W., Lorenz, W.J., Lorenz, A., Iffländer, H., Zabel, H.J., Kaick, G. v., Pfeiler, M.: Treatment of the Dunning prostate tumor R3327-AT1 with pulsed high energy ultrasound shock waves (PHEUS): growth delay and histomorphologic changes. J. Urol. 146, 1143–1146 (1991)

Debus, J., Peschke, P., Huber, P., Lorenz, A., Lorenz, W. J.: Pulsed high energy ultrasound – are the biological effects due to radical formation? Radiology 185, 202 (1992)

Huber, P., Debus, J., Peschke, P., Hahn, E.W., Lorenz, W.J.: In vivo measurement of ultrasonically induced cavitation by a fibre-optic technique Ultrasound in Med. and Biol. 20, 811–825 (1994)

6.5 Therapy Monitoring of Brain Tumors by Means of Magnetic Resonance Spectroscopy

by Peter Bachert and Thomas Heß

Low-grade astrocytomas are slowly growing tumors of the glial cells. Typically, they are not sharply delineated but infiltrate the normal brain tissue. Besides surgical removal, radiotherapy is a suitable means of treatment of these tumors. At the Deutsches Krebsforschungszentrum, a technique is applied that allows us to adapt the radiation fields to the irregular contours of the tumors. To optimize therapeutic efficacy, spatial precision (stereotactic) treatment planning with magnetic resonance tomography is employed. This procedure allows healthy brain tissue to be largely spared.

Up to now, the response of these tumors to radiotherapy has been evaluated by analyzing the changes in tumor size using imaging modalities. With these methods, however, early effects of radiotherapy in the tumor can only be detected after they have reached macroscopic dimensions. In a clinical study, we therefore elaborate a method of therapy monitoring by means of localized nuclear magnetic resonance spectroscopy. A noninvasive technique offers insights into the metabolism of tissues, i.e., into processes taking place at the biochemical level.

Nuclear magnetic resonance (NMR) is based on the intrinsic angular momentum of certain atomic nuclei, such as those of hydrogen (^{1}H, the proton), of the rarely occurring stable carbon isotope ^{13}C, and of phosphorus (^{31}P). Nuclear spin plus nuclear electrical charge produce a magnetic momentum which aligns with the orientation of a static external magnetic field and can be reversed by radiowaves of an appropriate frequency (called resonance or Larmor frequency). In returning to the ground state, the nuclear spin system emits a pulse-shaped radiowave field, the NMR signal. Analysis of the signal provides information on the interaction of the spins with their surroundings.

In 1888, Heinrich Hertz, who then worked at the University of Karlsruhe, was the first to generate electromagnetic radiation in the radiofrequency band. In much the same way as x-rays, radiofrequency waves are capable of passing through living tissue. However, the energy of the quanta of radiowave fields is approximately 12 orders of magnitude lower than that of x-rays, which makes it impossible to excite molecules or to break up chemical bonds: it is a non-ionizing radiation.

The most important property for the application of magnetic resonance spectroscopy is that the resonance frequency of a nuclear spin is proportional to the strength of the local magnetic field in which it sits. The local field depends, among other factors, on the distribution of electrons in the molecule. As a consequence, the frequencies of, e.g., the protons in water molecules and of the methyl protons of lactic acid differ slightly – by approximately 0.0003 percent. Protons in other chemical groups and compounds have still different resonance frequencies. Consequently, the nuclear spin resonance signal of living tissue, generated by the reorientation of the nuclear spins in a large number of different metabolites, is a complex mixture of frequencies. For analysis, the signal received a radiofrequency antenna is digitized and separated into its frequency components. This procedure is comparable to the action of a prism, which separates white light into the component spectral colors, and to that of our acoustic sense, which separates a sound mixture into individual tones.

Magnetic resonance spectroscopy hence makes it possible to identify chemical groups and metabolites on the basis of their characteristic frequencies or, as one could almost say, by their "color hue," with the intensity of the signals being a measure of the concentration of the emitting substances.

Since its discovery in the mid-1940s, magnetic resonance of atomic nuclei has been widely applied in analytical chemistry, in molecular and solid-state physics, and in biochemistry. Imaging techniques based on this phenomenon finally became established in radiological diagnostics in the 1980s. Magnetic resonance tomography uses the comparatively intense NMR signals from hydrogen atomic nuclei in tissue water and in fatty acids to obtain anatomic cross-sections from within the human body, offering excellent soft-tissue contrast (Fig. 56a and c). Although the wavelengths of radiofrequency waves are in the order of meters, which according to the classical theory of Ernst Abbe would not even permit the imaging of an animal the size of an elephant, their phase coherence and sharpness in frequency make it possible to resolve even structures in the sub-millimeter range.

If the spectral resolution is increased and the observed frequency range extended so that signals from other nuclei are also included, magnetic resonance opens a window to observe the metabolism of living tissue. For example, phosphorus (^{31}P) NMR spectroscopy allows us to measure the concentrations of important molecular carriers of energy in intact cells. The development of localized hydrogen (^{1}H) NMR spectroscopy at the end of the 1980s provided a tool for non-invasive examinations of the chemical composition of the human brain.

The protons of cell water provide by far the strongest ^{1}H NMR signal in vivo. Protons in macromolecules, such as proteins and nucleic acids, or in solid structures, such as the mineral substance of bones and teeth, do not normally contribute to the in vivo NMR signal. For less intense resonances to be resolved, the tissue water signal must be suppressed. Localized spectra obtained in this way from the human brain show resonance lines of extremely high resolution that belong to the following metabolites: N-acetyl-aspartate and N-acetyl-aspartyl-glutamate, NAA(G); creatine and phosphocreatine, (P)Cr; cholines, Cho; inositols. The characteristic ^{1}H NMR signal of lactic acid is seen in tissue with severe alterations of the energy metabolism (Fig. 56b and d).

Due to the small amount of quantum energy involved, magnetic resonance spectroscopy is a completely harmless technique. However, it is also very insensitive since it can detect only the coherent signal of an enormous number of nuclear spins. High concentrations of the metabolites to be detected are therefore required, with the result that for a typical acquisition time of 5 min for a localized ^{1}H NMR spectrum, the region in the brain to be examined must have a volume of at least one cubic centimeter.

Since it is possible to repeatedly measure the relative concentrations of certain metabolites of the brain tissue without any harm to the patient, ^{1}H magnetic resonance spectroscopy has been used for the assessment of the response of brain tumors to treatment. Such studies, however, have not yet been performed systematically. Some authors report isolated observations of different tumors at undefined times following radiotherapy. In planning the examinations, however, it must be taken into account that the total radiation dose is usually split into small single fractions which are applied daily over several weeks.

In our clinical study on the assessment of tumor response to treatment and follow-up, NMR examinations were performed at the beginning of therapy, after 1 and 2 weeks of therapy, as well as 6 weeks after the end of the treatment phase. In all cases, the tumor region to be studied by localized NMR spectroscopy was set to a volume of 8 cubic centimeters.

The results presented here are preliminary since our study was only conducted over a period of 2 years, and hence a correlation between the long-term effects of stereotactic radiotherapy on the tumors and the early changes seen in magnetic resonance spectra cannot yet be established.

A quantitative evaluation of the data from the 15 patients examined up to now show that all magnetic resonance spectra recorded prior to the beginning of treatment demonstrate a significantly reduced concentration of NAA(G) in the tumor tissue (Fig. 56b and d). A strong NAA(G) resonance, can be considered as a characteristic feature of ^{1}H NMR spectra of normal white matter. At the same time, we found an increased signal of Cho-containing compounds compared to the normal value in 11 of the 13 brain tumors studied (Fig. 56b). This agrees with the increase in phosphomonoester and phosphodiester signals frequently observed in phosphorus (^{31}P) magnetic resonance spectra of tumors and can be attributed both to the accel-

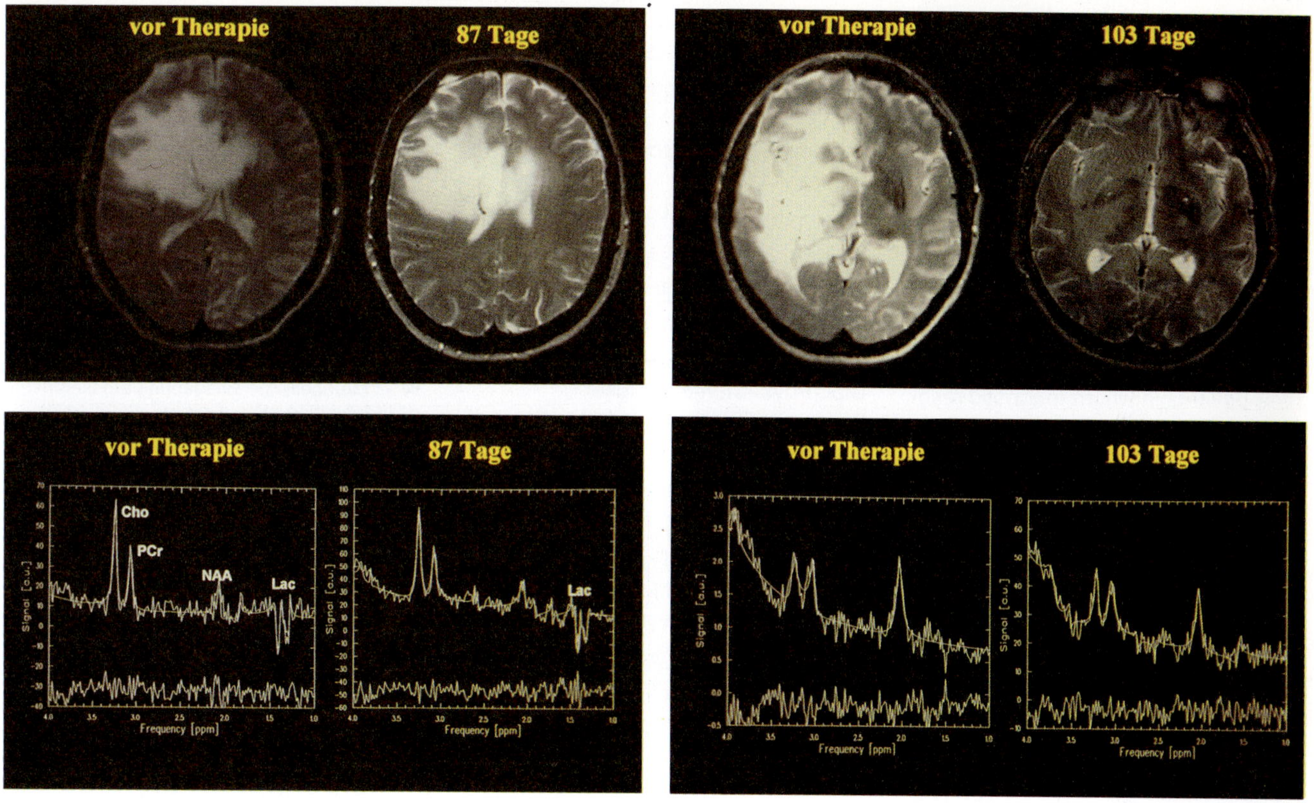

Fig. 56 a, b, c, d
Monitoring of response to radiation therapy in patients with low-grade astrocytomas. Figures a and c show the tumors before (left) and after treatment (right). Figures b and d show the respective magnetic resonance spectra. The tumor of the patient in Fig. 56 a did not respond to radiation treatment; there was no reduction in tumor size and edema. The hydrogen magnetic resonance spectra of tumor (b) show a consistently high-intensity choline signal. In figure c the patient's tumor has regressed completely. Assessment of the spectra in (d) shows a distinct reduction in the choline and N-acetylaspartate intensity during radiation treatment

erated turnover of membrane phospholipids in rapidly dividing cells and to necrotic cell decay.

Nine patients with a decrease of tumor size during the observation period showed individually differing changes in the relative concentrations of metabolites. A correlation between metabolic effects in the tumor detected in the early phase of therapy (i.e., spectral changes seen by quantitative evaluation of the NMR data) and conventionally defined therapeutic success was not identifiable, indicating that there are, in addition to the actual effects in the tumor, other unknown factors affecting the spectral pattern. In several patients a constant feature of abnormal spectra, i.e., eleva-ted values of the signal intensity ratio $I_{Cho}/I_{(P)Cr}$ and reduced values of $I_{NAA(G)}/I_{(P)Cr}$, was found despite a clear decrease in tumor size. This observation is compatible with the findings of
S. K. Szigety and co-workers, who in 10 patients found changes in the ^{1}H magnetic resonance spectra of irradiated tumor-free brain tissue that are similar to those of the tumors. These findings are relevant to our study insofar as they demonstrate that even healthy brain tissue undergoes what are presumably dose-dependent changes in

the relative concentrations of metabolites, and is hence only of limited value as reference tissue. However, these radiation-induced changes do not have imperative character. "Normalization" of the spectral pattern, i.e., a strong NAA(G) signal and a (P)Cr signal that is more intense than the Cho signal, was observed in one of the patients. This patient had a radiologically detected complete remission of the tumor.

The lactic acid signal was found in three patients in whom magnetic resonance tomography showed no shrinkage of the tumor. In two of the three patients this signal had already been detected before radiotherapy was started (Fig. 56b). The implication is that a high lactic acid concentration in the tumor, detectable by magnetic resonance spectroscopy before and during therapy, could be associated with a poor response to radiotherapy. Since a high level of lactic acid indicates that the tissue has a reduced oxygen supply, these findings would be compatible with the known worse response to irradiation of tumor cells in poorly perfused tissue. The important question arises as to whether tumors in which lactic acid is observed with magnetic resonance spectroscopy during or following therapy have a higher degree of malignancy.

Further investigations and follow-up studies performed over a period of several years and in a larger number of patients are required to confirm the preliminary findings presented in this article. Magnetic resonance spectroscopy may then gain acceptance as a non-invasive diagnostic technique capable of providing important clinical information not accessible with other diagnostic imaging techniques.

Dr. Peter Bachert
Division of Biophysics and Medical Radiation Physics

Dr. Thomas Hess
Division of Oncological Diagnostics and Therapy

Participating Scientists

Prof. Dr. Gerhard van Kaick
Division of Oncological Diagnostics and Therapy

Prof. Dr. Walter J. Lorenz
Dipl.-Phys. Clemens Müller
Division of Biophysics and Medical Radiation Physics

In collaboration with

Dr. Georg Becker
Institute of Clinical Radiology, Municipal Clinics of Mannheim

Selected publications

Bachert, P., Bellemann, M.E., Layer, G., Koch, T., Semmler, W., Lorenz, W.J.: In vivo ^{1}H, ^{31}P-{^{1}H} and ^{13}C-{^{1}H} magnetic resonance spectroscopy of malignant histiocytoma and skeletal muscle tissue in man. NMR Biomed. 5, 161–170 (1992)

Schad, L.R., Gademann, G., Knopp, M.V., Zabel, H.-J., Schlegel, W., Lorenz, W.J.: Radiotherapy treatment planning of basal meningiomas: Improved tumor localization by correlation of CT and MR imaging data. Radiother. Oncol. 25, 56–62 (1992)

Ende, G., Bachert, P., Kolem, H., Blankenhorn, M., Semmler, W., Knopp, M.V., Lorenz, W.J.: Metabolische Bildgebung am Gehirn des Menschen mittels lokalisierter in vivo ^{31}P-^{1}H-Doppelresonanz-Spektroskopie. Z. Med. Phys. 4, 14–20 (1994)

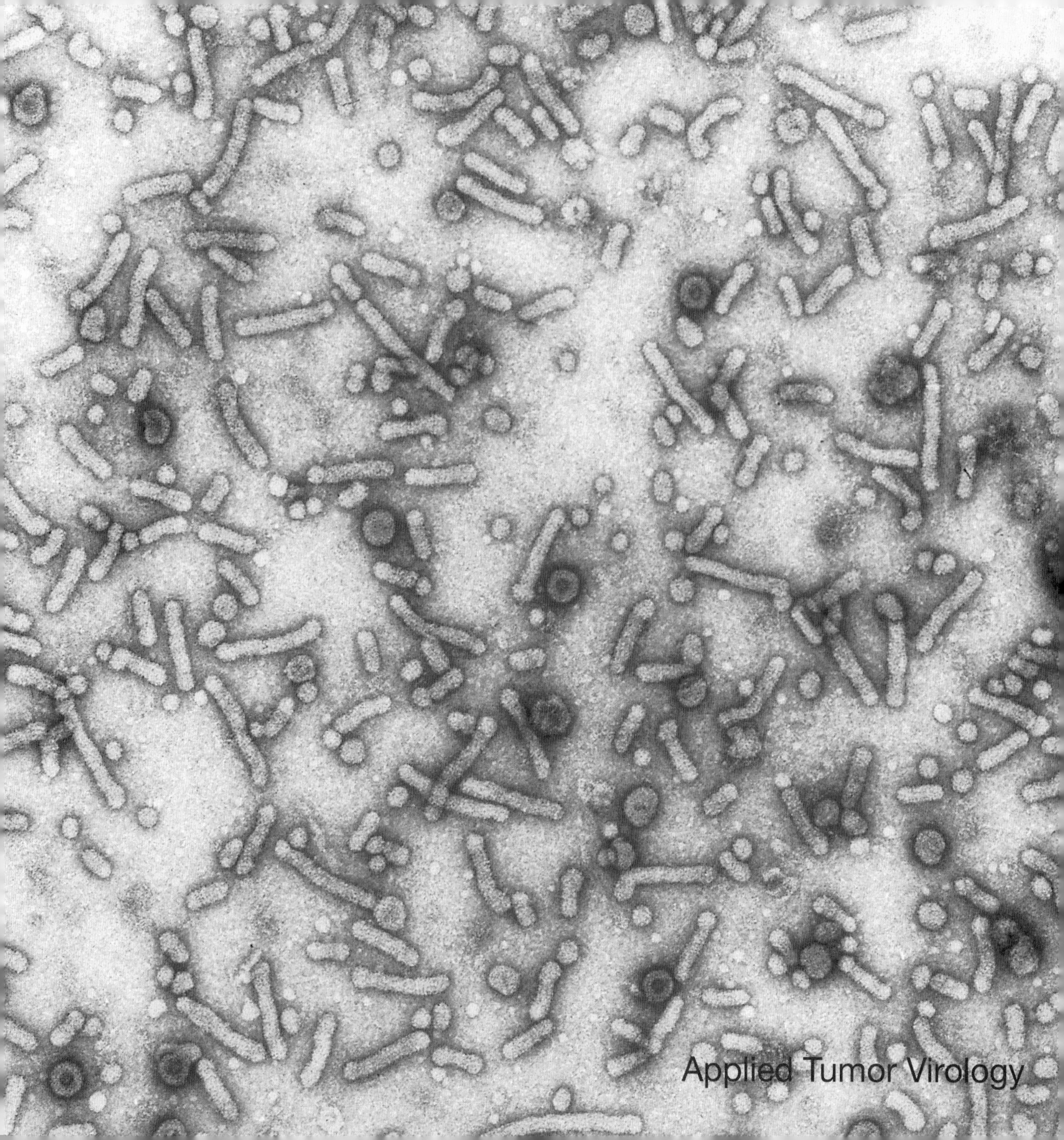
Applied Tumor Virology

7

Applied Tumor Virology

The Research Program Applied Tumor Virology investigates the role of various viruses in carcinogenesis and the possibilities for the application of this knowledge in fighting cancer.

One focus of work is the investigation of the relationship between development of genital cancer and infection with human papilloma viruses (HPV). How do the whole organism or individual cells react to an infection with certain papilloma virus types? When does the infection change the cell into a malignant one? Aside from these questions, much emphasis is put on epidemiologic studies on the frequency of HPV infections and investigations on the immune response as well as on the development of new tools for diagnosis. They will be the basis on which strategies for the prevention of or the fight against HPV infections will be developed.

The vital role played by the hepatitis-B virus (HBV) in the development of liver carcinoma was proven by epidemiologic studies. Researchers investigate certain viral genes to reveal how these viruses contribute to the malignant changes in liver cells, especially by the use of transgenic mice.

Epidemiologic studies have also indicated that still unidentified viruses may be related to the development of other tumors. These hints are subject to further research. Presently, for example, the researchers are investigating Hodgkin's disease, a malignant degeneration of certain hematopoietic cells.

Apart from studies on "classic" antiviral substances (such as for example interferons, i. e., messenger molecules of the immune system), scientists work on the development of new therapeutic concepts.

It has been known for some time that the smallest viruses, the parvoviruses, can inhibit cell growth. In epidemiologic studies and with molecular-biological methods the researchers are now attempting to unveil the basic mechanisms of this interaction. They are also trying to produce artificial virus particles which will serve as vehicles to introduce genetic information into cells.

Such transfer of genes into cells is a requirement for many forms of the so-called "gene therapy" for cancer and other diseases, as developed now by many international groups.

The lymphotropic papova virus belongs, together with the papilloma viruses, to the group of small tumor viruses, which contain a double-stranded DNA genome. Experimentally, they can mainly infect cells of Burkitt's lymphoma, a malignant disease of immune cells, which is particularly common among children and adolescents in Africa. The researchers are trying to find out which structures on the surface of the degenerated cells cause these cells to be preferentially infected by the virus. Papova viruses might also be suitable as gene transfer vehicles like the above-mentioned parvoviruses.

The Research Program also investigates the Human Immunodeficiency Virus (HIV), which is known to cause AIDS. The stages of infection may be the clue to developing a successful vaccine or therapy. Researchers are therefore investigating the role of the envelope protein in viral infection and cell damage. Using antisense RNA, they are elucidating the function of the various viral genes and attempt to selectively inhibit these genes. This work should be useful for the development of new forms of antiviral therapy.

Another research group concentrates on the characterization of genes that play a role in inherited human diseases that are frequently related to cancer.

Since cancer is mainly a disease of older people, the Research Program Applied Tumor Virology also investigates the molecular processes of aging from which it hopes to deduce information on the processes that lead to the development of cancer.

A new research group investigates the body's own defense against viruses and tumors. Special consideration is given to the recognition by the immune system of intracellular changes induced by tumors or viruses.

Coordinator of the Research Program:
Prof. Dr. Jean Rommelaere

Divisions and their heads:

Tumor Virology:
Prof. Dr. Jean Rommelaere

Genome Modifications
and Carcinogenesis:
Prof. Dr. Angel Alonso

Tumor Virus Immunology:
Prof. Dr. Hans-Georg Rammensee

Virus-Host-Interactions:
Prof. Dr. Claus H. Schröder

Characterization of Tumor Viruses:
Priv.-Doz. D. sc. Ethel-Michele de Villiers

Organization of Complex Genomes:
Dr. Peter Lichter

Retroviral Gene Expression:
Prof. Dr. Rolf Flügel

Immunosuppression by Viruses:
Priv.-Doz. Dr. Hans-Georg Kräusslich

Molecular Genome Analysis:
Dr. Annemarie Poustka

7

7.1 73 Papillomaviruses – the Many Faces of a Human Carcinogen

by Ethel-Michele de Villiers

Can cancer be caused by infection, although cancer is not infectious? Is that not illogical? As we will see, no.

For almost exactly 30 years, since the discovery by Epstein, Achong, and Barr in 1964 of the Epstein-Barr virus, the role of viruses in human cancer has intrigued scientists. Since that time research has come up with more and more surprises.

After the Epstein-Barr virus, which we now know is involved in the genesis of different human tumors, such as Burkitt's lymphoma, occurring mainly in Central Africa, cancer of the nasopharynx in Southern China, and cancers of the lymph nodes (lymphomas) associated with organ transplantations, the hepatitis B virus (HBV) started claiming scientific attention in the 1970s. Today we know that this jaundice-inducing pathogen is responsible for a high proportion of liver cancers, mostly occurring only 30 to 50 years after primary infection. At the end of the 1970s, the retrovirus HTLV 1 was isolated, which causes a form of blood cancer especially prevalent in the coastal regions of Southern Japan and in the Caribbean.

Another development taking place at almost the same time but with less media exposure was the analysis of papillomaviruses pathogenic to humans. This led to the discovery of what is certainly the most important group of tumor viruses known today. Papilloma or wart viruses were represented electron microscopically in normal cutaneous warts by an American group as early as 1946, although their infectiousness had already been known since the turn of the century.

In the mid-1970s, work by Freiburg virologists under Harald zur Hausen and by a study group at the Pasteur Institute in Paris under the direction of GÇrard Orth showed that the hitherto held assumption, according to which histologically distinct warts were caused by one and the same papillomavirus, was wrong. It was established to the contrary that different papillomavirus types, biochemically very distinct although morphologically indistinguishable, were responsible for the induction of different types of warts, thus proving the plurality of this virus group.

Seventy-three different virus types affecting humans are known today and present studies indicate that many more remain to be identified. Therefore, wart viruses should not be seen as just wart viruses. Some are found in normal cutaneous warts, others in genital warts and – more importantly – specific types are present in precursor lesions of genitourinary cancer, certain forms of cancer of the oral mucous membranes, and skin cancers. These precancerous growths have little in common with normal warts and mostly present themselves as relatively inconspicuous whitish and reddish blemishes on the skin or mucous membranes, scarcely contrasting with the background. Most of them disappear completely after a while. However, some of them stay for years or decades and have the potential to develop into malignant tumors.

Carcinogenesis is a kind of accident in the process of infection. The genetic material of the virus present in the precursor stage as a circular molecule, is integrated into the cell's genetic material prior to the development of cancer. The virus thereby loses part of its genetic make-up and is no longer capable of providing the information necessary for its own replication. From this moment

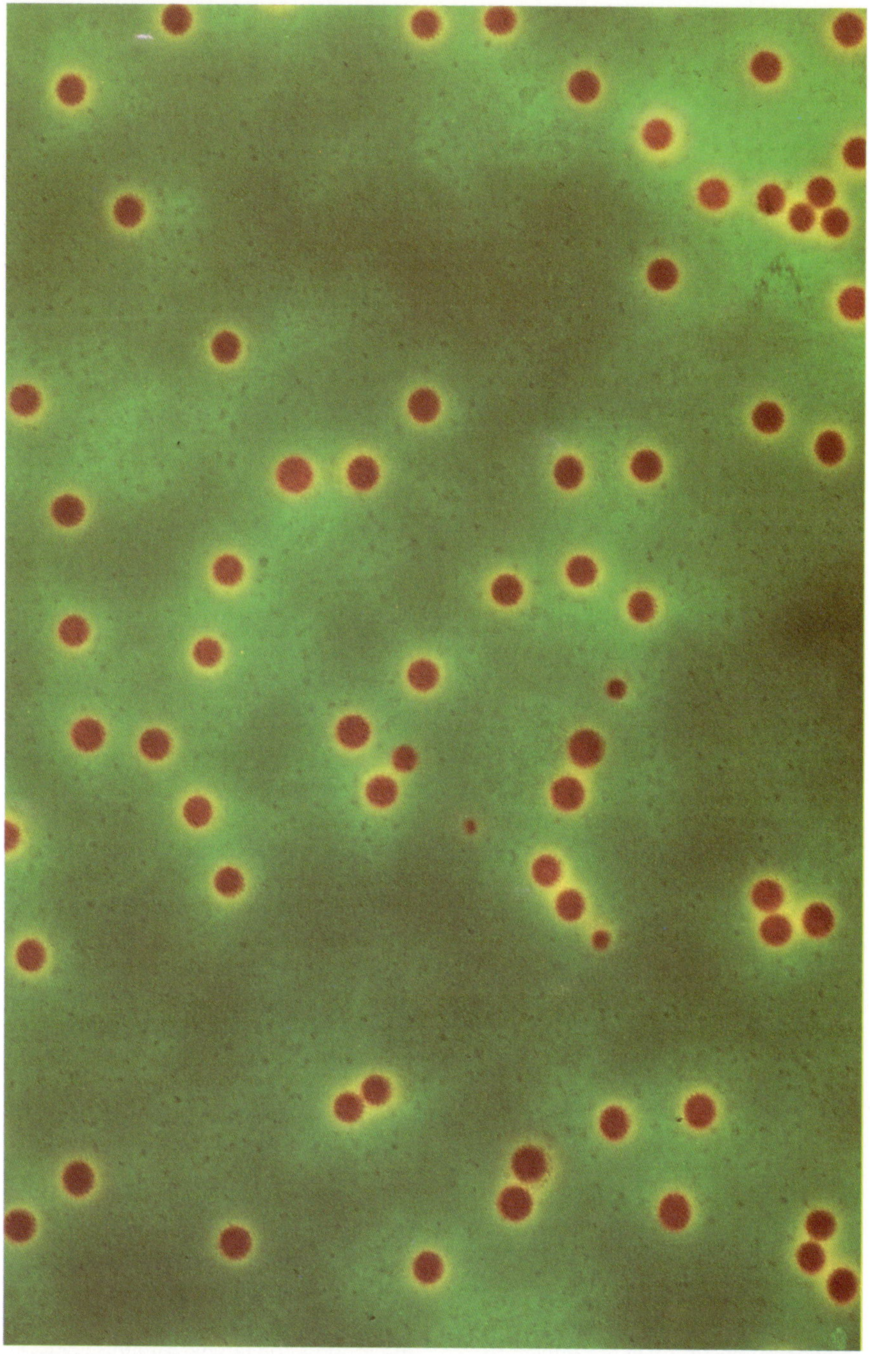

Fig. 57
Papillomaviruses seen on electron microscopy

on, it is no longer infectious. However, certain genes of the virus will always remain when the cell turns into a malignant tumor, namely the so-called E6 and E7 genes which under normal circumstances promote the growth of infected cells so as to increase the number of cells which will produce viruses later on. As we know today, their activity is essential for tumor growth. They are already deregulated by insertion into the cell's chromosomes and, due to an increase in their production, continuously cause alterations in the cell's genetic material (mutations). The latter is the basis for the inactivation of the natural controlling functions of the host cell itself and of adjacent cells, further enhancing the activity of viral genes. This eventually results in invasive growth of the altered cell into adjacent tissue and permits the establishment of secondary growths (metastases).

The genetic material of certain papillomaviruses is present in more than 90% of all cervical cancers, accounting for approximately one-third of genital cancers in women and cancer of the penis in men, and is identifiable in two-thirds of malignant tumors occurring in the anal region. Type 16 is the most prevalent virus present in these tumors, with types 18, 33, 45, 52, and 58 occurring less frequently and a number of other types being rare. Available results indicate that they are also the cause of these cancers. Today, scientists are mainly interested in understanding the exact mechanism underlying the interaction between virus and host cell. Cervical cancer ranks second in cancers in

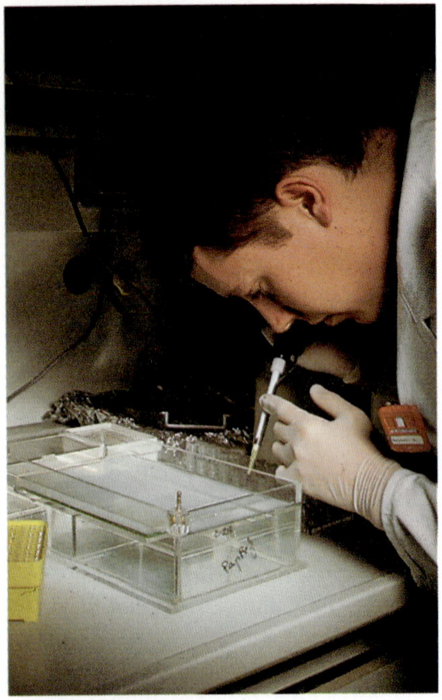

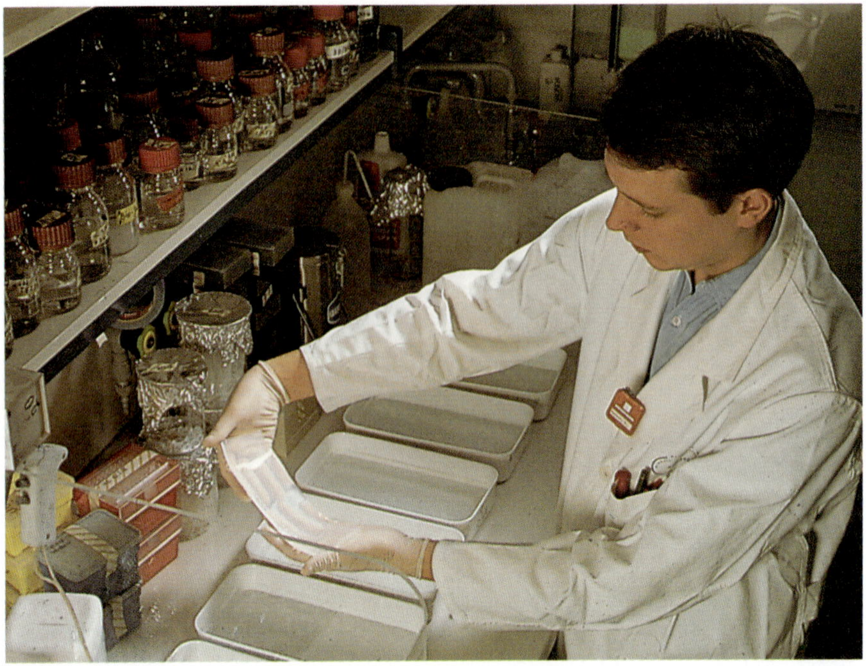

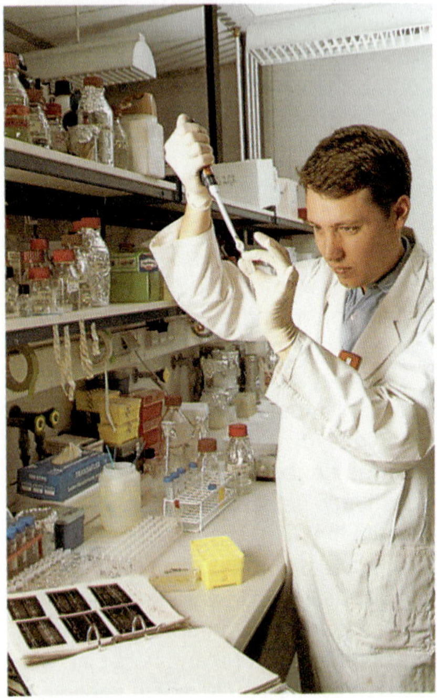

Fig. 58 a through c
A number of steps is required to investigate tissue samples for the presence of papillomavirus DNA. First of all, DNA from a number of known papillomaviruses is applied to a gel support medium and separated on the basis of molecular size. The HPV DNA in the gel is then denatured, transferred to a nylon membrane and fixed. Cellular DNA is extracted from the tissue sample in a number of steps, radiolabeled and applied to the membrane in solution. If the tissue sample contains a specific type of papillomavirus, this HPV DNA binds to the matching papillomavirus DNA on the membrane. Binding can be visualized on x-ray films as a black band

women worldwide. Elucidation of the factors involved in causing this type of cancer will represent a major scientific advance.

Papillomaviruses are not only involved in cancers occurring in the genital region but also in certain types of skin cancer. As early as the late 1970s, specific types (especially HPV 5 and 8) were detected in a rare hereditary form of papillomatosis of the skin (Epidermodysplasia verruciformis) in which warts at sites of the body exposed to the sun frequently develop into cancer. Emerging evidence suggests that certain new types play a central role in skin cancer which develops following organ transplantations, and possibly also in other types of skin cancer. Skin cancer is by far the most prevalent, but – except for melanoma – also the mildest type of cancer.

Papillomavirus infections of the oral mucosa, the larynx, and the nasal cavities also merit special interest. Especially in cancer of the tonsils, but also of the tongue, the larynx, and the nose, an increasing number of tumors have been found to contain the genetic material of papillomaviruses in their cells.

More and more evidence is accumulating to suggest that the many and varied viruses of this group may be the most important cancer agents in humans and as such warrant special attention. A normal wart is certainly no cause for alarm, since it generally contains harmless representatives of this virus group. Nor is the presence of the types associated with cancer an immediate cause for concern since only a small number of individuals develop the associated tumor years or decades after the initial infection. However, detection of such an infection should prompt affected individuals to have check-ups more frequently.

For the future we have reason to hope that more potent vaccines against these "secret cancer agents" will be made available. Several laboratories are doing interesting work but efficiency studies are so far lacking.

The Reference Center for Human-Pathogenic Papillomaviruses at the Deutsches Krebsforschungszentrum plays an important role in the identification and characterization of representatives of this viral group. New isolates from all over the world are transmitted to the Reference Center, where they are tested for their homology to HPV types already known and, if necessary, further characterized. The Center also examines numerous tissue samples from different types of tumors for the presence of papillomaviruses, an approach that has resulted in the identification and isolation of a whole series of new virus types.

Priv.-Doz. D. sc. Ethel-Michele de Villiers
Division of Characterization
of Tumor Viruses

Selected publications

de Villiers, E.-M.: Heterogeneity of the human papillomavirus group. J. Virol. 63, 4898–4903 (1989)

de Villiers, E.-M.: Human pathogenic papillomavirus types: An update. In: Current Topics in Microbiology and Immunology. Ed.: zur Hausen, H., Springer Verlag, Berlin, Heidelberg, 186, 1–12 (1994)

zur Hausen, H.: Molecular pathogenesis of cancer of the cervix and its causation by specific human papillomavirus types. In: Current Topics in Microbiology and Immunology. Ed.: zur Hausen, H., Springer Verlag, Berlin, Heidelberg, 186, 131–156 (1994)

7.2 Hepatitis B Virus as a Causative Agent of Liver Cancer – Elucidation of the Mechanism

by Claudia K. Rakotomahanina, Claudia Lamberts, and Claus H. Schröder

More than 200 million people worldwide are infected with the human hepatitis B virus (HBV). The health implications of this virus are not limited to liver inflammation; epidemiologic studies have demonstrated that patients with chronic infection carry a very high risk of developing liver cancer. Initial infection during birth or in early childhood is common. However, tumors usually develop after decades and are rare during childhood. The association between infection and the development of cancer has not yet been elucidated on the molecular level. Chronic liver inflammation on its own due to the virus might induce modifications in the genetic material via cell regeneration processes and thus favor tumor development. However, a large number of scientists postulate a direct role of the virus as a causative factor. A likely culprit is the viral transactivator Hbx since it both enhances the expression of a great number of cellular genes and influences cell growth per se.

Formation of viral factors is regulated by both free and integrated viral deoxyribonucleic acid (DNA) in the chronically infected liver. Forms can be expected to occur that possibly only possess carcinogenic characteristics due to changes resulting from integrational processes. For instance, the shortened form of a structural viral protein has been hypothetically linked to carcinogenesis as a transactivator. Viral oncogenes are possibly only formed in critical quantities following long chronic infection, i.e., due to several integration events. This would be consistent with the long periods of time observed between infection and tumor formation.

Strikingly, HBV-DNA integrated into the genome is regularly found in chronically infected liver tissue and tumor tissue. Even though the site of integration on the human genome appears to be purely random, similar structures are identified on integrated DNA. Transitions between viral DNA and cellular DNA are regularly found in a narrow region of the HBx gene termination. No other viral gene region presents a similar accumulation of transitions. RNA copies (mRNA) of HBx genes shortened in this way, also covering segments of adjacent cellular DNA, have already been detected before and are the basis of hybrid protein formation from HBx and cell proportions that differ from case to case. In the course of studies on the activity of integrated viral DNA, RNA copies terminating at a signal motif on the HBx gene, and thus only including HBx sequences, have been identified in our laboratory. This short RNA copy permits the formation of a short HBx protein (HBtx) which is identical in ev-

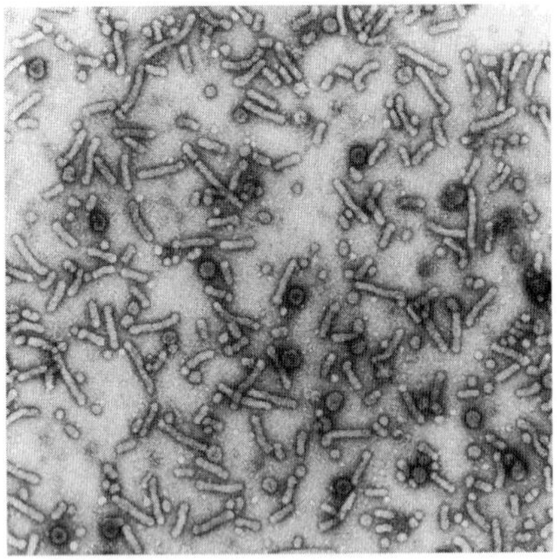

Fig. 59
Electron microscopic 12000-fold magnification of hepatitis B viral particles. The small spherical and filamentous particles are incomplete, lacking a nucleocapsid and viral genome

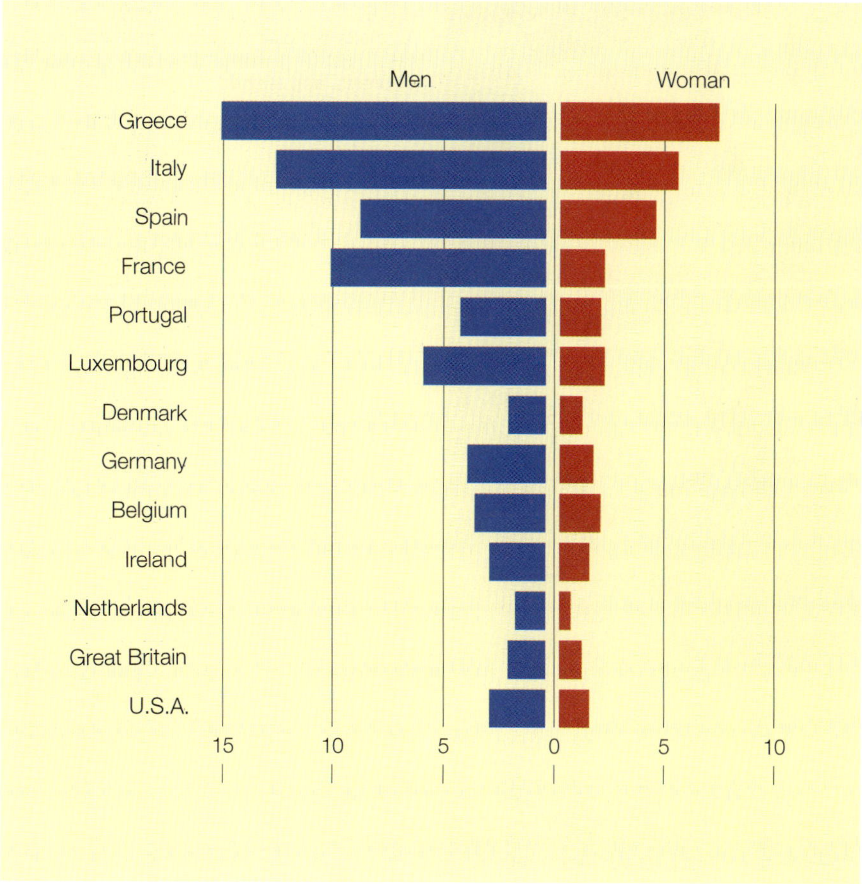

Fig. 60
A north-south divide with ominous implications: mortality from liver cancer is six times higher in southern Europe than in northern Europe for men and five times higher for women (Facts and Figures of Cancer in the European Community, IARC 1993)

ery case. First insights suggest that this predicted short HBx protein possesses, in contrast to the authentic Hbx protein, an increased ability to change the growth behavior of cells that can be cultivated in the laboratory. We have started comparative studies investigating the biological activity of HBtx and HBx. Identification of transcripts leading to the formation of a uniform viral factor HBtx supports the hypothesis that the hepatitis B virus is directly involved in the genesis of liver cancer.

The risk of developing liver cancer increases with the length of time chronic infection is present. The longer the virus is able to multiply in a cell and in daughter cells derived by cell division, the higher the probability that its genetic material will be integrated in the host genome and the higher the probability of integrated formation with HBx cell transitions. A uniform viral factor HBtx can be formed from the various integrates that, together with other cell modification, may contribute to tumorigenesis. It is conceivable that HBtx is not only active on the producing cell itself but also has an indirect growth activating effect on hepatic cells not capable of HBtx formation themselves.

Further outlook

Chronic infection appears to provoke changes in the liver leading to a steadily increasing disposition for tumor formation. This process would explain why tumor recurrence is frequently not attributable to the surgically removed tumor but of separate origin. One way to define the risk of liver cancer a patient carries may be to determine quantitatively the viral factor HBtx or its transcript. This may be investigated in a comparative study using liver tissue from patients with chronic infection, either suffering from primary liver cancer or free of any tumor. Elucidation of the mechanism underlying tumorigenesis by HBtx is certainly still a long way off. The most important thing from the point of view of the patient is to find ways and means of stopping the chronic viral replication leading to liver cell cancer. It may be possible to harness elements of the virus' own mechanisms to control replication as inhibitors.

Claudia Lamberts
Claudia Rakotomahanina
Prof. Dr. Claus H. Schröder

Division of Virus-Host-Interactions

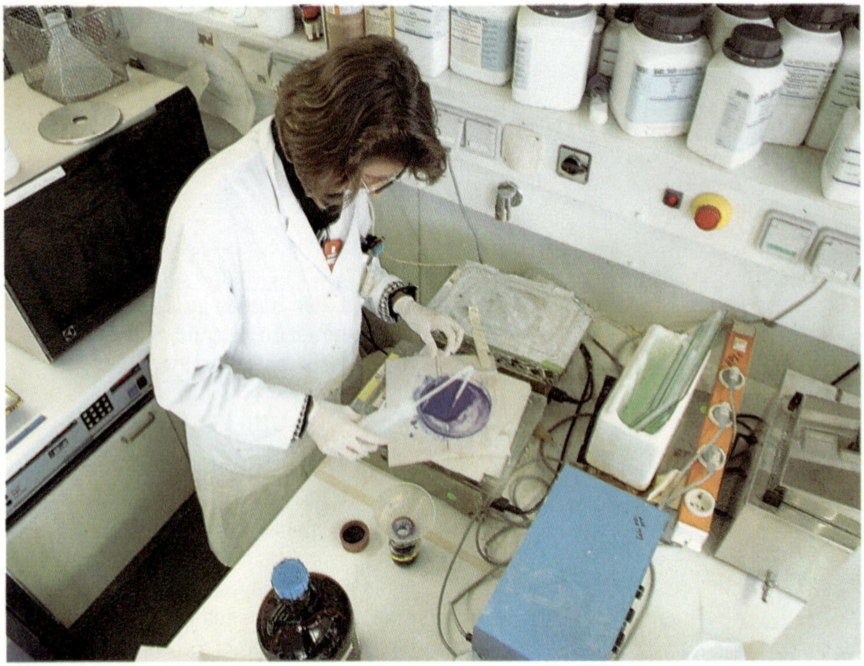

Fig. 61
To make proteins (e.g., viral proteins) visible, they must be isolated, separated by electrophoresis, and stained

Selected publications

Caselmann, W.H., Meyer, M., Kekule, A.S., Lauer, U., Hofschneider, P.H. and Koshy, R.: A transactivator function is generated by integration of hepatitis B virus preS/S sequences in human hepatocellular carcinoma DNA. Proc. Natl. Acad. Sci. USA. 87, 2970–2974 (1990)

Lee, T., Finegold, M.J., Shan, R.F., de Mayo, J.L., Woo, S.L.C. and Butel, J.S.: Hepatitis B virus transactivator X is not tumorigenic in transgenic mice. J. Virol. 64, 5939–5947 (1990)

Takada, S., Gotoh, Y, Hayashi, S., Yoshida, M. & Koike, K.: Structural Rearrangement of Integrated Hepatitis B virus DNA as well as Cellular Flanking DNA is Present in Chronically Infected Hepatitis Tissues. J. Virol., 64, 822–828 (1990)

Kim, C.M., Koike, K., Saito, I., Miyamura, T. and Jay, G.: HBx gene of hepatitis B virus induces liver cancer in transgenic mice. Nature 351, 317–320 (1991)

Lamberts, C., Nassal, M., Velhagen, I., Zentgraf, H., and Schröder, C.H.: Precore-mediated inhibition of Hepatitis B Virus progeny DNA synthesis. J. Virol. 67, 3756–3762 (1993)

Rakotomahanina, C. K., Hilger, C., Fink, T., Zentgraf, H. and Schröder, C. H.: Biological activities of a putative truncated hepatitis B virus x gene product fused to a polylysin stretch. Oncogene 9, 2613–2621 (1994)

7.3 How the Immune System Controls the Inside of Cells

by Hans-Georg Rammensee

The human body is made up of billions of cells, every one of which represents a complex microcosm with a variety of organelles equipped to perform functions as diverse as the transmission and storage of information, the production of energy, the supplying of raw materials, the production of proteins and other substances, and, finally, the almost complete recycling of waste. Each cell is surrounded by a membrane. Since large molecules do not easily traverse this membrane, unless special sluice-gates are provided, they are not able to simply invade the cell.

Antibodies are such large molecules. They are one of the most potent weapons of the immune system, as was shown by Emil von Behring and Shibasaburo Kitasato as early as 1890 in their work on diphtheria and tetanus. Antibodies are capable of recognizing and attacking any foreign substances that invade body fluids and in most cases can bring about their destruction. These foreign substances include diphtheria and tetanus toxins, snake venom, and freely floating organisms such as bacteria, parasites, and viral particles. However, antibodies are impotent against parasites that have already gained access to cells. Intracellular pathogens include all viruses, a whole range of bacteria, and some unicellular organisms, such as the causative agents of malaria. Naturally occurring antibodies are powerless in the face of cancer cells. Although certain tumor cells have modified surface structures compared to normal cells and are susceptible to recognition by antibodies, these slight differences between cancer cells and normal cells usually can only be found in the inside of the cell. Often, as in cervical cancer, the cancer cells may contain viral proteins not found in normal cells. However, even cancer cells which do not present detectable viral proteins contain proteins that are not found in other cells. For example, in tumor cells the tumor suppressor gene p53, normally able to prevent uncontrolled cell growth, frequently presents with an amino acid not found in healthy cellls. Furthermore, cancer cells frequently contain fusion proteins made up of two normally non-matching parts linked together by chromosomal bridges. Antibodies are powerless in the face of all these tumor-specific intracellular proteins.

The immune system has a specific and extraordinarily sophisticated defense mechanism to combat pathogens which have already invaded the cell and to cope with the changed intracellular protein situation characteristic of cancer cells. This defense system detects affected cells and destroys them together with parasites contained in the cells and genetic mutations. It functions as follows: All proteins occurring in the cell are subject to a steady cycle of synthesis and degradation. The ultimate products of protein degradation are the individual “building bricks” of proteins, the amino acids, with protein fragments, or peptides being the intermediate products. This also applies to parasite and tumor-specific proteins. Specific peptide receptors continuously pick up a small portion of the peptides occurring during this recycling process in the cell, carry them to the cell surface and display them on the outside of the cell. These peptide receptors are known as “MHC molecules” (or, to be more precise: Class 1 MHC molecules). The abbreviation stands for “Major Histocompatibility Complex,” a historical designation which does not elucidate the func-

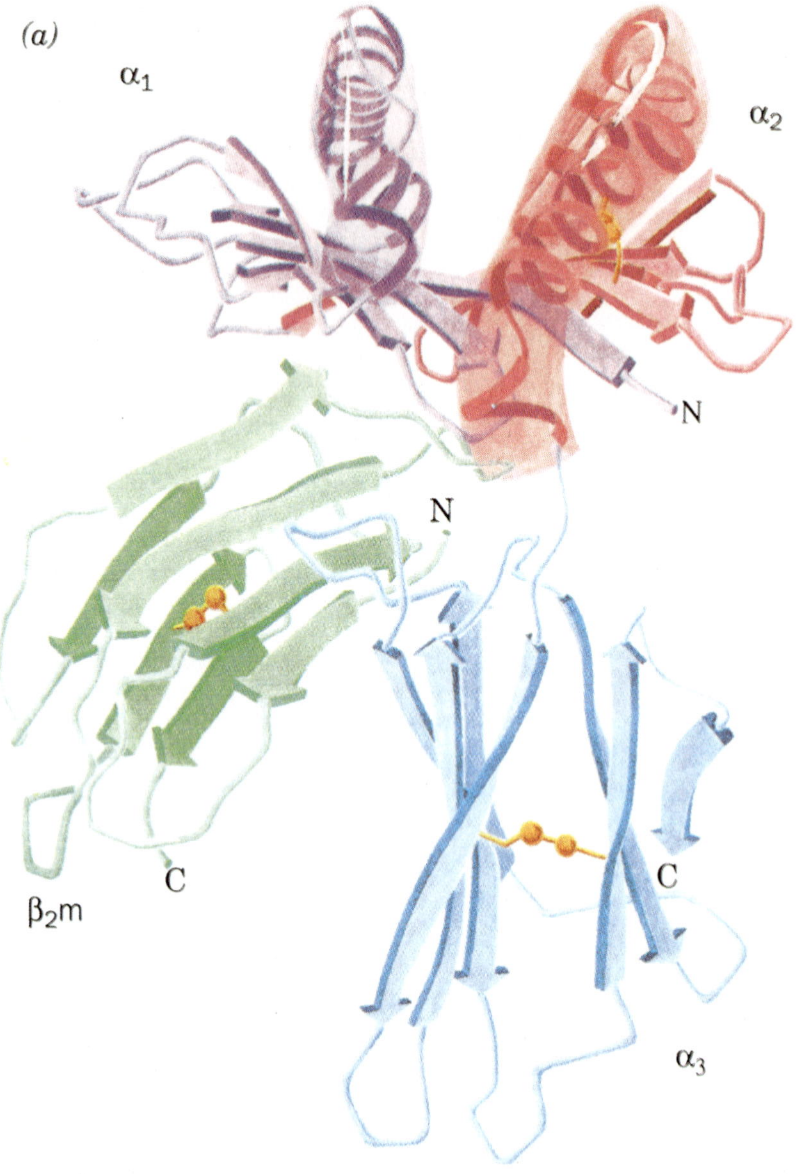

Fig. 62
Class I MHC molecules (the figure shows a structural model) bind protein fragments. Specialized immune cells are able to recognize these fragments and can tell whether or not they come from normal endogenous proteins. Any proteins that appear foreign to the immune cells are killed

tion of these molecules. The receptors pick up one or two fragments from each cellular protein which they carry to the outer surface of the cell, ensuring the permanent exhibition of small samples of each cellular protein on the cell surface. Specific defense cells of the immune system, the T lymphocytes, are capable of recognizing these samples presented by the MHC molecules and of establishing whether they originate from the body's own proteins. The T cells kill any cells not displaying normal peptides on the MHC molecules and any other peptides not recognizable to them. In this way the immune system can recognize and fight cells that have sustained any changes in their interior, even if these changes are invisible to antibodies.

The MHC molecules play a central role in this defense system: only what they collect in the inside of the cell – a process not guided by chance – can be subsequently detected by the T lymphocytes on the cell surface. The rules followed by MHC molecules for uploading peptides are thus critically important for the understanding of this defense system.

The research program of the Tumor Virus Immunology Division is devoting much effort to the elucidation of these rules and to the application of insights gained in the design of new treatment modalities for cancer in cooperative interaction with clinical study groups.

Investigation of these rules involves isolation of MHC molecules from a larger cell mass. Peptides bound to them are separated and analyzed. We have developed the techniques required for this and so have been able to find thousands of different peptides on a single cell, originating from all sorts of cellular proteins. All peptides isolated from the same MHC species have common fea-

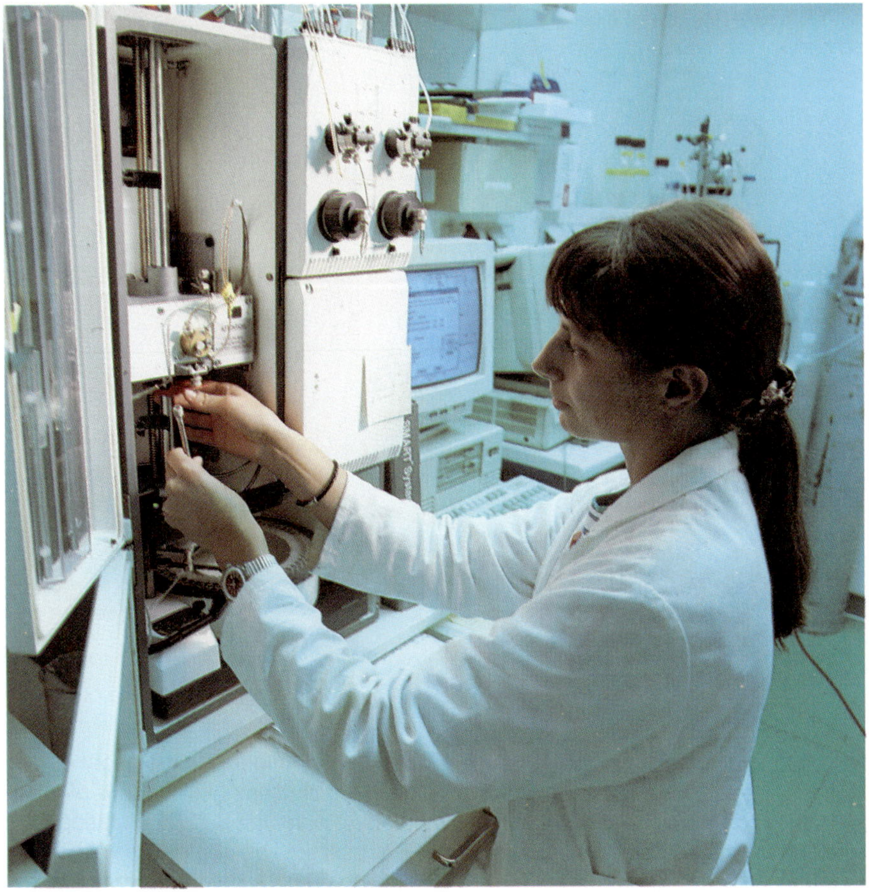

Fig. 63 a
The peptides taken from MHC molecules are separated according to their size and composition by forcing them under high pressure through a small column packed with a special material. The figure shows a column being changed

tures, however. Let us, for example, study an MHC molecule of the white mouse, the K^d-molecule. All peptides separated from K^d-molecules are exactly nine amino acids long and all of them possess the amino acid tyrosine (the one-letter code is Y) at position two and one of the aliphatic amino acids leucine (L), valine (V), or isoleucine (I) at position nine, i.e., at the last position. A peptide of the influenza virus isolated from K^d-molecules of infected cells shows for instance the sequence TYQRTRALV. Another peptide occurring on K^d-molecules of normal cells exhibits the sequence SYFPEITHI and is derived from a normal cellular protein, a protein tyrosine kinase. A tumor-specific peptide of the sequence KYQAVTTTL (isolated from a mutated protein) found on K^d-molecules of tumor cells is responsible for causing fatal cancer in nonimmunized mice and is recognized by killer T cells which destroy any tumor cells and protect immunized mice from cancer in this way.

For comparison, let us now look at peptides of another MHC molecule, the D^b-molecule of the black mouse: Again, all the peptides are nine amino acids long and all of them possess an asparagine (N) at position five and either methionine (M), isoleucine (I), or leucine (L) at position nine. For example, the peptide ASNENMETM isolated from the influenza virus is found on D^b-molecules of mice cells infected with influenza.

Thus, both MHC molecules contain peptides of a precisely defined length, namely nine amino acids. These peptides must have predetermined amino acids at two particular positions, all other positions being variable. Examination of peptides isolated from a great variety of MHC molecules revealed that each one has its own and unique peptide specificity. The term "peptide motif" is used to describe the rules governing this peptide specificity. Human MHC molecules are also known as HLA molecules, short for Human Leukocyte Antigen molecules. There is an 80% probability that each individual possesses at least one of the HLA molecules HLA-A1, HLA-A2, HLA-A3, HLA-B7, HLA-B8, HLA-B27. The rules of peptide specificity are of major importance to the immune system. All proteins represent chains of varying lengths consisting of the 20 different amino acids. The 20 building bricks of proteins can be abbreviated according to a single-letter code using all the letters in the alphabet, except B, J, U, X, and Z. It may

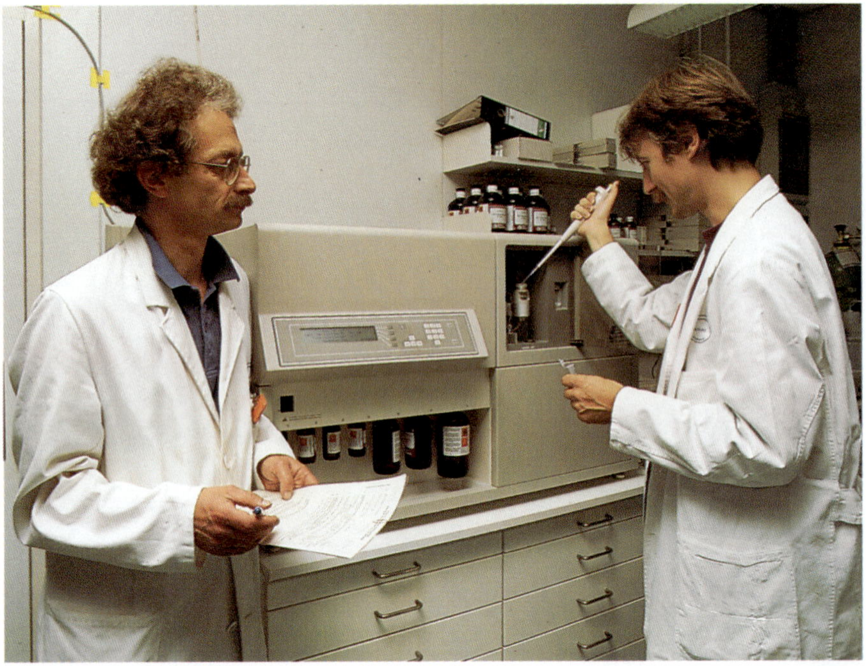

Fig. 63b
The amino acid sequence of the separated peptides is analyzed by Prof. Hans-Georg Rammensee and Dr. Stefan Stevanović in a peptide sequencer

therefore be useful to think of proteins in terms of strings of letters or texts, but it is important to remember that blanks and punctuation marks do not occur. Peptides would then correspond to individual words in these texts. A nucleoprotein from the influenza virus consists of 498 amino acids, corresponding exactly to the number of letters used to designate it.

This protein contains the already mentioned peptides TYQRTRALV and ASNENMETM at position 147–154 and at position 367–374 respectively. The K^d-molecule of the mouse hence selects a peptide from the starting third of the protein, whereas the D^b-molecule selects one from the terminal part. The HLA-B27 molecule present in roughly 5% of Central Europeans selects the peptide SRYWAIRTR from the terminal third and the HLA-A2 molecule selects the peptide KLGEFYNQM from the starting third. The MHC molecules there-fore comb the amino acid sequence of proteins for sites that exactly match their own peptide motive. They then carry the matching peptides to the cell surface and put them out for display. At a rough estimate, a given peptide motif finds its match once per hundred peptides of a protein, i.e., about three peptides of a protein consisting of 300 amino acids will fit a given MHC molecule. Only these peptides are recognizable to the T cells, the remaining protein sequence being invisible to them. This selectivity of MHC molecules has considerable implications for the understanding of the immune system and for potential targeted interventions in the body's immune response, for example in cancer, autoimmune diseases, and infectious diseases.

Since each individual possesses different HLA molecules and therefore recognizes different peptides from the proteins of a certain pathogen, a single peptide would not be useful to produce a potent vaccine for the whole population. The SRYWAIRTR peptide, for example, would be able to provoke killer cells against influenza in individuals with HLA-B27 but would be useless in anybody else. A vaccine based on peptides would therefore have to include a great number of peptides. Peptide selectivity of MHC molecules also has consequences for the pathogenic agents. An influenza virus might escape the clutches of killer cells of an individual with type B27 by mutating the R at position two of the SRYWAIRTR peptide. This mutation would not be any advantage in other people since killer cells in individuals without B27 ignore this position of the viral protein. A pathogenic agent can therefore elude the MHC molecules of a single individual by mutation but not the hundreds of MHC molecules occurring throughout the whole population. This is probably the reason why there is such a large number of different HLA types and why each individual possesses different HLA types. To be more precise, each individual possesses his or her own collection of up to six different HLA class 1 genes, with hundreds of different genes occurring in the population.

In autoimmune diseases the immune system attacks the endogenous substances by mistake. In many autoimmune diseases a reasonably specific relationship has been observed with specific HLA types. For example, ankylosing spondylitis is closely associated with HLA-B27 and multiple sclerosis correlates with HLA-DR2. (DR2 is a class 2 MHC molecule; class 2 molecules have slightly different properties than the class 1 molecules described so far.) In such cases, as detailed knowledge of the MHC function suggests, the T cells mistakenly consider a specific peptide from an endogenous protein displayed on the relevant HLA molecule as foreign and attack it. Such peptides, which in multiple sclerosis possibly originate from a myelin protein, could therefore possibly be considered as being the crux of autoimmune diseases. This is why we are at present endeavoring to identify such pathogenic peptides. The information obtained might be used to develop strategies for direct suppression of the self-reactive T cells and hence combat disease. Some encouraging results have already been reported in mouse models of autoimmune diseases.

Growth of a tumor is already an indication that the immune response has been inadequate. The reason for this inadequacy might be that certain tumor cells have no abnormal structures. In many cases, however, the body's immune system is not provoked into action even though tumor-specific antigens exist, for example, because the tumor-specific peptide is present in quantities too tiny to initiate T-cell activation.

This is where specific immunotherapy comes in. A much smaller quantity of antigen is required in already activated T cells for antigen recognition than is necessary for initial activation of these T cells. The approach is therefore to look for peptides on MHC molecules of tumors which differ from peptides of normal cells. We try to artificially provoke a T cell response against these tumor-specific peptides, as, for example, by immunization with the relevant peptide in an appropriate formulation. A Belgian study group under the direction of Thierry Boon has done important pioneering work in this field.

The scientists identified an HLA-A1-bound peptide from melanoma cells of a patient. The patient's killer cells recognized the peptide but were obviously not activated enough to kill all the melanoma cells. The same HLA-bound peptide is also seen on melanoma cells of other patients if they possess the HLA-A1 molecule. At present, efforts are under way to immunize type A1 melanoma patients with this peptide, thereby activating the relevant killer cells strongly enough to enable them to kill all melanoma cells. In addition, we are searching for other peptides in the melanoma-associated protein referred to as MAGE-1 – from which the HLA-A1-bound peptide originates – and which match other HLA molecules. Other research efforts are directed at using the MAGE-1 protein itself for immunization. The problem is how to infiltrate the protein into antigen processing in such a way as to provoke formation of the relevant peptides. We are also looking for peptides or proteins in other cancers amenable to similar procedures. As mentioned at the beginning of this article, candidates for such tumor-specific proteins include viral proteins, fusion proteins, and the mutated tumor suppressor protein p53. In the Applied Tumor Virology Research Program work is being done on tumor-specific proteins from the human papilloma virus.

A fundamental restriction on any approach to specific immunotherapy in cancer is imposed by the fact that a whole range of tumors inactivates the production of MHC proteins. A T-cell mediated immune response is irrelevant in these MHC-negative tumors since the T cells are only capable of recognizing their antigen on MHC molecules.

In many international centers – most of them outside Germany – scientists are trying to integrate genes for nonspecific immune activators, such as cytokines or cellular-adhesion molecules, into tumor cells taken from patients. After reintroduction of the modified tumor cells into the patient as a kind of "gene therapy," the cancer cells are supposed to be more visible to the immune system. This procedure is based on the consideration that cancer cells already contain tumor-specific antigens but that the immune system needs support in fighting the tumor. More detailed insights into the tumor antigens and MHC molecules involved will be of invaluable help in the purposeful planning of these new approaches to treatment.

Prof. Dr. Hans-Georg Rammensee
Division of Tumor Virus Immunology

Participating Scientists

Dr. Stefan Stevanović
Dr. Kirsten Falk
Dr. Olaf Rötzschke

In cooperation with

Prof. Dr. Günther Jung
Institute of Organic Chemistry,
University of Tübingen

Prof. Dr. Masafumi Takiguchi
The Institute of Medical Science,
University of Tokyo, Japan

Selected puplications

Falk, K., Rötzschke, O., Stevanović, S., Jung, G., Rammensee, H.-G.: Allelespecific motifs revealed by sequencing of self-peptides eluted from MHC molecules. Nature 351, 290–296 (1991)

Rötzschke, O., Falk, K., Deres, K., Schild, H., Norda, M., Metzger, J., Jung, G., Rammensee, H.-G.: Isolation and analysis of naturally processed viral peptides as recognized by cytotoxic T cells. Nature 348, 252–254 (1992)

Boon, T.: Teaching the immune-system to fight cancer. Scientific American 268, 82–89 (1993)

Rammensee, H.-G., Falk, K., Rötzschke, O.: Peptides naturally presented by MHC class I molecules. Ann. Rev. Immunol. 11, 213–244 (1993)

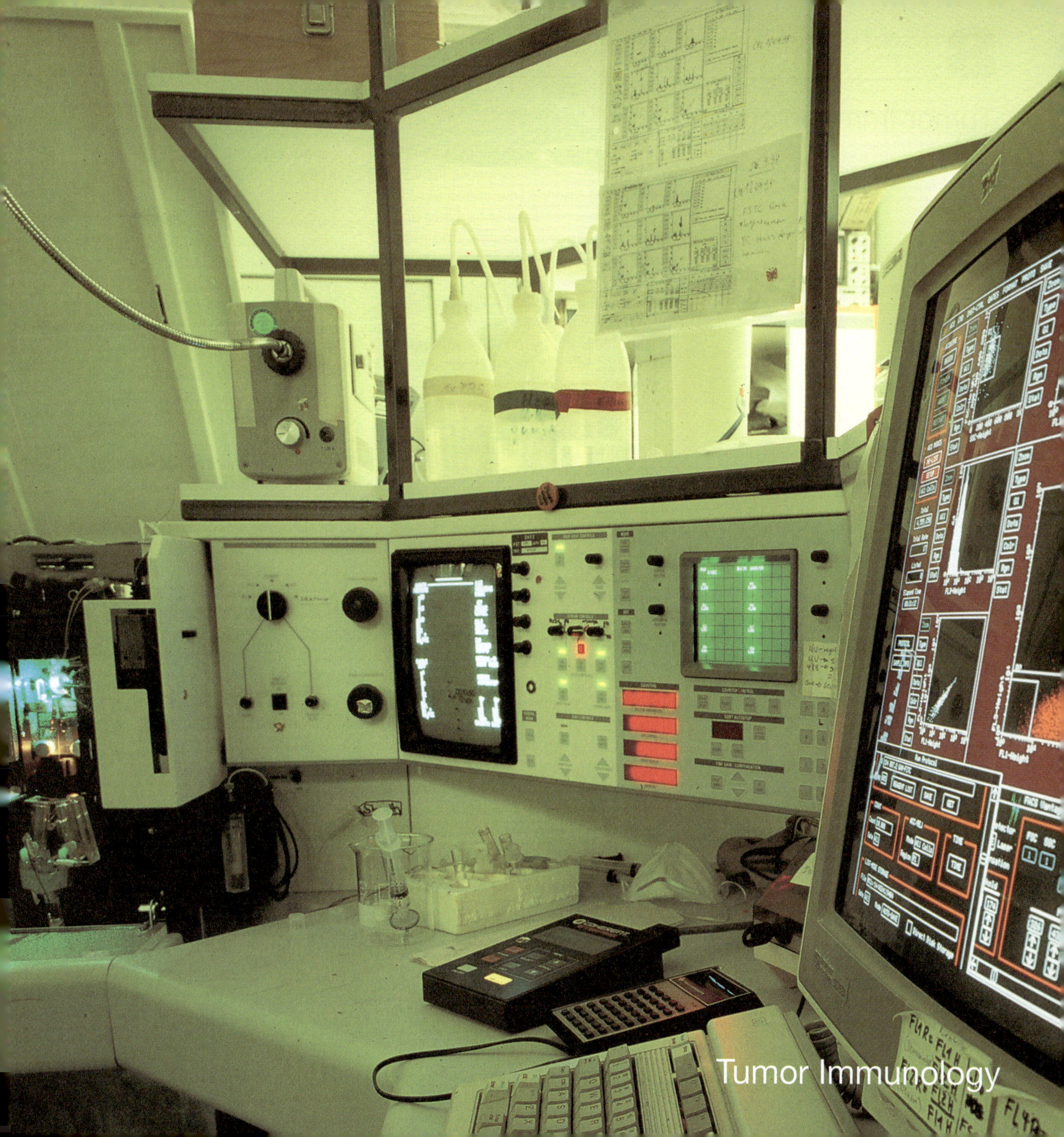

Tumor Immunology

8

Tumor Immunology

The work of the Research Program is concentrated on new immunological methods of tumor diagnostics as well as on immunological concepts for tumor therapy and the investigation of the biological mechanisms underlying processes of cellular interaction and metastatic spreading.

The priorities are in the following fields:

- Manufacturing of monoclonal antibodies against tumor-associated antigens and differentiation antigens for diagnosis and therapy of tumors.

- Expression of membrane antigens on cells. In this context, not only tumor-specific antigens, but also viral antigens and mainly histocompatibility genes are investigated. In particular, their role is being explored in the immunological struggle between the host and the tumor.

- Regulation of the immune system. This includes the investigation of immunoregulatory products of tumor cells, the identification and biochemical characterization of lymphokines, biochemical aspects of the activation and regulation of T-lymphocytes under normal and pathological conditions, investigations of mutagenized tumor cell lines as well as the structure of antigens and lymphokine receptors.

- Analysis of the immuno-pathogenetic mechanisms for cancer and HIV infection.

- In addition, the research program investigates the programmed cell death (apoptosis) and its significance in tumor research and in the immune system.
- Auto-immune disease models and immunological tumor models have been established in transgenic mice with histocompatible and other genes. These give important insights into the mechanisms of regulation and pathogenesis.
- Another focus of research is concerned with the mechanisms of tumor invasion and the development of metastases.

The development of new therapeutic concepts with an immunological basis is an important objective of research which is being worked on along various lines in all divisions. These investigations take into account that tumor cells are recognized by the immune system in many cases and also that they can potentially be eliminated. On the other hand, currently unknown regulatory mechanisms prevent resistance in terms of transplant rejection.

Coordinator of the Research Program:
Prof. Dr. Peter H. Krammer

Divisions and their heads:

Cellular Immunology:
Prof. Dr. Volker Schirrmacher

Immunochemistry:
Prof. Dr. Wulf Dröge

Immunogenetics:
Prof. Dr. Peter H. Krammer

Molecular Immunology:
Prof. Dr. Günter Hämmerling

8.1 Immune Tolerance and Cancer

by Bernd Arnold
and Günter J. Hämmerling

The task of the immune system is to selectively eliminate harmful pathogens, such as viruses and bacteria, while at the same time sparing endogenous structures so as to avoid provoking autoimmune disease. The capability of distinguishing „self" from „foreign" is due to specific recognition processes mediated by receptors located on the surface of B and T lymphocytes. One major question of tumor immunology is why the immune system is unable to fend off cancer cells even though the process of transformation from normal cells to tumor cells generally involves the development of new structures, such as oncogene or tumor suppressor gene mutations, which in principle should be recognizable to the immune system. The immune system should also be capable of detecting tumors associated with viruses, which usually express viral proteins that are clearly recognizable as foreign. These viruses include the hepatitis B virus implicated in liver cancer, for which an effective vaccine is available; human papillomavirus, linked with tumors of the genito-urinary tract; the Epstein-Barr virus, associated with Burkitt's lymphoma in Africa and nasopharyngeal carcinoma in the south of China; and human T lymphocyte virus 1 implicated in causing T cell leukemia in Japan.

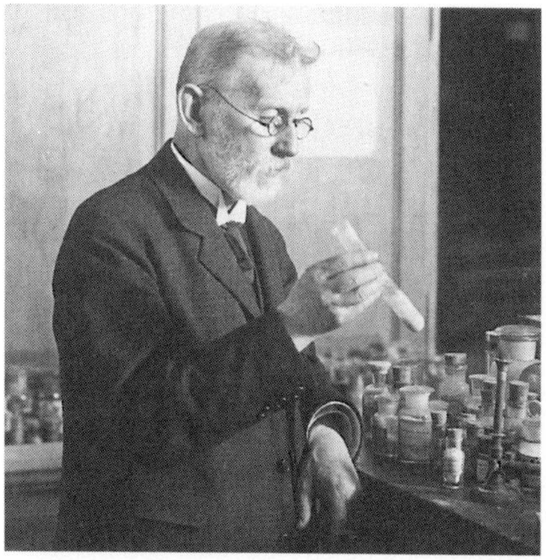

Fig. 64
The explanation for the immune system's ability to distinguish self from non-self has continued to elude scientists since the days of the great immunologist Paul Ehrlich. Only now are we coming close to finding an answer

Lymphocytes taken from tumor patients can be activated in tissue cultures to provoke a reaction with tumor cells, which shows that potentially tumor-reactive lymphocytes are in fact present. However, this antitumor response demonstrated in vitro evidently fails in vivo, i.e., in the patient. The question is, why?

Some of the many explanations for this phenomenon will be discussed in the following.

Down-regulation of target structure for immune responses

T lymphocytes do not recognize the tumor antigen as such but only fragments of it. These fragments or peptides bind intracellularly to major histocompatibility complex (MHC) molecules which ferry them to the surface of the cell, where they are recognized by T lymphocytes. In many studies, we and other working groups have often encountered tumors in humans and animals which had stopped synthesizing MHC-molecules, thereby evading the attack by killer cells.

Absence of adhesion molecules

Apart from the MHC-peptide complex, other molecules are required on the cell surface in order to bring about the en-

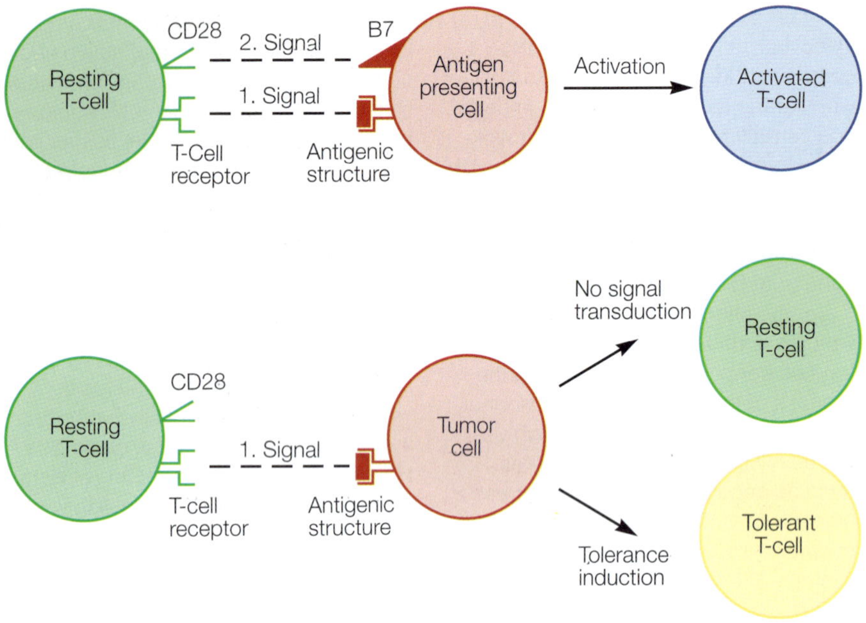

Fig. 65
Two signals are needed to activate T-lymphocytes. The first signal is triggered by antigen-specific recognition and the second by a non-specific adhesion process. If there is no second signal, the T-cell tolerates the non-self entity or ignores the antigen entirely. The result in both cases is that the tumor cell escapes attack by the immune system

counter between T cells and the tumor cell, which is indispensable for T cell activation. In the absence of the necessary adhesion molecules on cancer cells – because they were never present or because they were down-regulated – no activation signal is given and the T cells ignore the tumor cells.

Absence of the co-stimulatory signal

Alternatively, the encounter may well produce a signal – albeit the wrong one. It was discovered that two signals are required for the activation of T lymphocytes, one of which is mediated by the T cell receptor, and the other, a co-stimulatory signal, by specific cell interaction molecules. In the absence of the co-stimulatory signal, T cells are paralyzed when they encounter an antigen, and tolerance is induced. Later on, tolerant T cells no longer respond to normal activation signals (Abb. 65). In many tissues these co-stimulatory molecules were never present to start with. This prevents endogenous tissue from attack, thereby precluding autoimmune disease, but at the same time induction of tolerance makes it impossible to combat tumors originating in these tissues.

For the design of immunotherapeutic concepts, it is important to distinguish between these two possibilities since the conditions for activating quiescent T cells and those for overcoming the tolerance of inactivated cells are very different. The ultimate goal of immunological research is to use the body's own immune defenses for fighting tumors, an approach associated with less strain for the patient than conventional therapeutic modalities, such as radiation or chemotherapy. Before this goal can be reached, however, the complex mechanisms underlying the immune response must be elucidated.

The important aspect of how T cell tolerance arises and how it can be overcome in tumors is addressed in the following.

Tolerance in the immune system

The question as to how the immune system is capable of distinguishing between endogenous and foreign structures has intrigued scientists ever since they first began to systematically explore the immune system. The outstanding immunologist Paul Ehrlich raised the specter of „horror autotoxicus" as early as 1900. Only now, 90 years later, are we beginning to understand the rudiments of immune tolerance.

T lymphocytes originate from bone marrow cells and migrate to the thymus, where they mature. In this process many millions of T lymphocytes are produced that differ in the receptors they carry for potential antigens. Thus the immune system equips us with enough different T cell receptors to be able to recognize and eliminate any imaginable foreign structure. However, in the process of T cell development, T cells with a specificity for endogenous structures are also produced. These still immature thymocytes receive a signal to die when they encounter autoantigens in the thymus. In this manner, the thymus serves as a filter system for the destruction of autoreactive T cells. Of course, this negative selection only works if the autoantigen is present in the thymus. Since different tissues produce different proteins that are not all represented in the thymus, a second mechanism is required, namely the induction of immune tolerance in the periphery.

Peripheral tolerance

To find out which processes outside the thymus contribute to tolerance, we produced transgenic mice with an additional gene in their genome. This transgenic animal model allows us to study the impact of a single gene on the functioning of the organism. Expression of a gene can be focused to particular tissues by means of tissue-specific regulatory gene sequences. In this way we put a „foreign" MHC protein on liver cells or certain cutaneous cells of transgenic mice. Even though the Kb-antigen was not present in the thymus, these mice were tolerant and did not reject Kb-positive skin and/or tumor transplants. These findings proved for the first time that tolerance can be induced outside the thymus.

Transgenic animal models can also be used to directly follow the fate of T cells that encounter a protein in the periphery which is not present in the thymus. Only a very small percentage of cells in a T cell population is usually directed against a given antigen (0.01 to 0.1 percent) – a number too small for visualization. However, it is possible to transfer the genetic material for a foreign T cell receptor to mice so that all T cells carry the same receptor and can therefore be studied in the flow cytometer using suitable antibodies.

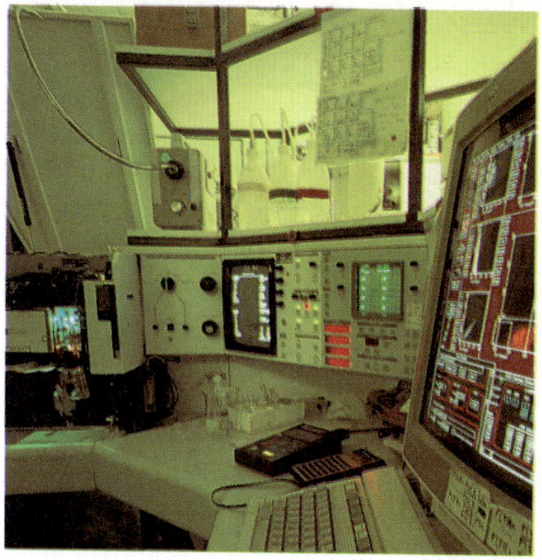

Fig. 66
A fluorescent cell sorter and console, used to visualize various surface markers of T-lymphocytes with antibodies coupled to different fluorescent substances. With this method the different cells can be distinguished by their color

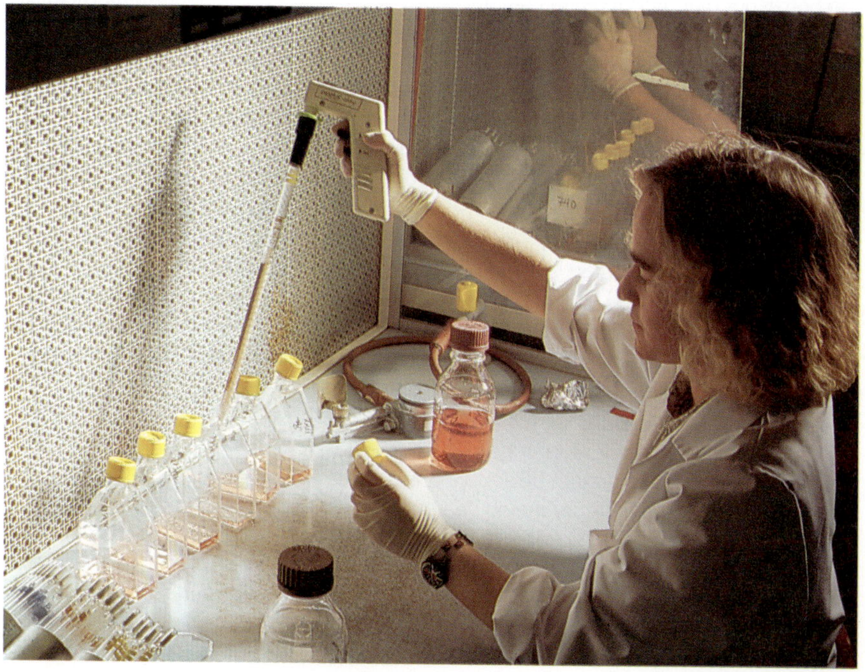

Fig. 67
Human tumor cells are diluted in culture medium on a sterile bench and transferred to several culture flasks. These tumor cells are challenged with T-lymphocytes to see if the latter are able to recognize specific features of the tumor cells

Several key insights were gained from these studies. On the one hand, interaction between young T cells and an antigen in the periphery can lead to the elimination of these autoreactive cells, which, of course, is the surest kind of selftolerance. On the other hand, the encounter may only cause inactivation, depending on the amount of antigen and the extrathymic tissue in which the antigen is present. The result is that these T lymophocytes are still present in the organism but cannot do any harm, i.e., they are not capable of causing autoimmune disease. Stimulation of these T cells in tissue culture shows that they are fully reactive. This is comparable with the behavior of tumor-specific lymphocytes from patients in tissue culture reported at the beginning of this article. Indeed, preliminary evidence exists to suggest that even a proliferating tumor may induce tolerance without the corresponding lymphocytes being eliminated. To activate the immune system into defensive action against the tumor in such cases, we have to learn how to overcome this type of selftolerance.

Overcoming tolerance

We thus considered how inactivation of Kb-reactive T lymphocytes could be overcome in the transgenic mice mentioned above. For this purpose we introduced either interleukin IL-2, a very powerful soluble T cell growth hormone, or B7, a co-stimulatory molecule, in Kb-positive tumor cells by gene transfection. We infected tolerant mice with the tumor cells altered in this way. This not only resulted in rejection of these tumor cells but also enabled the animals to reject both the unchanged Kb-positive parent tumor and the Kb-positive skin transplants.

These findings demonstrated for the first time that tolerance may be overcome systemically by simultaneous administration of antigen and IL-2. The co-stimulatory molecule B7 was not capable of overcoming tolerance of autoreactive cells. By contrast, following expression of B7 on a number of tumors, achieved by gene transfer, the tumors became highly immunogenic and were capable of activating normal T cells into tumor rejection. This reveals that the conditions under which normal and tolerant T cells are activated differ in important respects.

The findings on overcoming selftolerance in tumors obtained from animal experiments are very encouraging. However, as mentioned before, there are several possible explanations for a tumor's capability of evading control by the body's natural defenses. It is therefore important to investigate different tumor types to find out to what extent the absence of an immune response is due to T cell inactivation. In these instances, it can be expected that detailed insights into the mechanisms of overcoming selftolerance and of activating T lymphocytes against tumor antigens will contribute to the development of new immunotherapeutic approaches.

Dr. Bernd Arnold
Prof. Dr. Günter J. Hämmerling
Division of Molecular Immunology

Participating Scientists

Dr. Günther Schönrich
Dr. Judith Alferink
Dipl.-Biol. Andreas Limmer

Selected publications

Schönrich, G., Kalinke, U., Momburg, F., Malissen, M., Schmitt-Verhulst, A.-M., Malissen, B., Hämmerling, G.J., Arnold, B.: Downregulation of T cell receptors on self-reactive T cells as a novel mechanism for extrathymic tolerance induction. Cell 65, 293–304 (1991)

Arnold, B., Schönrich, G., Hämmerling, G.J.: Multiple levels of peripheral tolerance. Immunol. Today 14, 12–14 (1993)

Hämmerling, G.J., Schönrich, G., Ferber, I., Arnold, B.: Peripheral tolerance as a multi-step mechanism. Immunol. Rev. 133, 93–104 (1993)

Ferber, I., Schönrich, G., Schenkel, J., Mellor, A., Hämmerling, G.J., Arnold, B.: Levels of peripheral T cell tolerance induced by different doses of tolerogen. Science 263, 674–676 (1994)

Schönrich, G., Alferink, J., Klevenz, A., Küblbeck, G., Auphan, N., Schmitt-Verhulst, A.-M., Hämmerling, G.J., Arnold, B.: Tolerance induction as a multi-step process. Eur. J. Immunol. 24, 285–293 (1994)

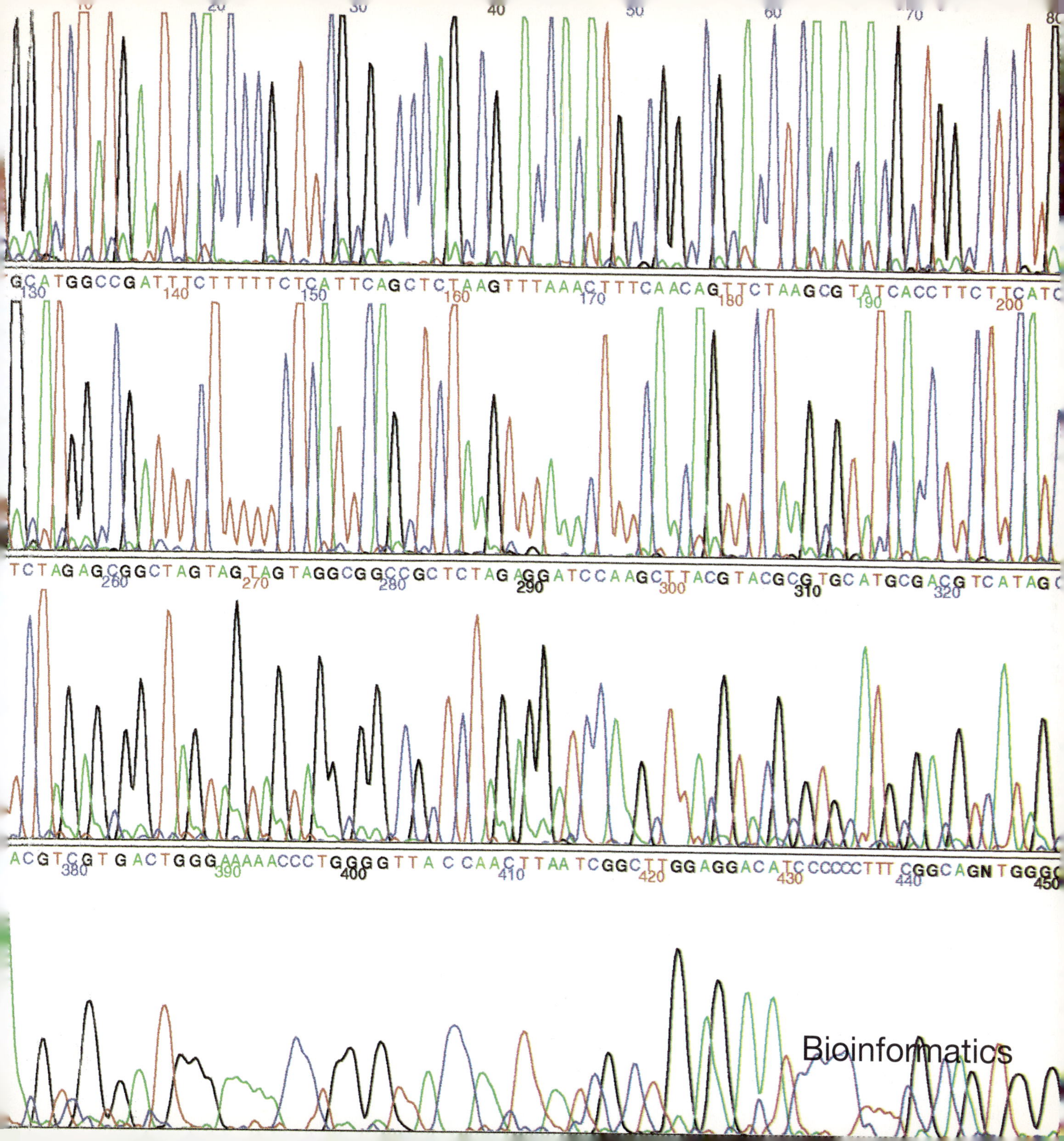
Bioinformatics

9

Bioinformatics

Although the term “informatics” (equivalent to “computer science”) was coined more than 30 years ago, a definition in due logical form still does not exist. For some scientists informatics is “a fuzzy semantic construct whose origin is intuitive usage which fills a communication need,” whereas for many others an operational definition may be sufficient: informatics encompasses numerous different disciplines which are in some way concerned with the analysis, application, acquisition and accessibility of information.

Bioinformatics at the Deutsches Krebsforschungszentrum has a broad spectrum, comprising the activity of four basic domains of research, namely, biomedical informatics, biophysics, biostatistics, and mathematical biology. In all four disciplines there is a “continuum” between the fundamental research for new knowledge and the application of current knowledge to a specific practical problem (“application research” or, in technical language, “engineering”). For example, the “engineering” aspects of bioinformatics would involve the design, creation, and development of new information methods and systems in biology and medicine.

One example for application research included in the Program “Bioinformatics” is computational statistics, which aims to improve the existing statistical software, to explore new algorithms for complicated statistical problems and to include the “expert knowledge” in the analysis of collected data.

Another “engineering” work in the Program will be the “scientific visualization”: it designates the application of graphic and imaging techniques to computational science and will encompass all our research domains, from molecular structural design to medical imaging and spatial reconstruction.

Perhaps the best recent example of the continuum between application and fundamental research is given by the activity in genome informatics. In the Deutsches Krebsforschungszentrum there exist different experimental groups doing molecular research, and they require information about homologous DNA and protein sequences. The quantity (there is a “deluge” of sequence information) and importance of such data make it essential that the data be collected in easily accessible and current databases. The database work (data collection, handling, data distribution) is (and remains) the primary practical aim of the applied research in genome informatics at the Center. Within GENIUSnet at the Deutsches Krebsforschungszentrum there has been established the German base of a European network for the distribution of molecular biology data. In addition, the Division of Molecular Biophysics has also actively participated in the creation of an integrated genetic database management system.

In quite a rough and general formulation, the research themes of the Program Bioinformatics at the Deutsches Krebsforschungszentrum would include:

1) dynamics of genes and molecules,

2) cell population dynamics, and

3) clinical informatics.

In short, the unifying concept is modeling processes and structures.

Indeed, one part of the first topic is devoted to the study of molecular dynamics of macromolecules of biological interest: it has practical applications in problems related to, e.g., mutagenesis and drug design. Molecular dynamics simulation represents the most informative method for obtaining detailed descriptions of atom fluctuations in biopolymers and of the variation with time of their structural parameters. Other methods are used to predict three-dimensional protein structures.

The second topic of the Program Bioinformatics consists of a variety of mathematical, statistical, and computer models trying to describe (and to understand) the growth of normal and malignant cell populations. This aim is related to the investigation of the cell cycle and its control, as well as of other significant events throughout the cell's life, e.g., differentiation, adaptation and survival. In the framework of probability theory, the above cell populations can be considered as large random systems, specifically "spatial random systems with interactions," an interpretation which introduces new concepts (interaction, cooperative phenomena, stability and metastability, complexity, etc.) and allows to re-formulate some biological questions about the heterogeneity of cell populations, the effect of small random perturbations, the existence of different biological time scales, the influence of spatial dimension on the qualitative behavior of cell systems, etc. As it is known, this analysis of large stochastic systems requires the extrapolation from the microscopic level at which the systems are defined, to a macroscopic level at which the laws governing the behavior of interacting cell systems are formulated. Actually, the problem of the integration of local mechanisms into a global structure is the central problem of biology: morphogenesis as well as carcinogenesis are the best, but most complex examples.

A special class of models deserves mention in view of their correlation to current experiments in chemical carcinogenesis and risk assessment. These models may be divided into three groups:

1) "physiologically based" pharmacokinetic models describing the biotransformation of a putative carcinogen,

2) compartment models for tumor incidence and mortality, and

3) "tumor incidence models" that describe the apparition of a malignan clone through a directed chain of events (including such cellular events as, e.g., DNA damage and repair).

The last theme deals with practical developments in clinical informatics, and more precisely with the elaboration of new medical information systems. As it is known, MIS is defined as a set of formal arrangements by which facts concerning the health and health care of individual patients are stored and processed in computers. The project DILEMMA will provide an integrated technology to support decision-making and information management in all phases of cancer care, including support for distant care (by general physicians) and home care. Also, the project HELIOS (Hospital Object Software Tools) is devoted to the creation of fully integrated medical software required for building critical parts of a Ward Information System.

Coordinator of the Research Program:
Prof. Dr. Claus O. Köhler

Divisions and their heads:

Medical and Biological Informatics:
Prof. Dr. Claus O. Köhler

Molecular Biophysics:
Priv.-Doz. Dr. Sandor Suhai

9.1 Artificial Neural Networks in Genome Research

by Martin Reczko and Sandor Suhai

Genome research and genome informatics

The primary goal of genome research is the analysis and characterization of entire genomes of complex organisms, including humans, with the aim of uncovering basic mechanism of genome expression, modification, and evolution. The understanding of these basic biological phenomena will certainly contribute also to our capabilities in diagnosing, curing or avoiding several diseases including many forms of cancer. As opposed to traditional molecular genetics based on the analysis of single genes, genome science necessitates the characterization and analysis of large quantities of genetic material and the extraction of complex information from genomes as large as several billion nucleotide bases. Many researchers anticipate that the results from large genome projects will form the basis of a profound revolution in biology and medicine. Walter Gilbert has argued that genome projects are effecting a change in the paradigm by which biologists do experiments and extend knowledge of biology. Heretofore, biology has been an experimental, descriptive science. With knowledge of the genome nucleotide sequence of the organism, in the new paradigm, biologists will use this information, and other database information, to begin with predictive conjectures, followed by experiments. In this way, they will be able to design more sophisticated experiments more rapidly, as the hypotheses, based on the expanding databases of genomic information and formulation of more general principles, become more precise and sophisticated.

Of course, information in addition to the genetic information will be required to formulate and answer such predictive questions. The rules by which the genome information is expressed must be known, as must the regulatory mechanisms used by the organism. A solution to the folding problem of proteins must be delineated, so that once the protein sequence will be translated from genomic DNA, its three-dimensional structure and its function can be accurately predicted. Both of these two problems (localization of regulatory signal sequence patterns on the genome and uncovering the rules determining the evolution of spatial folding patterns for a protein molecule) form part of the research program of the Molecular Biophysics Division at the Deutsches Krebsforschungszentrum.

Beyond genomic information, details of how the organism interacts with its environment must be determined, including cell-cell interactions and interaction with the environment external to the organism. Such knowledge is still very incomplete for any organism. Nevertheless, the firm beginnings of biology as a predictive science are there, and the directions to proceed and the problems that need be solved are at least partly clear. In the biological description of a given organism on the basis of its genome, the way in which the information will be presented and manipulated will be restricted in the beginning to database descriptions. These databases are computerized software tools for manipulation of the information contained in the first principles.

The role of genome informatics

As first step toward a predictive description of higher organisms, the current objective of several national and international genome projects is to delineate genetic and physical maps of the total DNA complement, ultimately yielding the total nucleotide sequence of this DNA. These projects will produce enormous amounts of information. For comparison, the March 1994 version of the EMBL Nucleotide Data Library, the result of 12 years of diligent data collection, contains 150 megabases of sequences, i.e., 3% the size of the human genome. A major effort of the human genome initiative is development of much faster methodologies for DNA sequencing, the result of which will be dramatic increases in the rate at which DNA sequences are obtained. This rate, currently exponential with a doubling time of about 2 years, is already creating significant bottlenecks in user accessibility and usage. Geneticists will not only easily access all the information available for an organism in different databases (in some cases distributed currently over three continents), they also want to transform it into other useful information more relevant for their actual problem. Simple examples of such transformation include the localization of signals controlling gene expression, the translation of DNA sequence to protein, the prediction of the three-dimensional molecular structure of the gene products, etc. Currently, there are four main areas of active informatics research to develop new computational tools that will be able to cope with the expected volume of experimental genomic data: computer-based (automated) laboratory notebook, integrated genomic data bases, nucleic acid sequence analysis, and protein structure prediction.

Genome laboratory notebook

The first area of genome informatics includes the development of general informatics tools to describe experimental protocols and collect descriptive data including how the data were generated, statistics regarding the precision and accuracy of the data, and information concerning the distribution and fate of the data items. Examples of such items are the specific cosmid and yeast artificial chromosomes (YACs), sequence-tagged sites (STSs), key restriction sites, and genes. Descriptive data, for example, those for a cosmide, include the construction information, restriction map and other mapping information, genetic data associated with the cosmid, where the cosmid is stored, distribution information, and so on. Several such computerized laboratory notebooks have been developed during the past years, primarily to serve the demands of certain, organism-specific genome projects.

Genomic databases

Database activities factually became an integral part of all running genome projects. They are concerned with appropriate storage of all relevant information associated with experimental items as well as related descriptive and logistic data, genomic sequences and their features, three-dimensional structural information, etc. The most important genomic databases will be housed, maintained, and updated in national and international research institutions, accessible to users by remote login from around the world. Examples of such are the EMBL Nucleotide Data Library collected in Heidelberg, the Genome Data Base (GDB) and the Online Mendelian Inheritance in Man (OMIM), maintained at Johns Hopkins University in Baltimore, the Protein Information Resource (PIR) collected in Bethesda and Munich, and the Brookhaven Protein Data Base (PDB) containing the atomic structures of several hundred biopolymers. Besides such specialized databases concentrating on a particular type of genomic information, there are several international efforts to develop comprehensive systems integrating very different kinds of genomic data (genetic and physical mapping, sequence, structure, disease data, etc.) into a unified software framework including powerful analytic tools. Three years ago, the Molecular Biophysics Division of the Deutsches Krebsforschungszentrum initiated a European collaboration to design and implement such an environment (called Integrated Genomic Database, IGD) in Heidelberg.

DNA sequence analysis

The third general area of genome informatics, DNA sequence analysis, includes analysis of raw sequence data, compilation of the final sequence with appropriate confidence level statistics on the sequence determination, gene and site identification, translation to protein sequence, search of international databases for sequence similarities, secondary structure analysis of RNA sequences, and so on. Many of these types of analyses are standard tasks found in comprehensive software packages including HUSAR (Heidelberg Unix Sequence Analysis Resources) developed in the Molecular Biophysics Division of the Deutsches Krebsforschungszentrum. One of the most demanding computational problems in genomic sequencing is the identification

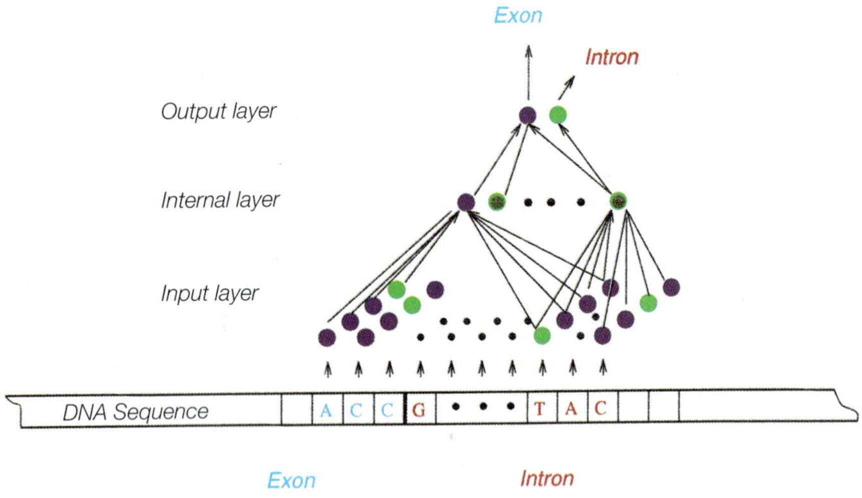

Fig. 68
A neural network is able to identify the exons in DNA sequences. Exons are those sections of a gene which contain information on protein structures

of protein-coding regions in raw genomic DNA. Though the use of efficient software based on artificial neural networks is a promising avenue to seek for a solution of this problem (as it will be discussed in a subsequent section), alternative approaches prefer computer hardware: dedicated “sequence analysis chips” are under development containing a “hardwired” version of popular database search and sequence comparison algorithms. Beyond the analysis of “signals” in DNA sequences (genes, restriction sites, protein binding sites, transcription and translation signals, etc.), new informatics approaches use more general linguistic and cryptology methods, with the aim of discovering new “signals” or “words” or “paragraphs” in the DNA language.

Protein structure prediction

Once a gene is found and translated, one wishes to know the structure, function, and molecular evolution of the resulting protein. Sequence similarity algorithms often yield valuable clues concerning structure and function of a new protein sequence, and multiple alignments of homologous protein sequences provide the basis for evolutionary studies (through the construction of molecular phylogenetic trees). The most ambitious goal of this fourth research field of genome informatics is concerned with the reconstruction of the three-dimensional molecular architecture of proteins from the linear (one-dimensional) sequence of amino acids. The research activities of the Molecular Biophysics Division of the Deutsches Krebsforschungszentrum aiming to contribute to the solution of this problem, often called the second genetic code, will be reviewed in the last section of this chapter.

Artificial Neural Networks

The interconnections of natural nerve cells have been used as a model for constructing artificial systems ever since cybernetics has tried to construct universal computing machines. The foundation for this approach is the knowledge gained about neurophysiology over the past 10 years. It was found out that the processing of information in nervous systems is almost solely based on the transfer of electric activities between many neurons. The activities are conducted from one neuron to another via connections called synapses. Depending on the type of a synapse, the activity of a neuron can excite or inhibit the activity of another neuron. The effect and spreading of the activities in a neural network depends on the connectivity between the neurons and the type and strength of all the synaptic connections.

Artificial neural networks simulate these effects using simple processing units. Each of these units only performs the computation of a single number corresponding to the activity. The synapses are modeled using weighted connections to other processing units. In order to calculate the activity of a processing unit, the activity of all processing units is multiplied with the weights of the connections leading to this processing element. These products are summed up to get the internal activity of a unit. This is the most simple model of the dentrits in natural neurons where synaptic influences are integrated into a stimulus for the neuron. The internal activity is transformed into an activity visible to other processing units using a threshold function. This should reproduce the transport of an activation along the axon of a nerve cell. In the simplest case, the activity value is only 1 if the internal activity exceeds the threshold and 0 otherwise. It was shown in 1943 that every logical expression may be computed using these binary processing units.

Around the same time the hypotheses was made that learning capabilities of higher organisms can explained by changes in the synaptic strength between the neurons. The assumption is that synapses between neurons that are activated simultaneously are amplified and synapses that are rarely used are weakened. An artificial neural network is also capable to change the synaptic weights in response to external stimulus if learning rules according to these natural phenomenons are applied. To achieve this the processing units are defined to be either input or output neurons. These networks can simulate simple processes in perception mechanisms. The input activities represent sensory impressions, the concepts of the perceived objects correspond to the activities of the output neurons. Different input patterns are presented to the input neurons one after another. Each of them should then be associated with a certain pattern of the output neurons. The activity of each output neuron is computed by adding the activities of the input neurons weighted by the synapses leading into the output neuron. These activities are compared with the output patterns used as training examples. Each synapse of the network is changed by the learning rule so that the output activities get closer to the desired training output patterns. Different training examples are processed repeatedly by the network until the network output matches the training pattern sufficiently.

Artificial neural networks trained with these learning algorithms have been used successfully in applications in robotics, speech recognition and synthesis, signal processing and classification. It was also shown that these networks can be applied reasonably in complex pattern recognition tasks in biotechnology and for the prediction of important features of biological objects and sequences.

Predicting funtional sites on genomes using artificial neural networks

Databases for genomic sequences are constantly expanding. Apart from that, there is a steady increase in efficient methods available in mathematics and computer science to predict and analyze functional sites on nuclear acids. The recognition of defined sites on nuclear sequences, i.e., binding sites for restrictive enzymes, is traditionally based on the construction of a consensus sequence which can be found in newly sequenced DNA. Considerably more information about the binding mechanism can be found in a table consisting of a compilation of various possible sequences which shows the frequency at which bases occur at each position on a binding site. The information in these tables can be easily generated using neural networks. Furthermore, neural networks are able to recognize signals which are only defined by a combination of various partial characteristics. These characteristics are difficult to discover when only using existing statistical or rule-based methods. There is extensive genetic evidence for context-dependent and/or compensatory mutations in regulatory genome sequences. In order to be able to fully understand and analyze this, methods are needed which accept them in their entirety and use all the available information. In other words, a method which is capable of cross-correlating each position with the others.

Recognition of promoter sequences on genomic DNA

The starting point of genes on DNA is marked by specific DNA sequence patterns. These sequence segments are called promoters, and enzymes bind here to copy DNA. The statistical analysis of the bacteria *Escherichia coli* promoter sequences led to the identification of two very constant sequence fragments, the TATAAT and the TTGACA boxes. They are situated, respectively, at the positions −10 and −35 upstream from the starting point of the transcription. It has not been possible to find any exact rules for the requirements of promoter sequences. This is probably due to the large variability of the sequence on these segments. We have developed a time-delay-network which identifies promoter signals in bacterial DNA very accurately. The network can recognize 100% of the promoters in an independent test of the complete gene of a bacterial plasmid. Only 0.1% of the tested positions are classified false positive. The system is, therefore more suitable for analyzing larger amounts of sequence data than the best of the former promoter identifi-

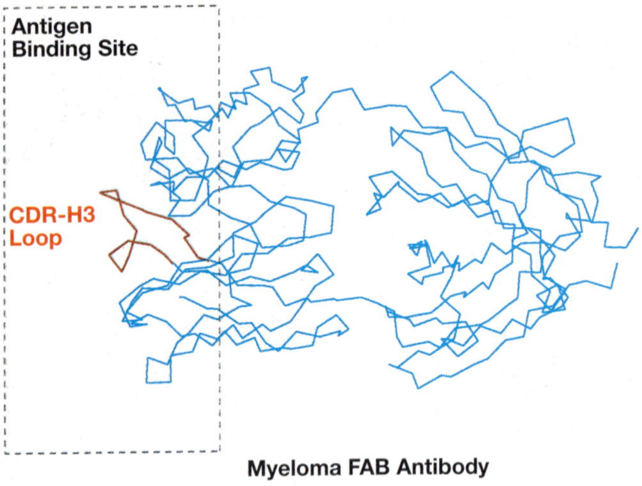

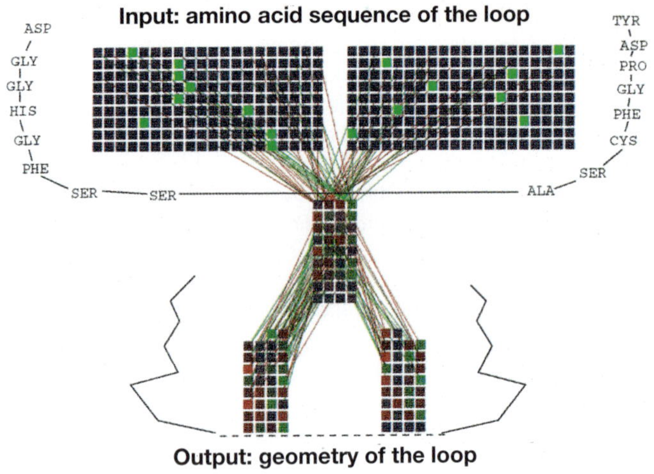

Fig. 69
A three-dimensional representation of an antibody. The neural network predicts the geometry of an important part of the antigen binding site, here highlighted in red

Fig. 70
If the amino acid sequence of the binding loop is known, the geometry of the loop can be estimated using the data stored in the network

ers. In the same test sequence they gave a false positive classification about 10 times more often for the complete identification of all the promoters.

Identifying coding regions in genomic DNA

After sequencing large pieces of DNA which have been taken from higher organisms, the gene should be identified. To do this, the regions which code the sequence of a protein into gene products have to be identified. These regions which are known as “exons” interchange with “intron” sequences which do not code amino acid sequences. The transition point of these regions shows special partial sequences. Particular enzymes are able to bind themselves to the RNA copy of DNA and cut out pieces which are not translated into an amino acid sequence. The identification of splicing sites is an important step in differentiating exon and intron regions.

In work of our group, a neural network was trained in which splicing sites were presented. As a counterexample, partial sequences which are not found on splicing sites were used. The networks could identify and classify all the splicing sites of test genes which each consisted of over 25 000 base pairs. The false positive rate was only 0.1%. Together with the prediction of exon regions in the DNA sites, the networks are an important tool when first analyzing DNA sequences.

Predicting structural characteristics of proteins

One of the most successful applications of neural networks is the prediction of the secondary structure of proteins which have a known amino acid sequence and an unknown structure. For each amino acid of a protein, the secondary structure defines whether it is part of a larger regular structure or not. The typical substructures of a protein take either the form of a helix or extended sheet. The shape of a multitude of these structures is determined solely by the local amino acid sequence which makes up the structure. 72% of the amino acids in a test sequence of a protein can be correctly classified as belonging to either the helix, sheet of other structure class. This is about 5% more accurate than the secondary structure prediction using the best non-neural method.

An important application of protein structure prediction is determining the geometry of antibody binding sites. Of the six variable loops which define the surface of an antibody protein and hence the potentially binding antigens, the CDR-H3 loop has the largest variability with respect to the length and structure of the loop. Existing prediction methods only allow short CDR-H3 loops to be predicted. In collaboration with Andrew Martin of the University College London, England, a special neural network architecture was developed. The architecture predicts the structure of CDR-H3 loops which contain up to 17 amino acids. It is possible to improve the binding affinity and hence the effectiveness of many antibodies by combining classical approaches with the networks. This leads to a drastic reduction in the number of required experiments.

In order to determine the function of a protein which has a known sequence and an unknown structure, more detailed information is required about the structure than merely the position of the helices and sheets. An important observation is that from the 400 protein structures which are currently known, some distinct folding patterns occur repeatedly. It is thus possible to group all proteins into a limited number of fold classes. Many proteins are, therefore, grouped together in the same folding class although their sequences are not very similar. This implies that a multitude of alternative sequences may fold up to the same structure. A possible explanation for this is that only a limited number of structures are able to fulfil the distinct function of a protein. The evolutionary pressure limits the number of possible protein structures, but not the number of sequences which make up these structures. We have developed a neural network which enables the fold class of a protein to be determined, even when, apart from the amino acid sequence, no other information is known. It has been trained to identify one out of 45 well-defined fold classes. 77% of the test proteins with a very low sequence similarity to the proteins used for training were classified into the correct fold class. The wrongly classified proteins were almost always assigned to fold classes where the structure was very similar. The neural network provides a reliable tool for predicting the fold class when only the protein sequence is known. Traditional methods of detailed structure determination can be applied much more effectively once the fold class has been identified. All biological researchers who have access to the Internet can use this tool.

Conclusion

In the field of Molecular Biology, artificial neural networks have proved to be useful in many ways. The networks complement existing statistical and analytical methods in classification and system identification. There are two main criteria for the application of neural networks. The first one is the presence of a large amount of data which has been derived from experiments, and the second is the assumption that there are correlations between observations which cannot yet be described analytically. As a large amount of biological data, especially in the field of genome research, is available, the criteria have been met. We hope that we will soon be able to model the complex relations found in molecular biology with the help of the steady increase in neurobiological knowledge and increasingly complex artificial neural network systems.

Dipl.-Inform. Martin Reczko
Priv.-Doz. Dr. Sándor Suhai
Division of Molecular Biophysics

Participating scientists

Dipl.-Inform. Artemis Hatzigeorgiou
Dipl.-Inform. Frank Herrmann

In collaboration with

Dr. Henrik Bohr
Center for Biological Sequence Analysis, Technical University of Denmark, Lyngby, Denmark

Dr. Andrew C. R. Martin
Biomolecular Structure and Modelling Unit,
Department of Biochemistry and Molecular Biology,
University College London,
England

Prof. Dr. Paul Levi
Dipl.-Inform. Niels Mache
Prof. Dr. Andreas Reuter
Dr. habil. Andreas Zell
Institute for Parallel and Distributed High-Performance Systems,
University of Stuttgart

Prof. Dr. Jens Reich
Dipl.-Math. Jens Hanke
Bioinformatics Research Center,
Max-Delbrück-Centrum,
Berlin-Buch

Prof. Dr. Shankar Subramaniam
Department of Physiology and Biophysics,
Beckman Institute,
University of Illinois,
Urbana, Illinois, U.S.A

Dr. Rebecca Wade
European Molecular Biology Laboratory,
Heidelberg

Selected publications

Reczko, M.: Protein Secondary Structure Prediction with Partially Recurrent Neural Networks, SAR and QSAR in Environmental Research, 1, 153–159 (1993)

Reczko, M., Bohr, H.: Recurrent Neural Networks for Protein Distance Matrix Prediciton, In: H. Bohr, S. Brunak (Eds.), Protein Structure by Distance Analysis, IOS Press, 87–97 (1994)

Reczko, M., Bohr, H., Subramaniam, S., Pamidighantm, S., Hatzigeorgiou, A.: Fold Class Prediction by Neural Networks, In: H. Bohr, S. Brunak (Eds.), Protein Structure by Distance Analysis, IOS Press, 277–286 (1994)

Reczko, M., Suhai, S.: Applications of Artificial Neural Networks in Genome Research, In: S. Suhai (Ed.) Computational Methos in Genome Research, Plenum Press, 191–208 (1994)

9.2 The Genome Project

by Annemarie Poustka

Knowledge of the human genome would be of immense value for our understanding of human diseases. The recent dramatic progress in recombinant DNA-technology allows the systematic analysis of the human genome which will enable us to solve a plethora of formerly unsolved problems in biology and medicine. The goal of the genome project is, therefore, to analyze the entire genetic information of the human genome. From the beginning, the „Human Genome Project“ was conceived to especially provide data for medical research, and worldwide, approximately 300 million U.S. dollars) are required annually to finance this global project.

The human genome contains 3 x 109 base pairs (bp), which are represented on 44 autosomes and two sex-chromosomes. In contrast to the number of base pairs, the exact number of genes, the functional units in the genome, is not well known. According to the latest estimations, there are around 60,000–80,000 genes in the human genome. Changes in these functional units, each of them coding for a separate peptide, are directly or indirectly responsible for many human diseases. In genetic diseases with defined genetic traits a single aberrant peptide may lead to a severe phenotype such as Chorea Huntington, cystic fibrosis or the fragile X syndrome.

In addition to these relatively rare „classical“ genetic diseases, a strong genetic component has been demonstrated for a large number of common diseases such as diabetes, cardiovascular diseases and many of the mental disorders. Genidentification for these diseases with complex genetics is difficult since several genes and/or nongenetic factors (e.g. environmental factors) are involved. Cancer is another good example of a complex disease with a well demonstrated genetic predisposition. Interestingly, genetic „cancer-predisposing“ germ-line defects are usually the same as those found in somatic mutations (non-hereditary) in the tumor itself.

The elucidation of these genetic defects, which lead to cancer and other human diseases, will thus open far-reaching possibilities for the diagnosis, prevention and therapy of these diseases.

Background

The „human genome project“ started in the U.S.A. at the end of the eighties. In a written editorial by the Nobel laureate Renato Dulbecco it was suggested that the fundamental problem of cancer could be resolved by analyzing the entire sequence of the human genome. The costs for the entire sequencing were estimated at three billion U.S. dollars. Even though this sum appears to be extremely high for a biological project, it is nowhere near the costs for a space station and is considerably cheaper than a particle accelerator.

In spite of its scientific value, sequencing of the entire human genome has not yet been undertaken. Current concepts are limited to the analysis of functional sequences of the genome by combining genetic and physical mapping techniques with direct analysis of genes expressed in different tissues.

Genome mapping, establishment of a catalog of all genes

Genome mapping approaches include three different types of maps: The

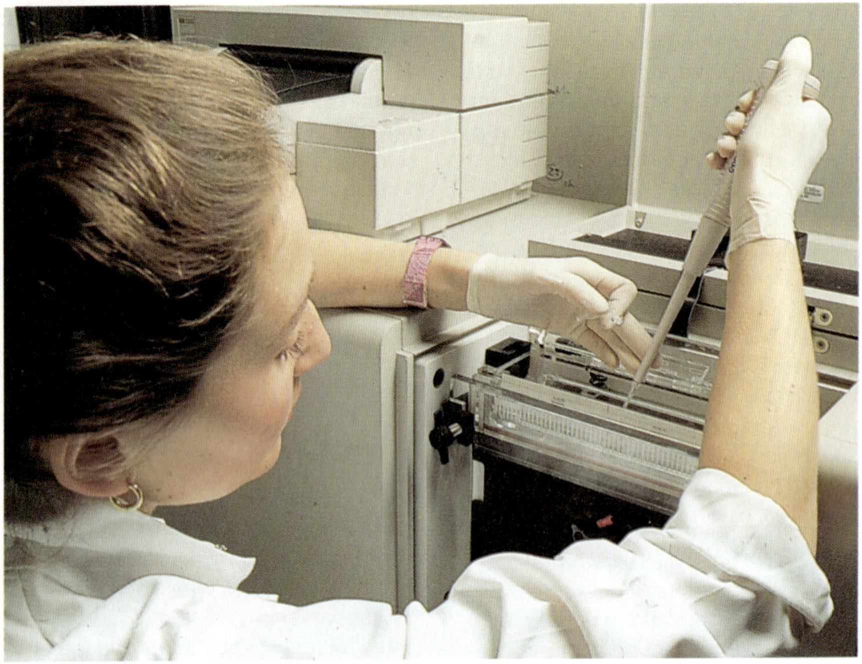

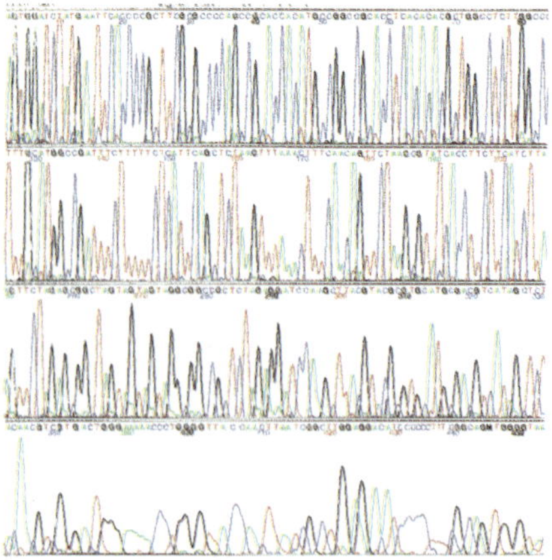

Fig. 72
The human genome is three billion bases long. The ultimate goal of the genome project is to determine the entire sequence. A segment of around 450 bases is shown here. The letters A, T, C and G stand for the four bases in the genetic code

Fig. 71
Since the advent of automatic sequencers scientists can analyze the DNA sequence much quicker than with the conventional laboratory methods formerly used

physical-, the genetic- and the transcription map. Due to the very recent and rapid technological progress the physical map is the most advanced. In physical mapping, genomic DNA is split into fragments and reordered according to its original chromosomal order. The correct arrangement of cloned DNA enables then the analysis of genes and regulatory sequences. Most of this work was accomplished by Généthon, a French research center, founded by the French muscular dystrophy association. Ordered YAC (yeast artificial chromosomes) libraries covering most of the human genome are expected to be completed within the next two to three years. Technically more suitable cloning systems, e.g. P1 & cosmid clones are likely to partly replace the YACs to allow a rapid molecular analysis of the cloned genomic regions.

Physical mapping of the genome is paralleled by another program, which is conducted to improve a genetic map, i.e. by isolating DNA sequences required for genetic localization of disease-genes. Jean Weissenbach at Généthon has already developed over 2,000 highly polymorphic probes. These probes are used for genetic linkage analysis. Linkage studies allow the identification of a defined genetic region which co-segregates (links) with a certain phenotype, thus allowing the localization of „pathogenic" genes that follow a simple hereditary pattern. In addition, we expect that with the availability of a high resolution genetic map, diseases with more complex heredity pattern will be localized to defined chromosomal regions. In order to clone and analyze the respective genomic region co-segregating with a certain disease, it is essential to align the polymorphic genetic markers of the genetic map to the physical map. In general this is accomplished by hybridization- and PCR- (Polymerase-chain-reaction) based methods.

As a final step of the first phase of the human genome project, some laboratories started to sequence the peptide coding sequences (cDNAs). Partial sequencing is used to directly identify genes expressed in different tissues. Since conventional gel-sequencing is slow and expensive, new sequencing strategies are now being developed to speed up the sequencing efforts. These technically demanding experiments are expected to provide detailed information on the frequency of expression of individual transcripts in different tissues. The ultimate goal is to identify representative cDNA clones for each of the 60.000 to 80.000 genes expected in the human genome and to establish a catalog listing all existing genes. This catalog will provide access to all functional units present in the human genome and will thus ease the identification of putative disease-genes. After completion of the genetic and physical maps and the identification of the genes, these genes have to be exactly localized on the physical and genetic map, resulting in an integrated genetic physical and transcriptional map.

The final steps of the human genome project, the entire sequencing of all genes listed in the catalog and finally of the complete human genome will further simplify the identification of disease-genes. Furthermore, this information will be the basis for a systematic analysis of a great number of biological processes. In comparison to the genome of other organisms, such as yeast (genome size: 15 megabases) or the roundworm Cenorhabditis elegans (genome size 100 megabases) the sequencing of the entire human genome is a gargantuan task, not only because of the enormous complexity of the human genome but also because of the relative abundance of interspersed repetitive sequences, impeding the assembly of short sequence stretches. Nevertheless, due to the rapid development in recombinant DNA-technology, we expect that partial sequencing of genomic regions will be used for diagnostic purposes in the foreseeable future.

Clinical implications

Over the next couple of years we expect an enormous increase in the number of identified disease-genes and a burgeoning of the information on the function of these genes. These insights in molecular medicine will certainly be applied to improve and facilitate diagnosis on the basis of DNA. We will be able to precisely distinguish between diseases with similar symptoms but different causes, thereby helping physicians to improve their decisions on correct treatment. Great hopes are placed in the possibility of diagnosing common disorders with a genetic compound such as Alzheimer's disease, diabetes, arteriosclerosis, and rheumatism even before the occurrence of symptoms – a development which will also have important economic implications.

Once a gene product and its biochemical function are known, specific therapeutic procedures can be designed. Thus, it will be possible to design drugs capable of interacting with the target gene product or with the proteins interacting with this gene product. Any drugs of this type could be highly specific in their effects.

Especially for the development of new therapies, the use of animal models, which can often be constructed based on cloned disease genes, is important not only for the analysis of the function of the mutated gene, but also for the development and testing of both conventional therapies and somatic gene therapies. For example, the mouse model for cystic fibrosis provided encouraging results for the development of a specific gene therapy for this relatively common disease that has already been applied in patients. The rapid advances, which are being made in the genome project, are likely to further accelerate the advancement of molecular medicine, and this will certainly have a major impact on medical practice.

National genome projects

Analysis of all the information contained in the mammalian genome is important for further advances in medical and biologic basic research. Insights obtained can be used by many application-oriented research areas (medicine, the pharmaceutical research). For this reason a number of European countries (France and Great Britain in particular) and non-European countries (U.S.A, Canada, and Japan in particular) have been intensively promoting the analysis of the genome structure and sequence. Major methodological advances have meanwhile led to the use of fairly uniform concepts and technologies in the different projects, enabling the integration of large parts of the work in national research institutions. Due to their size, these large research facilities have the capacity to efficiently process massive amounts of data generated in genome analysis. An especially successful example is the French research center Généthon: with an annual budget of approximately twenty-five million marks (approximately fifteen million dollars), provided by the French muscular dystrophy association and the French government. It has made major advances in human genome mapping, the development of genetic probes, and partial sequencing of cDNA clones. A similar institution was established by the Wellcome foundation in Cambridge, England, under the direction of John Sulston. This research facility plans the entire sequencing of major regions of the human genome and model genomes. The annual budget is comparable with the budget of Généthon (about 15 million dollars). In the United States, the National Institute of Health (NIH) and the Department of Energy (DoE) are the sponsors of governmental genome research. Part of the annual budget of 200 million dollars is distributed among individual centers focusing on the analysis of a particular chromosome or several chromosomes, the development of technology, and the establishment of databases. In addition there are research institutions sponsored by industry. One of these institutions under the direction of Craig Venter analyzes cDNA sequences by partial sequencing („tag sequencing"), operating on an annual budget of seventy million dollars.

The large spectrum of institutions interested in genome analysis reflects the potential range of applications, including the identification of marketable substances for use in cancer research, the clarification of complex, genetically determined disorders, and geriatric research.

The German genome project?

Although German scientists have made major, internationally acknowledged, contributions to genome research, a coordinated, data-generating, central project has not been established.

A suitable scientific goal for a German genome project would be the large-scale study of gene expression at the messenger ribonucleic acid (or cDNA) and protein level, based on clone maps already established in other national projects. It should be used to develop new techniques for global analysis of expressed genes and to analyze their expression in different tissues and developmental stages. A long-term goal of this work should be the establishment of a complete „catalog" recording genes expressed in different tissues and developmental stages, their sequences, their position on the genetic and physical map of the organism and, as far as possible, the identity and function of their gene products. Available technologies (partial sequencing of cDNA clones) and automation techniques (robots for clone isolation, DNA amplification, DNA preparation) could be used for this. An intensive program to improve existing techniques and devices would also be required to speed up the pace of research.

Such a project can only be performed on the basis of large-scale use of automation, bioinformatics, molecular biology, and constant further development of the techniques applied. There is a need to establish structures analogous to the national centers of other genome programs, permitting a highly integrated and large-scale method of working. Only with the help of a central project designed to rapidly and cost-effectively generate the required data and provide it to interested working groups from different areas, can we be sure that we will not be left behind, as huge advances are made in a field of research that is of such central importance to biology, medicine, and industry.

The German Federal Ministry of Education, Science Research and Technology has recently taken up the issue and is now in the process of developing a research program to support genome research in Germany.

Dr. Annemarie Poustka
Division of Molecular Genome Analysis

Selected publications

Dulbeccco, R.: A turning point in cancer research sequencing the Human Genome. Science 231, 1055–1056 (1986)

Davis, B.D.: Human Genome project: is „Big Science" bad for Biology? Yes, it bureaucratizes, politicizes research. The Scientist 4, 13–15 (1990)

Lehrach, H., Drmanac, R., Hoheisel, J., Larin, Z., Lennon, G., Nizetic, D., Monaco, A., Zehetner, G., Poustka, A.: Hybridization Fingerprinting in Genome Mapping and Sequencing. In: Genome Analysis Volume 1. Ed.: Davies, K. E.. Cold Spring Harbor Laboratory Press, pp. 39–81 (1990)

Korn, B., Sedlacek, Z., Manca, A., Kioschis, P., Konecki, D., Poustka A.: A strategy for selection of transcribed sequences in the Xq28 region. Hum. Mol. Gen. 4, 235–243 (1992)

Collins, F., Galas, D.: A New Five-Year Plan for the U.S. Human Genome Project. Science 262, 43–46 (1993)

Sedlacek, Z., Konecki, D., Kioschis, P., Siebenhaar, R., Poustka A.: Direct selection of DNA sequences conserved between species. NAR 21, 3419–3425 (1993)

Sedlacek, Z., Korn, B., Coy, J., Kioschis, P., Siebenhaar, R., Konecki, D., Poustka, A.: Construction of a transcription map of a 300 kb region surrounding the human G6PD locus by direct cDNA selection. Hum. Mol. Gen. 2, 1856–1871 (1993)

Coy, J., Kioschis, P., Sedlacek, Z., Poustka, A.: Identification of tissue specific expressed sequences in Xq27.3 to Xqter. Mammalian Genome 5, 131–137 (1994)

Dietrich, W.F., Miller, J.C., Steen, R.G., Merchant, M., Damron, D., Nahf, R., Gross, A., Joyce, D.C., Wessel, M., Dredge, R.D., Marquis, A., Stein, L.D., Goodman, N., Page, D.C., Lander, E.S.: A genetic map of the mouse with 4,006 simple sequence length polymorphisms. Nature Genetics 7, 220–245 (1994)

Gyapay, G., Morissette, J., Vignal, A., Dib., C., Fizames, C., Millasseau, P., Marc, S., Bernardi, G., Lathrop, M., Weissenbach, J.: The 1993–94 Généthon human genetic linkage map. Nature Genetics 7, 246–339 (1994)

9.3 Image Processing in Medicine: From Basic Research to Routine Clinical Use

by Uwe Engelmann, Manuela Makabe, and Hans-Peter Meinzer

Since Wilhelm Konrad Röntgen discovered x-rays approximately 100 years ago, physicians have been able to see what the body looks like inside without having to open it. The classical x-ray method has since been continuously refined and expanded by new imaging techniques. Today we cannot imagine medicine without ultrasonography, computer tomography (CT), and magnetic resonance imaging (MRI), techniques that also play an essential role in the diagnostics and therapy of cancer. An important task of such techniques is to detect and classify tumors, and monitor the patient's response to therapy.

Digital imaging processing is designed to improve image quality and to process relevant information so as to assist the physician in making a diagnosis and deciding on treatment. Today new techniques permit the computation of three-dimensional views of the inside of the body and the presentation of these to the physician in a comprehensible way. The image on the right in Fig. 73 is an example of a three-dimensional representation of the brain, computed from a series of two-dimensional MR sectional images. The image was calculated using the „Heidelberg Raytracing Technique" developed by us.

To represent individual organs – for instance the brain – with this method, the

Fig. 73
The picture on the left is a magnetic resonance tomographic image of a human skull, the one on the right is a three-dimensional reconstruction of a brain as generated by the Heidelberg raytracing method

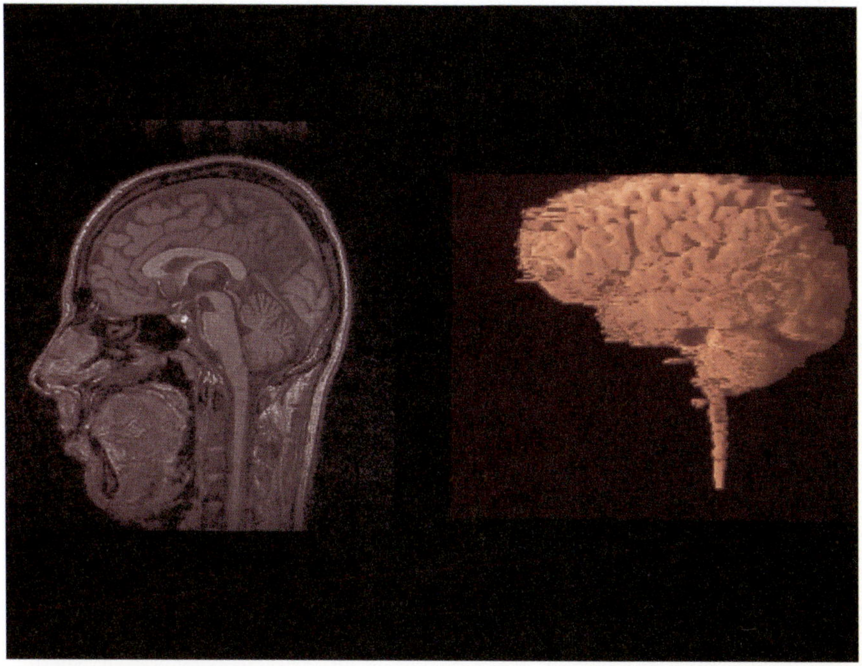

relevant image segments have to be separated from other image areas. The technical term for this is segmentation. Segmentation is indispensable for three-dimensional representations.

Research into and the development of suitable techniques for segmentation (and also organ identification) is therefore our main field of research.

One problem we are confronted with is that the computer „sees“ images differently than humans. Computed images are represented as gray value matrices in which relevant regions (i.e. organs in general) are detected applying mathematical methods. By contrast, humans combine visual information with existing knowledge and expectations about the image and patient when looking at an image. Humans thus use symbolic, abstract information for image interpretation.

The objective of our current research is to include existing knowledge of images and represented objects in computational image processing. In addition we intend to teach the computer to identify objects and relevant characteristics which distinguish an object. In recent years we have managed to elaborate some elements for the combination of knowledge and numeric processing. In 1993 these efforts were awarded the Olympus prize by the Deutsche Arbeitsgemeinschaft für Mustererkennung (German working group for pattern detection).

As mentioned above, we intend to teach the computer human abilities. To this end we have developed a technique enabling the computer to distinguish between certain regions, for instance organs, without prior information on how the represented regions differ. The technique is called „self-learning topological map“. The approach is taken from digital language processing and was developed by the Finn Teuvo Kohonen. We have adapted the technique to analyze images and further developed it for use in segmentation today.

If we want to communicate with the computer in such terms as „up“, „next to“, „between“ we first have to develop techniques allowing the „computation“ of these symbolic concepts from the image. Unfortunately hardly any previous work exists in the fields of artificial intelligence and image processing, with the result that we have to do the groundwork in these areas, too. We call the new field „topo-analysis“. The findings permit us to input previous knowledge on anatomy such as „The brain is located in the skull“ into automatic object detection programs.

Meanwhile it has become feasible to generate several images from one and the same body region. The images may represent the structures at different times or show different physical / chemical properties of the imaged tissue. Such data sets are called „time variant“ and/or „multimodal“. We have elaborated segmentation techniques which evaluate any available images of the same body region simultaneously and not successively, as is usually done. A typical example of such multimodal images are the modalities T1, T2, and proton density in magnetic resonance tomography. The findings in organ detection are more precise with this type of evaluation than with sequential evaluation.

Classical image processing techniques only include the relationship of pixels in the same image section to adjacent regions. However, medical imaging data are frequently whole image volumes (data cubes). For this reason adaptation of two-dimensional techniques to adjacent regions is required. This is another technique to improve the precision and reliability of our segmentation procedures.

There are two ways of identifying an object (for instance an organ). One way is to find the whole object as an area with certain characteristics and the other way is to look for an edge and / or the contour of the object. However, classical contour detection techniques have one major limitation: either the contours found are interrupted at many sites or so many contours are obtained that the problem arises as to which is the correct one. One procedure that does not have these limitations is called „active contours“. These contours are comparable to a rubber band. The rubber band is placed in the image (manually or automatically) and follows its tendency to contract until strong changes in brightness form an effective counter-force and prevent further contraction of the rubber band. The advantage with this method is the integrity of the resulting contours compared to other contour detectors.

After successful detection, the object/organ is represented in a three-dimensional image. Today, the generation of three-dimensional images from the inside of the body takes anything from several minutes to hours with the computers available. We have therefore been developing a specific computer in cooperation with the University of Mannheim, permitting the generation of three-dimensional representations almost in real-time (10 images per second). The objective of the cooperation is to develop a device which the physician may use on his / her own without the help of an information technologist so as to be able to generate three-dimensional images of relevant structures with a single key stroke and from any orientation.

Cooperation with hospitals

The findings from basic research can only be applied effectively by transfer into clinical settings. Performance of projects in cooperation with hospitals is therefore a major step in testing the techniques in routine hospital practice and stimulating further steps in basic research at the same time.

The projects typically involve three partners: clinicians formulate medical problems and provide anatomic and diagnostic knowledge required to evaluate findings. Radiologists generate images which are subsequently analyzed in the Division of Medical and Biological Informatics of the Deutsches Krebsforschungszentrum.

A basic prerequisite of a hospital project is communication and discussion between the groups involved. Communication with radiologists and feedback to the clinician are indispensable if one wishes to obtain images of a satisfactory quality and consequently satisfactory analytical results.

The clinical projects frequently require large amounts of data to be exchanged between the (external) radiological department and the Center. Transmission of data via floppy disk and magnetic tape is not feasible due to the enormous amounts of data. In a project with Deutsche Telekom we have therefore tested data exchange via the public phone network using ISDN. This was shown to be feasible and cost-effective and is now in routine use.

Detection and representation of suspicious regions in the female breast is a very important task of digital imaging processing which we have performed in cooperation with the Gynecological Hospital of Heidelberg University and the Joint Radiology Practice of the ATOS Praxisklinik in Heidelberg. The

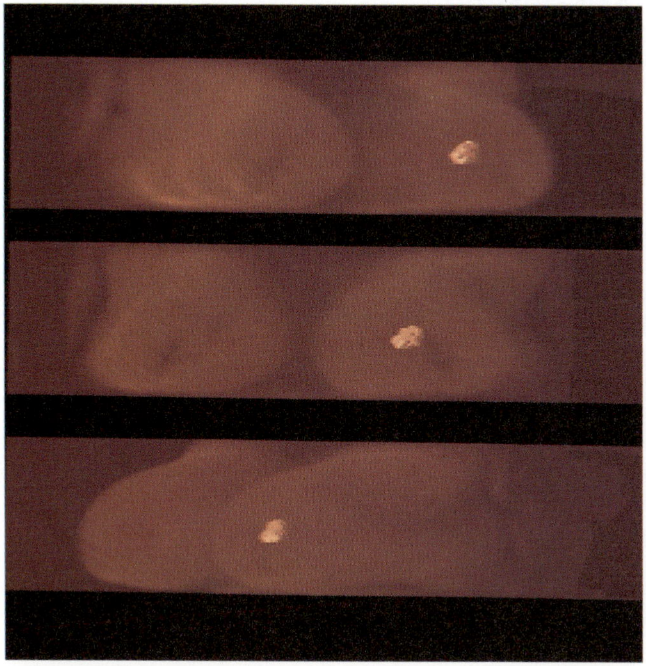

Fig. 74
Three-dimensional reconstructions of a female breast. A region of suspected malignant growth has been highlighted

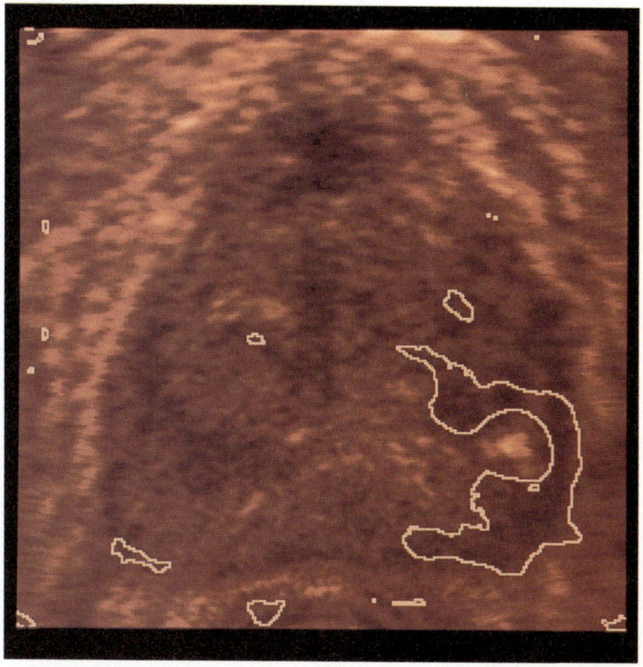

Fig. 75
Representation of regions of suspected malignant growth in the prostate as shown by automated detection techniques

technique we have developed for the detection of potential tumors is based on magnetic resonance images taken at different times following contrast agent administration. Fig. 74 shows a three-dimensional reconstruction of a breast with a suspicious region marked. In addition to the support from the radiologists involved, the potential role of MRI tomographs with low field strength in mammography is being investigated. If it is established that these small and cost-effective tomographs, which can also be used in private radiologists' practices, are as effective as the few expensive devices, the examinations can be carried out on a much larger number of devices in a cost-effective manner.

A common disease in men is prostate cancer. In cooperation with the Urology Clinic of Heinrich-Heine-Universität in Düsseldorf we are investigating the automatic differentiation of prostate tissue in ultrasonic images and have developed a technique capable of detecting differences in texture of healthy and diseased regions and which can classify the regions with the help of a classification procedure (discrimination analysis). Figure 75 shows a result of automatic detection of potential cancer regions.

In collaboration with the Institute of Anesthesiology and Surgical Intensive Medicine and the Institute of Clinical Radiology of the Mannheim Municipal Clinics we have been working on a solution for problems occurring in intensive care. Monitoring of patients with trauma requires daily measurement of intracranial pressure. We have developed a technique which evaluates routine computed tomography images of the patient in a three-dimensional manner by detecting cerebrospinal fluid and representing it in a three-dimensional image.

In a joint project with the Department of Cardiac Surgery of the Surgical University Hospital in Heidelberg we computed three-dimensional representations from magnetic resonance images of the heart, providing the cardiac surgeon with insights into anatomical structures before opening the heart. The work was awarded the 1992 Ernst Derra prize of the German Society for Thoracic, Cardiac and Vascular Surgery.

Integration in the hospital setting

One drawback of the clinical projects presented here is that they do not automatically ensure wide distribution of valuable research findings in clinical practice. Our work in recent years has demonstrated that digital image processing techniques are not only important in radiology where images are generated, assessed and processed. Physicians and nursing staff also require the images for their respective jobs. To ensure the smooth application of techniques for display and evaluation of images they must be incorporated into the clinical environment and the work flow of the medical staff. We therefore decided to tackle integration of our research findings into routine clinical systems in a European Union project. The task of the promotion program „Advanced Informatics in Medicine" (AIM) of the Commission of the European Union is to improve quality and standardization in medical informatics in Europe. HELIOS-2 is a project included in the promotion program in which, in addition to the German Cancer Research Center, six other European partners from five countries participate.

The objective of the project is to facilitate the establishment of ward information systems for European hospitals. It is hoped to achieve this by developing software development tools with which the hospitals' medical information technologists can relatively easily establish information systems for their own specific needs.

Our task within the project is to establish image processing components. In addition to representation routines, programs for simple manipulations of two-dimensional images are provided. Furthermore, the findings from basic research, tested before in hospital projects, are integrated into the HELIOS environment.

In principle we have been developing three different image processing components. The „Basic Image Processing Service" enables the user to display medical digital images of the patients on the screen, to perform simple evaluations and carry out measurements on the image. The „Advanced Image Analysis Service" includes the latest findings from the basic research for segmentation described above, for instance with regard to organ detection. The „Digital Director" is used for the establishment of three-dimensional views of routinely established CT or MR data. In addition we used segmentation functions from basic research and the „Heidelberg Raytracer".

The components permit the hospital's application software programmer to establish integrated systems which, in addition to images, contain other relevant information on the patient. The systems may be tailored to specific tasks that must be solved in hospitals and at the departmental level.

The „Basic Image Processing Service“ referred to above has been clinically tested at the Fox Chase Cancer Center in Philadelphia in the U.S.A. The center has a hospital information system permitting the input and use of patient data on more than 160 graphical displays (X-terminals). The displays are located in hospital wards, consulting rooms, and other medically relevant sites. Since the American system is based on the same standard as HELIOS we were able to integrate our image processing system within a very short time. For instance, system users may work on CT and MR images of out-patients and in-patients in combination with other information displayed on any of the 160 screens.

In the future we intend to develop „more intelligent object detection systems“, oriented at the human visual system and cognitive abilities. We will continue to actively work on the integration of our research findings into clinical routine. This will not be possible solely on the basis of scientific work of individuals but only by way of cooperation of scientists and physicians from different fields and specialties.

Deutsche Telekom supported the works in the ISDN project MEDICUS. The company Digital Equipment supports our work in their European External Research Program and Alpha Innovators program. The work referred to in the HELIOS project is sponsored by the Commission of the European Union in the promotion program Advanced Informatics in Medicine (General Direction XIII).

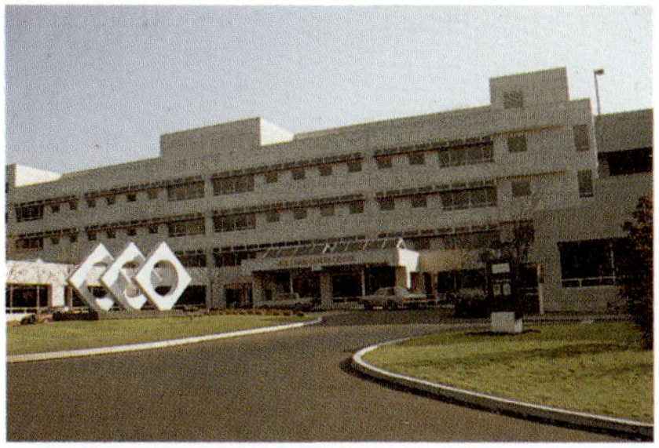

Fig. 76
The Deutsches Krebsforschungszentrum collaborates closely with the Fox Chase Cancer Center, Philadelphia, on a hospital information system

Dr. Uwe Engelmann
Dipl.-Inform. Med. Manuela Makabe
Priv.-Doz. Dr. Hans-Peter Meinzer
Division of Medical and Biological Informatics

Participating scientists

Dr. Hans Jürgen Baur
Athanasios M. Demiris
Dipl.-Inform. Med. Harald Evers
Dipl.-Inform. Med. Jochen Frey
Dipl.-Phys. Gerald Glombitza
Dipl.-Inform. Med. Ulrike Günnel
Irmhild Kocks
Dipl.-Inform. Med. Achim Mayer
Dipl.-Inform. Med. Kirsten Meetz
André Schröter
Thomas Wolf

In cooperation with

Prof. Dr. Patrice Degoulet
Dr. Christophe Jean
Hôpital Broussais
Paris, France
Dr. Jack London
Daniel Morton
Fox Chase Cancer Center,
Jefferson Cancer Center
Philadelphia, U.S.A.

Prof. Dr. Siegfried Hagl
Priv.-Doz. Dr. Christian Vahl
Department of Cardiac Surgery,
Surgical University Hospital of Heidelberg

Dr. Rüdiger Heicappel
Urology Clinic
Heinrich-Heine-Universität Düsseldorf
Dr. Wolfgang Lederer
Dr. Stefan Schneider
Dr. Wolfgang Wrazidlo
Joint Radiology Practice
ATOS Praxisklinik GmbH
Heidelberg

Prof. Dr. Reinhard Männer
Chair for Informatics V
University of Mannheim

Prof. Dr. Horst Cotta
Priv.-Doz. Dr. Hans-Martin Sommer
Dr. Alexander Rümelin
Orthopedic University Hospital,
Heidelberg

Prof. Dr. Klaus van Ackern
Priv.-Doz. Dr. Dr. Hans-Joachim Bender
Institute for Anesthesiology and Surgical Intensive Medicine,
Hospital Center of Mannheim Municipal Clinics

Prof. Dr. Max Georgi
Dr. Reinhard Loose
Institute for Clinical Radiology,
Hospital Center of Mannheim Municipal Clinics

Selected publications

Meinzer, H.P., Meetz, K., Scheppelmann, D., Engelmann, U., Baur, H.J.: The Heidelberg Raytracing Model. IEEE Computer Graphics & Applications, Vol. 11, No. 6, 34–43 (1991)

Engelmann, U., Schäfer, M., Schröter, A., Günnel, U., Demiris, A.M., Meinzer, H.P., Jean, F.C., Degoulet, P.: The Image Related Services of the HELIOS Software Engineering Environment. In: Proceedings of MIE 93, Eds.: Reichet, A., et al., Freund Publishing House, London, 703–707 (1993)

Frey, J., Scheppelmann, D., Engelmann, U., Meinzer, H.P.: A parallel topological map for image segmentation. In: Proceedings of MIE 93, Eds.: Reichet, A., et al., Freund Publishing House, London, 332–337 (1993)

London, J.W., Engelmann, U., Morton, D.E., Meinzer, H.P., Degoulet, P.: Integration of HIS Components through Open Standards: An American HIS and a European Image Processing System. In: 7th Annual Symposium on Computer Applications in Medical Care SCAMC 1993, Ed.: Safran, C., McGrawHill, New York, 149–153 (1993)

Schäfer, M., Engelmann, U., Scheppelmann, D., Meinzer, H.P.: Multimodal Segmentation of MR Images. In: Proceedings of MIE 93, Eds.: Reichet, A., et al., Freund Publishing House, London, 338–342 (1993)

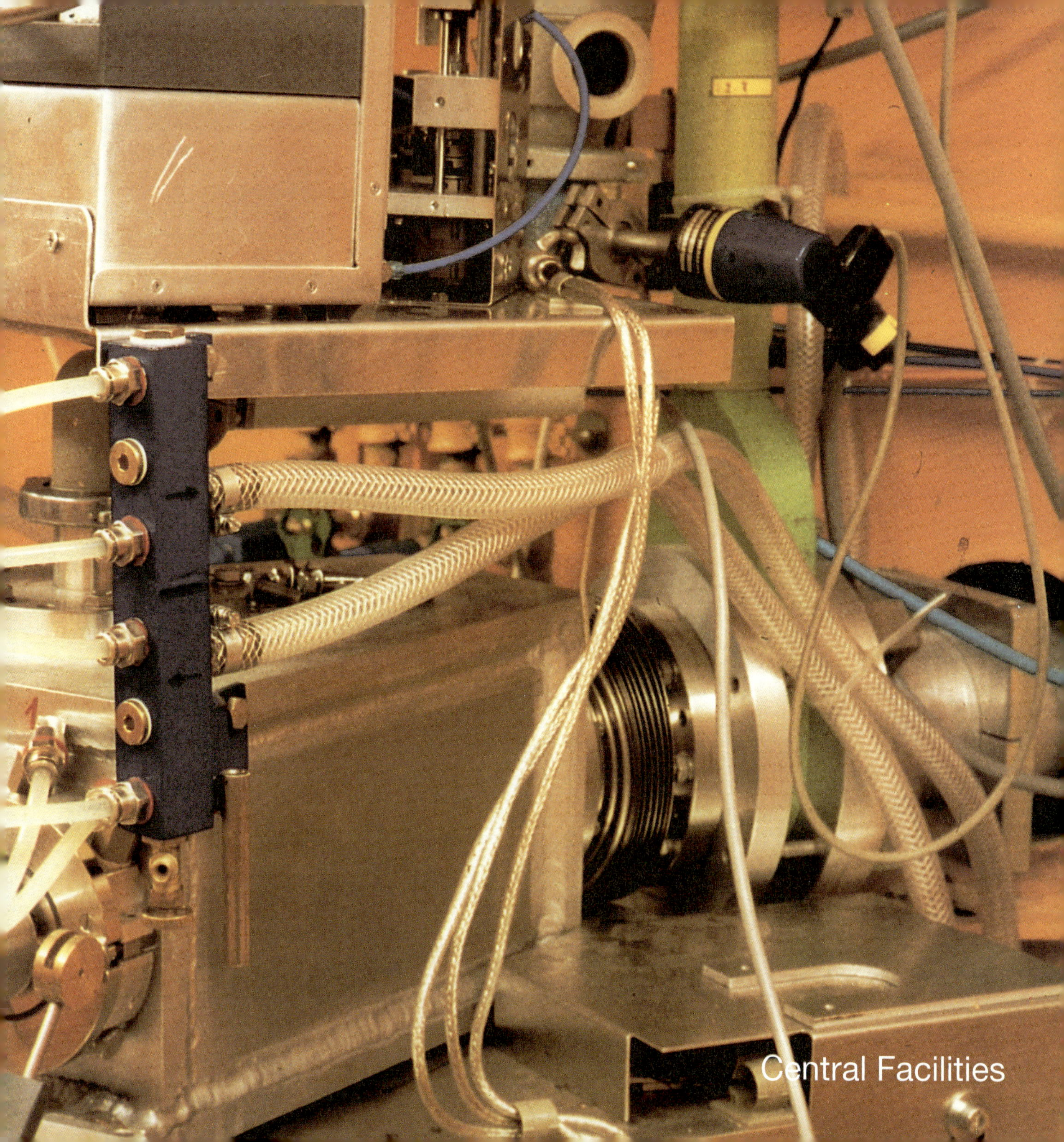

Central Facilities

10

Central Facilities

Central Library

The Central Library collects, catalogs, and provides scientific literature for the Deutsches Krebsforschungszentrum. In addition, it looks after the eight libraries of the research programs that exist in the Center.

The library is not only accessible to the staff of the Center, but also to guests. Due to its location in the vicinity of the University of Heidelberg's natural sciences and medical institutes and to the University Clinic, it is also much used by University members, especially students and physicians. The Central Library also provides services for the Tumor Center Heidelberg/Mannheim and for the Cancer Information Service (KID).

In accordance with the Center's working program, the library focuses on literature on tumor biology, mechanisms of carcinogenesis, cancer risk factors, cancer prevention, and research on cancer diagnosis and therapy. The library contains about 68 000 volumes and subscribes to 850 journals. The eight departmental Institute libraries contain an additional 14 000 monographs and 300 journals.

The classified arrangement of books makes it possible to find the literature without using the library's catalog. By open access shelving about 80% of the literature are freely accessible to employees of the Center and to guests.

Fig. 77
In the Center the international data banks Cancerlit, Medline and Scisearch are accessible on compact disk (CD). The databases on oncology, biomedicine and natural sciences comprise 14 gigabytes. The picture shows the CD-ROM server in the Central Library

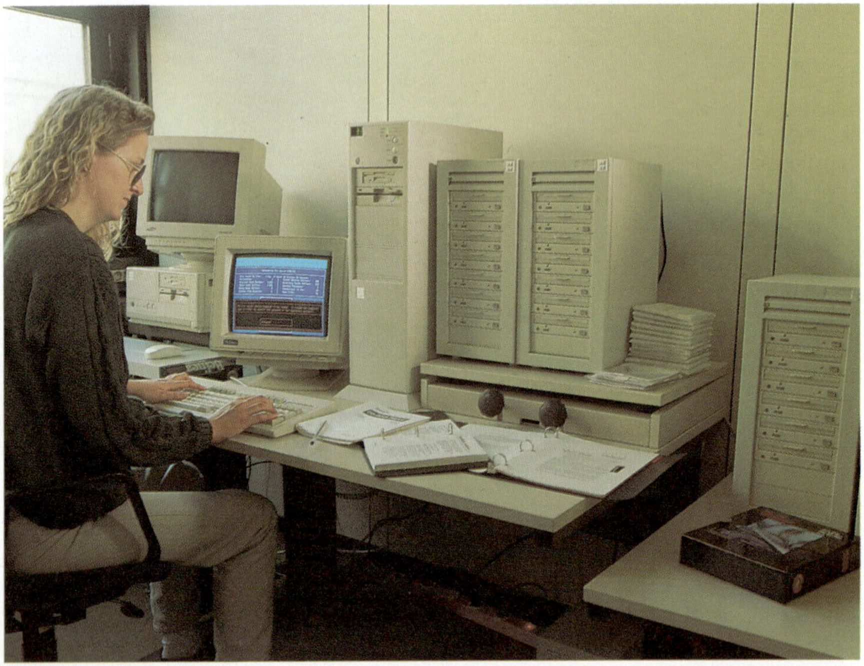

Only older literature is placed in the closed storage. The reading room has more than 80 workplaces. Books can be borrowed for 2 weeks for use within the Center. Journals cannot be borrowed, but copying machines are available. Its main aim being to assist research, the Center's Central Library is a reference library.

The menu-guided, on-line (OPAC) catalog, which is a special catalog on cancer-related issues, is accessible from the Center's terminals and thus from almost all workplaces within the Center. The connection of the Center's central computer to the postal data net (Datex-P) and to the German Research Net (DFN) allows out-of-house scientists to access the Center's data base.

The Information Center, which is part of the Central Library, supplements the in-house means for literature information by providing on-line access to several international biomedical and scientific data banks such as Medline and Scisearch. About 60 data banks, including factual data banks that give direct information without recourse to the literature, are presently being used. The on-line connections comprise (besides CD-ROM data bases for end-user searching) the data base supplier Data-Star in Bern, the Dialog Information Service in Palo Alto (U.S.A.), the DIMDI (German Institute for Medical Documentation and Information) in Cologne, and the STN (Scientific and Technical Information Network) in Karlsruhe.

Head:
Wiss. Bibl. Rolf-Peter Kraft (temporary)

Deputy:
Dipl.-Bibl. Gabriele Daume

Selection of the data bases available in the information center

Data base	Specialty
BIOSIS (Biosciences Information Service)	entire biological sciences
CA Search (Chemical Abstracts Search)	chemistry, biochemistry
Cancerlit (Cancer Literature)	oncology
Cancer Compact Disk – for end-user searching	oncology
Embase (Excerpta Medica Data Base)	biological sciences, pharmacy
FSTA (Food Science and Technology Abstracts)	nutrition and food sciences
INIS (International Nuclear Information System)	nuclear medicine
Medline (Medical Literature Analysis and Retrieval System Online)	biological sciences
Medline Compact Disk – for end-user searching	biological sciences
Scisearch Compact Disk (Science Citation Index Search) – for end-user searching	total exact sciences, multidisciplinary
Toxline (Toxicology Information Online)	toxicology, environmental research

Central Animal Laboratory

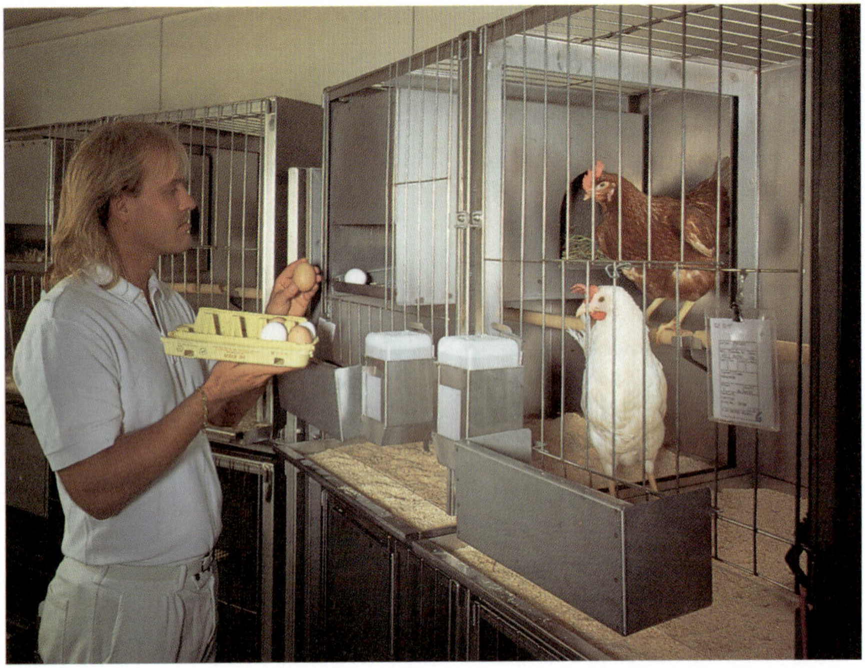

Fig. 78 a
The living conditions for hens in the Central Animal Laboratory follow current knowledge of animal behaviour. The hens are kept in groups of two and have bedding for scraping and dust baths, perches, laying nests, and a lot more space than hens kept for commercial egg production. The hens at the Center do the same as hens all over: they lay eggs. The egg yolks are used to obtain antibodies for scientific purposes

Progress in biomedical research is the cornerstone to improvement in health, the quality of life, and life expectancy. Despite the fact that alternative methods are being developed, animal experiments are still indispensable for the classical disciplines. The use of animals for research, though, has been reduced to an absolute minimum. There can be no doubt that animal experiments have made a major contribution to our knowledge of biomedical interactions and helped to shed some light on the extremely complex nature of cancer. Animal experiments continue to play an important role, especially in basic research, where animal models are used in the development of methods for the improved diagnosis and treatment of tumors and to gain insights on ways to prevent cancer.

The Central Animal Laboratory, or rather the centralized animal laboratory, consists of five barrier units, an isolator station divided into five subunits, and a conventional (open) animal area which, however, is steadily declining in importance. The main task of this central facility is to ensure that all the laboratory animals, whatever the species (largely mice and rats, but also rabbits, guinea pigs, chickens, marmots, and amphibians), are housed, fed, cared for, and given medical treatment in accordance with modern-day standards (animal protection laws, ethology). In general we do not breed our own animals. If possible, we buy all the diverse animal strains we need from selected and reliable breeders. The laboratory is authorized to issue instructions to the users of the animal laboratory with respect to all aspects of user and animal hygiene and the keeping of experimental animals. The animal laboratory is run and operated by a team of professionals comprising veterinarians specialized in laboratory animal science and microbiology, administrative personnel, diagnostic technicians and laboratory animal technicians, the majority of whom have been trained and examined in our center.

In accordance with the recommendations of the Deutsche Forschungsgemeinschaft (German Research Association), the head of the laboratory and his deputy are directly responsible to the Management Board of the Center and personally responsible for the enforcement and observance of national and international laws, regulations, and directives concerning the keeping of laboratory animals. They also supervise the internal regulations governing the rights and duties of operators and users. Apart from running the animal laboratory and supervising the general care of the animals, one of the duties of the staff is to know the characteristics of the different experimental animal species and advise on suitable animal models. The staff is also involved in the planning and technical conduct of animal experiments. It is an important objective of the Central Animal Laboratory to pass on knowledge and skills associated with laboratory animals and animal experiments. Thus, since 1990 we have offered a basic course on laboratory animal science and animal experimentation for postgraduate students in biology, veterinary medicine, and human medicine. Successful completion of this course is a prerequisite for admission to, and employment in, the animal laboratory. Since 1989 veterinarians wishing to further specialize in experimental animal science have trained at the Central Animal Laboratory.

Animal studies requiring official approval from the authorities can only be conducted after the necessary applications have been approved of by inhouse and external review boards (Regierungspräsidium Karlsruhe).The biostatistics working group may be required to establish a biometric study protocol on the basis of which subsequent detailed statistical analysis of the results gained from animal experiments is performed. The Internal Animal Protection Commission assesses the scientific benefit of projects involving animal experiments. Animal welfare officers are involved at all stages of an animal study – starting from the drawing up of the application for approval through to the end of the follow-up period – as advisers and supervisors who are not bound by directives. At the Deutsches Krebsforschungszentrum each of the divisions performing animal experiments receives additional assistance from one of six animal welfare officers performing this function in addition to their main duties. Three of them belong to the staff of the Central Animal Laboratory.

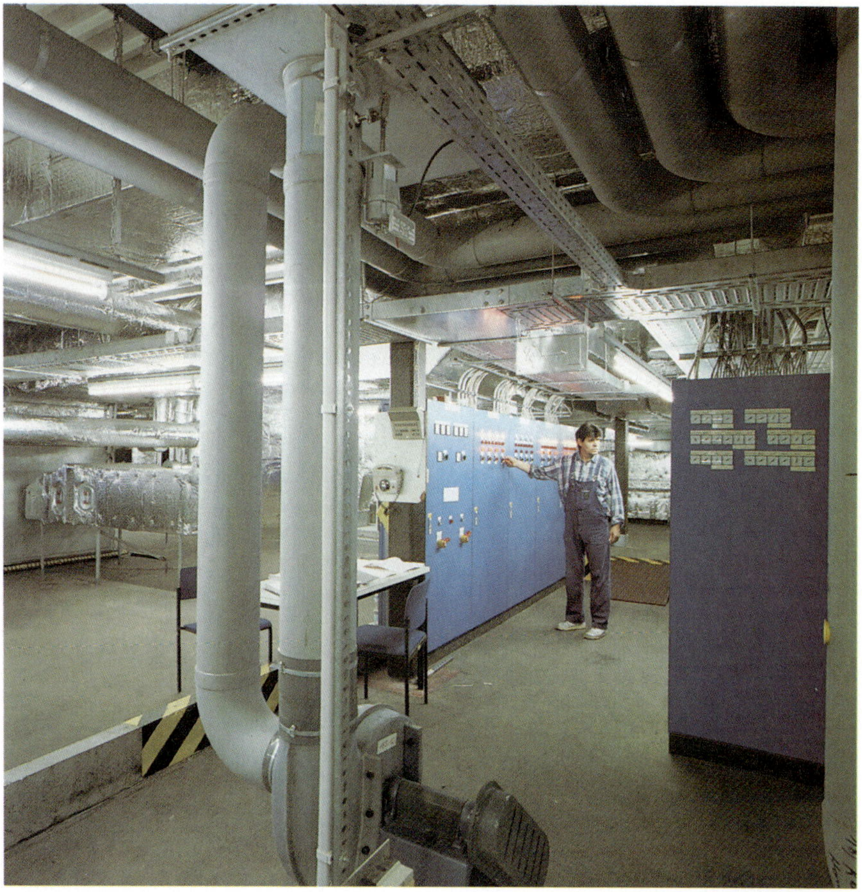

Fig. 78b
Considerable technical effort is required to maintain the right environment for all the various animal species. This system ensures a continuous supply of filtered fresh air at a constant temperature and humidity of the animals kept under barriered conditions

Many environmental factors may influence the biology and physiology and thus the reactions of the animals. To ensure that the experimental animals – the „material“ used to measure particular effects – are as far as possible standardized, it is crucial to minimize physiological deviations from the norm by maintaining consistent and exactly defined environmental conditions. Only then can reliable results be achieved from the smallest possible number of animals and unnecessary repetition of experiments be avoided.

Elaborate technical equipment in the animal laboratories ensures that a standard climate appropriate to the species is maintained. Lighting conditions that are independent of the outside world, with 12 hours of simulated daylight and 12 hours of darkness or twilight, reduce seasonal influences. All this together with the administration of a balanced diet appropriate to the species as well as personal care from qualified staff (trained and examined experimental animal technicians only) has brought us very close to the goal of a total standardization of the environment. Apart from the environmental and genetic standardization ensured by the breeders of the experimental animals, microbiological standardization of the animals is of particular importance. Once introduced into stocks, pathogens may spread and infect a large number of animals. The permanent objective is therefore to protect the animals from all microorganisms likely to impair their health (and/or that of the staff) and adversely affect their life span or physiological characteristics. The aim is not only to keep the animals healthy but also to keep them free of pathogens that could affect the experiments in which these animals are used, without actually causing disease in them. For this reason, we keep only so-called „specified-pathogen-free" (SPF) animals in our laboratory as far as possible. The term is used to denote animals shown to be free of defined pathogens or other microorganisms likely to influence their health or experimental results. Like humans, these animals have a normal physiological microbiological flora. To keep up these high standards, it is not sufficient to monitor the animals for the absence of clinical symptoms. The desired microbiological status, i.e., the absence of specific pathogens, is ensured by regular examinations using sensitive laboratory techniques.

To avoid infections, the introduction of pathogens into stock must be prevented. For this reason, newly acquired animals and all substrates that cannot be disinfected and may constitute a source of infection, for instance tumor tissue and serum, are examined for the absence of undesired microorganisms. In addition, a screening program has been developed which allows the early detection of infectious agents introduced into stocks. Random sampling is carried out at regular intervals using appropriate techniques. This screening for infections is carried out in our laboratory, which is equipped to perform state-of-the-art diagnostic techniques for the direct and indirect detection of bacterial pathogens, viruses, and parasites. The microbiological status of the experimental animals at the Deutsches Krebsforschungszentrum is therefore known at all times and can be taken account of in the evaluation of animals studies.

The aim followed by the conversion of animal laboratories from open to closed (standardized) experimental animal units was to minimize the variability of the physiological and pathophysiological variables measured in experimental animals and, thus, to enhance the quality and reliability of the experimental results. In this way the total number of animals required has been reduced by more than two thirds. The cost of keeping such SPF animals is considerable, but the benefits in terms of good science and animal protection justify the expense.

Head:
Dr. Uwe Zillmann

Deputy:
Dr. Werner Nicklas

Central Spectroscopy

The Central Spectroscopy department provides all other departments of the Deutsches Krebsforschungszentrum with analytical, spectroscopic service. The tasks range from routine analysis and quality control to the identification and structure elucidation of complex molecules. In addition, in long-term cooperative research activities, the newest analytical techniques are introduced and further developed, e.g., in vivo NMR spectroscopy or electrospray HPLC-mass spectrometry. The computer-based methods of molecular modeling (three-dimensional geometry, dynamics, structure-activity relationships) are also being pursued in this department. We offer the following analytical techniques.

– Mass spectrometry can be performed using various ionization schemes such as electron impact (EI), fast-atom bombardment (FAB), chemical ionization (CI), and electrospray; a coupling with gas chromatography (GC) or high-performance liquid chromatography (HPLC) is also possible.

- Infrared (IR) und Ultraviolet spectroscopy (UV).
- Nuclear magnetic resonance spectroscopy (NMR) is routinely performed for the natural isotopes ^{1}H, ^{13}C, ^{19}F, and ^{31}P using a magnetic field strength of 5.8 Tesla (1H resonance at 250 MHz). The more difficult analytical problems and the so-called two-dimensional NMR experiments are handled with the 11.7 Tesla research spectrometer, which is also used for the analysis of biological samples such as urine, blood plasma, and cultured cells. A third spectrometer with a 7.0 Tesla magnet which features a 15-cm bore is used primarily for research projects in the area of in vivo spectroscopy and imaging on the living mouse or rat.
- Modeling of the three-dimensional structure and the dynamic characteristics of a molelcule and its interaction with other molecules or with its binding site in a ligand-receptor complex.

The Central Spectroscopy department is dedicated to applying the most modern spectroscopic techniques to biochemical and biological problems in cancer research. Some of the current cooperative research projects are listed below.

- Structure elucidation and quantification of cancer-causing or tumor-promoting agents in biological samples.
- Structure elucidation of oligosaccharides, oligopeptides, fatty acids and their metabolites.
- Determination of the three-dimensional structure (conformation) and dynamics of peptides and oligosaccharides in solution.
- Analytical support for the synthesis and structure elucidation of new pharmaceuticals with anti-tumor activity.

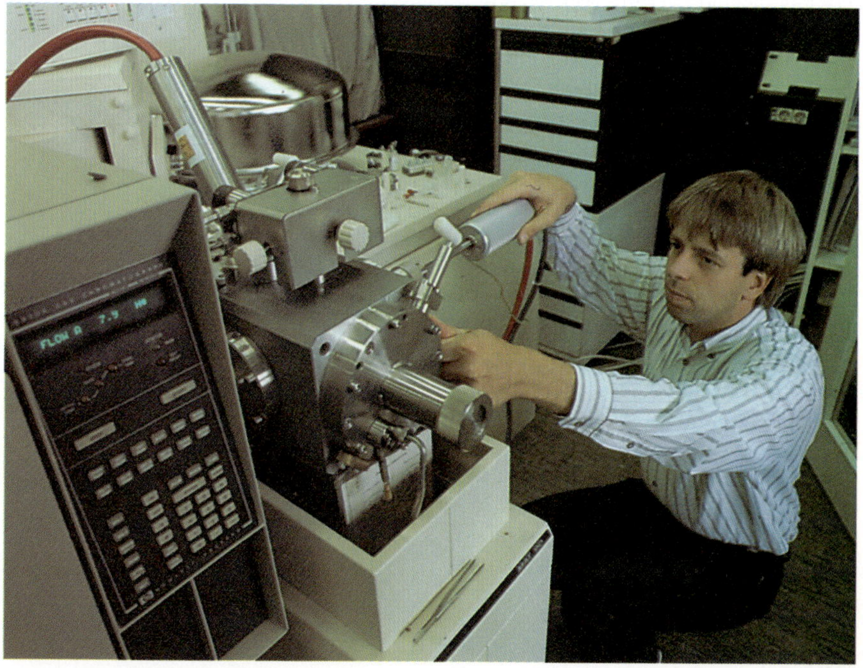

Fig. 79
During tumorigenesis minute amounts of oxidized fatty acids are released. These can be detected by mass spectrometry

- Determination of the pharmacokinetics and metabolism of pharmaceuticals.
- Study of the metabolism, e.g., phospholipid metabolism, of living tumor cells during growth and after various therapies.
- NMR imaging of tumor-bearing mice in order to study tumor growth, the appearance of metastases, and the effects of therapy.

The purpose of these projects is to provide precise analytical data at the molecular level, which should lead to a better understanding of tumor metabolism and help in the development of better tumor therapies with less side-effects.

In addition to collecting spectroscopic data, the Central Spectroscopy department is active in the further development of effective techniques for the archiving and analysis of spectra using our computer-based information system, SPEKTREN II. This relational data bank system has many thousands of entries containing mass spectra, infrared spectra and 13C-NMR spectra, as well as physical data and the corresponding two-dimensional structure representation. With the help of search algorithms, one can instruct the computer to look for spectra that correspond to a given molecular structure or for structures that are consistent with a measured spectrum. The spectroscopic data can also be coupled with other data banks (e.g., three-dimensional x-ray crystal structure or toxicological properties). In our department, methods are being developed which allow the three-dimensional structure (stereochemie) and conformational characteristics of a molecule to be stored (encoded) in a form that is compatible with a computer-based data bank.

A comprehensive software package, which can be thought of as a molecular construction set, has been put together in our department and is being continuously extended. The energy of a particular structure or conformation can be calculated, and the flexibility or molecular dynamics can be simulated. The modeling of the interaction between an effector molecule and its receptor is also very important for the understanding of the biological activity and for the rational design of new drugs. These computer-based methods are a useful addition to the modern techniques of molecular biology.

Head:
Dr. William E. Hull

Deputy:
Prof. Dr. Wolf-Dieter Lehmann

Radiation Protection and Dosimetry

The great variety of research performed at the Deutsches Krebsforschungszentrum requires the use of a number of radioactive labeled compounds. Sophisticated systems and devices are also necessary to generate radioactive substances for research, diagnostic, and therapeutic purposes and for radiotherapy. Handling and operating permits are required for the equipment and apparatus. A Central Service of Radiation Protection with specially trained staff is in charge of obtaining the permits and implementing statutory radiation protection regulations in the different areas, including the radioisotope laboratories, the irradiation equipment, the cyclotron, and the nuclear research reactor. The authorized licenses for the work in the radioisotope laboratories and for operating the irradiation equipment and for the cyclotron are issued by the „Staatliches Gewerbeaufsichtsamt Mannheim" pursuant to the „Strahlenschutzverordnung"; the authorized license for the nuclear research reactor is issued by the „Ministerium für Umwelt Baden-Württemberg" pursuant to the „Atomgesetz". These bodies also have a watchdog function.

In recent years a number of permits have had to be newly applied for, including for instance the permit for the cyclotron and the permit for the handling of radioactive substances in all radioisotope laboratories at the Center.

At the end of 1991 a permit for trial operation was granted for the new cyclotron that will mainly be used to produce positron emitters for nuclear medicine and fast neutrons for radiobiological research, and the final operating permit was granted in February of 1993following the installation and successful operation of the system. A number of radiation protection measures had to be introduced to obtain the permit, including for example radiation protection shielding and measurement of ambient radiation doses to test the efficacy of the shielding, the enforcement of a staff safety system for entering the area, and the safeguarding of the immediate environment.

The „Strahlenschutzverordnung" (Radiation Protection Regulations) of 1989 led to a number of permits being invalidated, including the comprehensive permit for the handling of radioactive substances in the entire cancer research center. Since this permit covers both the molecular biological and biochemical radioisotope laboratories and

Fig. 80
Inspection of the imaging quality and radiation dose of an x-ray machine used by the Radiological Diagnostics and Therapy Research Program

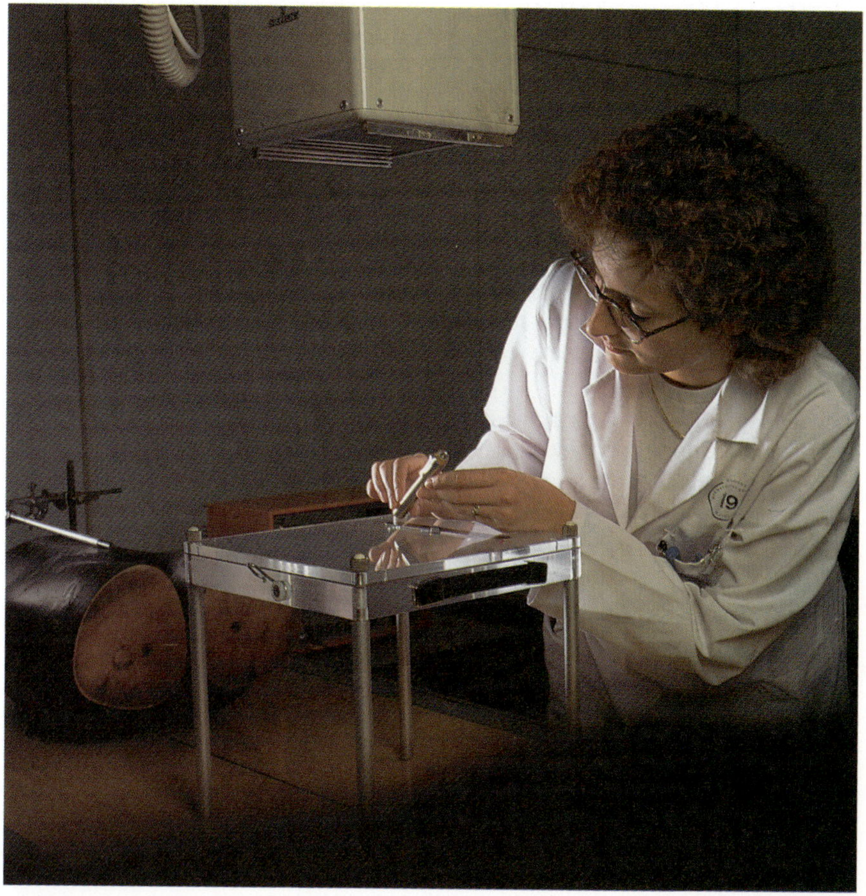

the radioisotope laboratories for experimental and clinical nuclear medicine with so many different radionuclides and applications, a practical means of applying the permit to the job on hand had to be established in cooperation with the authorities for each of the divisions concerned. Where necessary, smaller working units were also given their own set of operating procedures, as was the recently set up K. H. Bauer training laboratory. These specifications include such details as which laboratories handle which radionuclides, the maximum activities of the radioactive substances, special remarks on safety measures, and the names of the radiation protection officers in charge. The main content of the relevant specifications is also displayed at each radioisotope laboratory. This comprehensive reorganization and the installation of the necessary additional equipment in the radioisotope laboratories were completed in late 1993.

The Central Service of Radiation Protection and Dosimetry performs a number of routine radiation protection duties that include the following:

- personnel dosimetry, radiation protection monitoring and the counseling of staff at the workplace;
- advising staff on radiation protection, establishing radiation protection regulations;
- setting up workplaces operating with radioactive substances;
- radiation protection monitoring in the immediate environment of the DKFZ;
- monitoring and documentation of the purchase and production of radioactive materials;
- monitoring and dosimetry of experimental therapeutical devices;
- quality control of X-ray devices for medical radiography and their image processing;
- central collection and storage of radioactive waste;
- separation into radioactive waste and waste that is no longer radioactive as determined by measurements of the activity; delivery to the officially licensed depot and/or companies;
- reporting to the authorities.

The Central Service of Radiation Protection and Dosimetry must in particular cases intervene in work on hand in order to enforce the statutory laws, thus exposing itself to accusations of hampering research. However, the work of the Service in dealing with authorities and in coordinating the implementation of radiation protection regulations considerably relieves the divisions and greatly enhances research with radionuclides and ionizing radiation at the research center.

Some clue as to the diversity of radionuclides and the amount of their activity is given by the following facts: The major radionuclides used in experiments in the molecular biological-biochemical radioisotope laboratories are beta-emitting, in some cases long-lived radionuclides, such as Tritium, Carbon-14, Phosphorus-32, and Sulfur-35, and radionuclides emitting gamma radiation or characteristic X-rays in addition to beta radiation, such as Chromium-51, and Iodine-125. Expressed in terms of activity, the current annual requirement of common radioactive materials is 10 gigabecquerel (GBq) for Tritium and Carbon-14, respectively, 40 GBq for Phosphorus-32 and Sulfur-35, respectively, and approximately 20 GBq for Chromium-51 and Iodine-125. The main substances used in nuclear medicine are Technetium-99m, Iodine-131, and the positron emitters Carbon-11, Nitrogen-12, Oxygen-15, and Fluorine-18 with short half-lives. The total annual requirement is approximately 1,000 GBq for the generator-produced radionuclide Technetium-99m, approximately 100 GBq for Iodine-131, and the total daily requirement is 50 to 100 GBq for the short-lived positron emitters that have to be produced daily with the cyclotron.

Using the neutrons produced in the nuclear research reactor TRIGA HD II, individual radionuclides and entire radionuclide classes can be produced, for instance for applications such as radiochemistry and tracer detection, or neutrons can be used directly for quality control of neutron detectors. It is the Service's job to maintain the radiological safety of the research plant and ensure that the radionuclides produced and the resultant radioactivities are within the authorized limits. In addition the Service is responsible for regularly reporting the results obtained in radiation protection measurements to the relevant authorities and for implementing the obligatory repeat checks of the extensive radiation protection instrumentation in the presence of independent experts.

Nine persons are employed in the Central Service of Radiation Protection and Dosimetry. Another staff member is being trained as a radiation protection engineer under the dual training system. The division also trains young people on work placement schemes.

Head and Radiation Protection Officer:
Dipl.-Phys. Otto Krauss

Deputy:
Dipl.-Phys. Dr. Wolfgang Kübler

Research Reactor TRIGA in Heidelberg

On August 26, 1966, the first research reactor, TRIGA Heidelberg I, was put into operation at the former location of the Deutsches Krebsforschungszentrum on Berliner Strasse.

From 1972 to 1978 the research reactor TRIGA Heidelberg II was built in the new building of the Deutsches Krebs-for-schungszentrum with newly designed reactor safety systems and peripheral devices. The fuel elements were transferred from TRIGA Heidelberg I and are still being used. TRIGA Heidelberg II was put into operation on February 28, 1978 in the new building of the Deutsches Krebsforschungszentrum in the Neuenheimer Feld. TRIGA Heidelberg I was shut down and disposed of.

TRIGA reactors are very reliable irradiation devices and have a very low susceptibility to disturbances. The Center's reactor is operated and maintained by a team of three staff technicians. Repairs are carried out in the reactor cyclotron machine shop. Regular inspections according to the German Nuclear Power Law are conducted in collaboration with the Technical Control Board South-West. Since 1978, seven malfunctions were reported, but only the repair of the rotary irradiation system required a significant interruption of the reactor operation. All other malfunctions could be eliminated by exchanging electronic devices.

The reactor is mainly used for neutron activation, both in medical and biological research, as well as for material testing. In general, only neutron activation can detect small traces of metals in samples. In contrast to atomic absorption, neutron activation makes it possible to detect several elements simultaneously. In general, neutron activation analysis requires irradiation times of 50 hours and more.

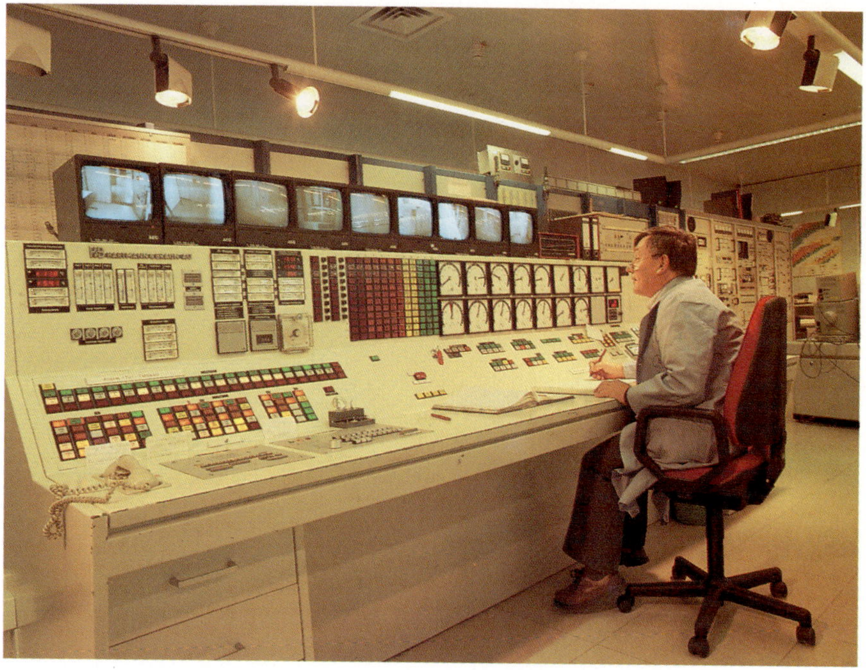

Fig. 81
The console of the TRIGA research reactor. The reactor is primarily used to make isotopes and for analytical trace determination in in-house and external research projects

The in-core irradiation positions are primarily used for operations that require a high neutron flux, such as the production of radionuclides for examinations in nuclear medicine. Since August 1966, about 12 500 experiments have been conducted with TRIGA Heidelberg II. TRIGA Heidelberg I and II have produced 5900 MW and 8200 MW in thermal energy, respectively, making a total of 8200 MW. Since 1978, about 38 000 samples have been irradiated in TRIGA Heidelberg II. During the past 16 years, the daily radiation time has increased continuously from about 5 to about 9.2 hours per working day. On average, the reactor has been operated 180 days per year; 30 days are required for reliability checks and tests, and 20 days for maintenance and repair.

The general trend has shifted to longer irradiation times and more irradiation samples per experiment. TRIGA Heidelberg II may also be used by scientists of the University of Heidelberg, the Nuclear Sciences Research Center in Karlsruhe, and the University of Karlsruhe. In special cases, experiments have also been conducted for universities outside the region and for several industrial companies.

General manager:
Prof. Dr. Walter Lorenz

Operational manager:
Dr. Wolfgang Maier-Borst

Deputy operational manager:
Dipl.-Phys. Otto Krauss

Cyclotron

How fast and to what extent does a kidney resume functioning after transplantation? Is the myocardium threatened by infarctation and, if so, to what extent? Which part of the lung is blocked by a carcinoma, and how aggressive is the tumor growth? Will chemotherapy succeed? Does a tumor respond to a specific therapy? All these questions can be addressed directly and without delay with the help of radioactively marked ("radiolabeled") substances.

Nuclear-medical function diagnosis, i.e., the in vivo detection of radiolabeled biomolecules and their metabolism, makes it possible to quantify physiological processes non-invasively and highly specifically and sensitively. Images of the distribution of radioactivity within the organism (scintigrams) show the temporal process of tracer accumulation and diffusion in the examined region. These scintigrams are the basis for the physician's assessment of the organ's functioning and of the kind and extent of pathological alterations.

A radioactive nuclide with specific physical and chemical properties serves as the "label" of its host molecule, the "chemical spy". Upon decaying, the nuclide must emit an energy quantum which is within the sensitivity range of the available detection devices (80 to 500 keV), the chemical process of integrating the nuclide into the host molecule must be fast, and the nuclide must not change the typical metabolic behavior of the host molecule. In addition, it must decay rapidly, i.e., its half-life must not be long compared to the duration of the examination. This makes sure that the patient's exposure to radiation remains small and that several examinations can be carried out in short intervals.

Some of these short-lived radionuclides with half-lives of minutes or a few hours decay so fast that they have to be produced at the site of their use. The most effective production technique is the transformation of stable isotopes by irradiation with charged particles, in most cases with protons and deuterons, which are the nuclei of the light and the heavy hydrogen. In order to be able to overcome the repulsive forces of the target nucleus, these subatomic projectiles have to be accelerated to high energies. Only then are they able to penetrate the target nucleus and to alter its structure in such a way that it becomes unstable (radioactive). Later, the radioactive nucleus spontaneously decays into a stable state, a process which is accompanied by the emission of positive or negative electrons and hard electromagnetic radiation (gamma rays). These rays can be detected outside the body.

The atomic projectiles are produced in small electromagnetic circular accelerators, so-called compact cyclotrons. The

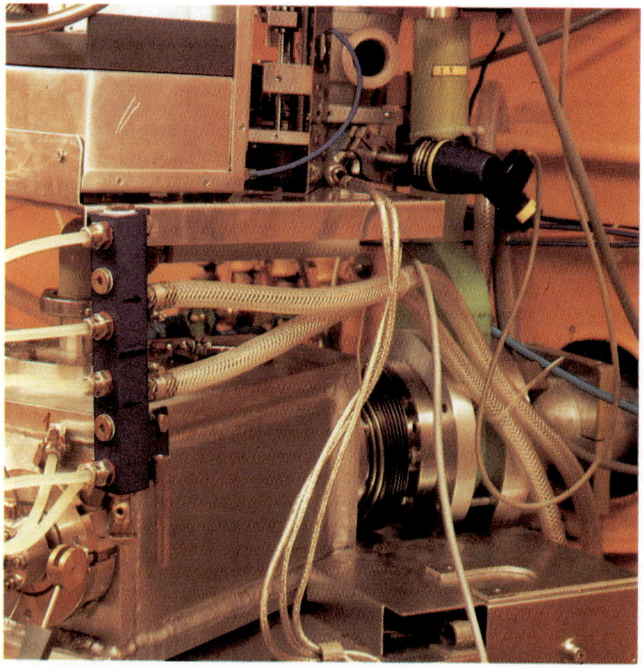

Fig. 82
The cyclotron supplies protons for producing the isotope fluorine-18. This isotope can be used to investigate tumor metabolism and the response to treatment in positron emission tomographic scanning. The proton beam is directed through a pipe into a pivoted vacuum chamber fitted with two targets

first cyclotron was built in 1930 in Berkeley, California, by the American physicist Ernest Lawrence. Five years later, his brother, the physician John Lawrence, and his colleague, Joe Hamilton, conducted self-experiments to study the distribution of the vital element potassium in the body using radioactive potassium-38 that had been produced by the then largest cyclotron of the "third generation". These experiments marked the beginning of nuclear medicine.

The advantage of nuclear transformation with charged particles is the fact that the product of the reaction is an isotope of another chemical element, which can be separated chemically from the irradiated original substance, the target. It is then available with a high grade of purity, i.e. with high specific activity. It is thus possible to effectively radiolabel extremely small, non-toxic amounts of specific pharmacons.

Since the late 1960s, there have been available compact cyclotrons especially designed for the production of radionuclides. Inside a cyclotron a strong magnetic field forces hydrogen or helium nuclei to move on helical paths; several times per cycle the particles are accelerated by a strong radiofrequency. The highest energy of the projectiles is mainly given by the diameter of the magnet – the larger the magnet the higher the energy, which is measured in millions of electron volts (MeV).

In 1968, the Volkswagenwerk Foundation gave a 22 MeV compact cyclotron to the Deutsches Krebsforschungszentrum; commissioned in 1971, it was in use for almost 20 years for the production of radionuclides as well as for the dosimetry and radiobiology of fast neutrons and charged particles.

After 28 months of construction, a new and stronger cyclotron was put into operation on April 25, 1991. It produces 32 MeV protons and 15 MeV deuterons (nuclei of heavy hydrogen) with higher ionic currents than its predecessor. The new cyclotron is a negative ion cyclotron – the first one capable of accelerating deuterons.

The new cyclotron is mainly used for producing known radionuclides that are suited for investigating the metabolism of tumors and their behavior after therapy on the basis of an innovative diagnostic technique, the positron emission tomography (PET). Among the radionuclides produced are the "physiological" radioisotopes, which, due to their specific nature or their chemical bond, do not change the metabolic behavior of the radiolabeled substrates: carbon-11, nitrogen-13, oxygen-15 and, above all, fluorine-18. The higher energies provided by the new cyclotron will result in a significantly higher yield and a longer life of the target system, in particular, in the case of the most important positron emitter, fluorine-18. Higher initial activities are of long-term importance, since the process of radiolabeling highly specialized biomolecules is becoming ever more complicated and thus slower, and since the degree of chemical purity needed today requires complex purifying processes. The loss of radioactivity during these processes has to be compensated for by higher initial activities.

In addition, higher energies and beam currents make it possible to develop long-lived radionuclides for the detection and tracing of slow biological processes (for example, with radiolabeled antibodies) for research purposes and, eventually, for application in medicine.

In 1993, a fast neutron facility for experimental purposes was built consisting of two beryllium targets of different thickness and hence different energy spectra, together with a so-called neutron collimator.

The charged particles, as well as the fast neutrons produced with their help, also serve as tools for radiobiologic investigations. The activation analysis with ions or neutrons offers numerous new possibilities in applied research, which might be of interest for scientists within and outside of the Deutsches Krebsforschungszentrum.

As a brief summary, it can be said that higher particle energies and currents lead to higher yields of the traditional radionuclides for development of new radiolabelling methods of higher specificity and purity. They also have a higher operational reliability and offer a broader potential for further research areas.

Guest scientists are invited to make use of the existing technologies. Thanks to this new cyclotron we are able to supply clinical partners in our region with short-lived radionuclides for development of their own diagnostic techniques, such as in positron emission tomography.

Head:
Prof. Dr. Walter Lorenz

Operating Manager:
Dr. Gerd Wolber

Central Data Processing

Almost all divisions of the Deutsches Krebsforschungszentrum use programs and the computing capacity of central computers which are accessible directly via terminals, personal computers or work stations. The spectrum of applications comprises the following focal points:

- Recording of laboratory data, e.g., by digitalization and storage in a form appropriate for data processing.
- Running of data banks, e.g., for DNA sequences, for spectra, experimental animals, and literature.
- Statistical analysis, e.g., of laboratory and animals trials.
- Image processing, e.g., for cell and organ sections.
- Simulations and calculations, e.g., for models of cell division and interactions between molecules.
- Presentation of the results by text processing, graphs, and diagrams.

The Department of Central Data Processing (ZDV) supports users in their data-processing applications by adaptation of instrument interfaces for recording of laboratory data with microcomputers, by transport of data to the appropriate evaluation computer or terminal via a local area network (LAN), by the operation of centrally available computers, and by provision of programs for user groups. Additionally, the tasks include training and counselling in the use of data processing, programming, and result presentation. Users who wish to employ personal computers in order to carry out individual data-processing independently are supported by the ZDV in the selection, configuration, and operation of their computer.

The central data-processing is carried out with IBM and Convex computers with the operating systems VM/CMS and Unix. 60 decentralized computers and about 500 terminals and personal computers in the Deutsches Krebsforschungszentrum are connected via a local computer network.

External, directly connected users are institutes and clinics of the University of Heidelberg via the data networks of the Federal Post Office (Datex-L, Datex-P). Access to the computers of the Deutsches Krebsforschungszentrum is also available to other authorized users.

In addition, by the connection of a computer to the Internet computer network and to the science networks WIN/ and BeLWü a worldwide exchange of data and information is possible for all users, especially with other research facilities and universities. There are high-speed computer connections to the University Computer Centre and to the Centre of Molecular Biology in Heidelberg.

The program languages available on the computers of the ZDV are C, APL, PL/1, and Fortran. The following generally recognized software packages are implemented: for statistics: SAS; for data banks: Sybase, Superbase, Informix; for graphics: Designer, Harvard Graphics; for word processing: Winword, Word. The Deutsches Krebsforschungszentrum's own developments are being used very intensively, e.g. for DNA sequence analysis: Husar.

The Central Data Processing gives support to all scientific research activities and service facilities in the Deutsches Krebsforschungszentrum in the use of the computer as a tool of modern research and is therefore organized as a central facility.

Head:
Dr. Kurt Böhm

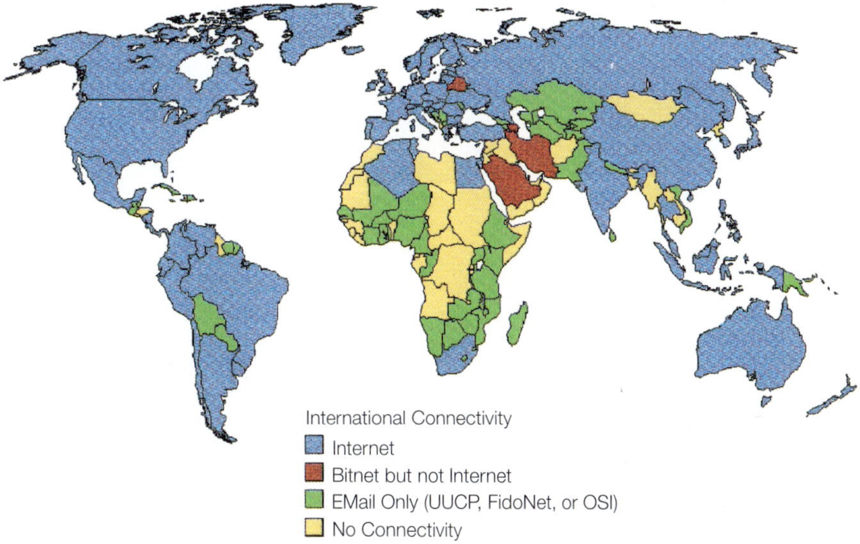

Fig. 83
International computer networks link the five continents. Today it is possible to exchange information electronically between most countries across the globe

Appendix

Evaluation of Results and Main Research Objectives

For the last 10 years, internal presentations of the scientific work within the individual divisions and external assessments of the whole Research Program with its divisions have alternated at regular intervals. The internal presentations of the research activities take place regulary and are supervised by the Scientific Council, the Coordinators of the Research Programs, and the Management Board. Here, the researchers from one division report on their work and their results and present concepts and prospects for future research. As a rule, each division presents its work every 2 years to the other staff of the Center and every 5 years to an expert panel consisting of the members of the Scientific Committee of the Board of Trustees and external experts from Germany and abroad. These assessments may result in a redefinition of scientific priorities, a redistribution of resources, an exchange of staff, an increase or reduction of working space, further investments or the establishment of special working groups or new divisions. The results of the presentations and the external assessments are discussed by the Scientific Council and implemented in agreement with the Board of Trustees and the Management Board. In 1992 and 1993 four Research Programs were assessed and 20 internal presentations took place.

In the period covered, several new divisions have been set up. In addition to these newly established divisions, further research focuses have been defined within the framework of a continuous reorientation and have been set up as temporary divisions.

Furthermore, with the arrival of a new generation several division heads have retired. Their fields of research have been superseded by new scientific challenges.

The appointment procedures for the clinical cooperation units at the University Pedriatric Hospital and the University Medical Hospital and Outpatient Clinic in Heidelberg have been completed. Priv.-Doz. Dr. Klaus-Michael Debatin leads the clinical cooperation unit with the Heidelberg University Pediatric Clinic, Priv.-Doz. Dr. Rainer Haas leads the Unit with the Medical Hospital and Outpatient Clinic.

Research sponsorship organizations both in Germany and abroad are funding a large number of projects for which scientists at the Deutsches Krebsforschungszentrum have applied and which have been judged worthy of support by the relevant expert boards. In 1991, 216 projects were approved (DM 20,424,700), in 1992 the number was 230 (DM 23,700,800), and in 1993 it was 265 (DM 23,434,500). There has been a noticeable increase in funds provided by the European Union. In the above years EU funds alone amounted to DM 1.17 million in 1991, DM 3.62 million in 1992 and DM 4.42 million in 1993.

The publication of the scientific results of scientists of Center in leading specialist journals in Germany and abroad is another element of the continuous evaluation of results.

New divisions and project groups

In the period 1991–1993, the Deutsches Krebsforschungszentrum established seven new divisions. Two existing ones were taken over by new heads and four project groups were given division status.

Dr. Peter Lichter, head of the new division "Organization of Complex Genomes," working in collaboration with Dr. Thomas Cremer from the Institute for Human Genetics and Anthropology of the University of Heidelberg, has developed a technique for visualizing segments of the chromosomes forming the human genetic material. With the help of fluorescent dyes, single pieces of DNA are labeled and then introduced into the chromosome sets of human cells. Here, they hybridize with the chromosomal DNA and provide light signals at the position of their complementary partner pieces. This technique enables chromosomal modifications, such as those causing cancer or hereditary diseases, to be localized many times faster than with conventional radioactive-labeling methods.

The division "Virus-Host Interactions," under the direction of Prof. Dr. Claus Hobe Schröder studies the subject of virus-induced carcinogenesis based on the cases of the papillomavirus in humans (cervical cancer) and the hepatitis-B virus (liver-cell cancer). Interest is focused on virus factors known as oncogenes which has been connected with the modification of the growth behavior of cells. For papillomaviruses it has become clear that there are two oncogenes which are regularly involved in carcinogenesis. In contrast, for the hepatitis-B virus a variety of different virus factors and mechanisms have been discussed in various cases. With a view to characterizing further cell factors, work is in progress to further develop an experimental system that can selectively switch on and off the responsible oncogenes. In addition, epidemiological studies of papillomavirus infection are being carried out in collaboration with Argentinean scientists. Progress in diagnostic techniques now makes it possible to search efficiently for papillomavirus markers in both benevolent and malevolent defects of the genital and the ear-nose-throat regions. Furthermore, a case-control study is yielding information on the risk factors that are responsible, together with infection by papillomaviruses, for the development of cervical cancer.

Priv. Doz. Dr. Ethel-Michele de Villiers is head of the new division "Tumor-Virus Characterization". The pathogens studied here are tiny, and their structure only becomes visible under the electron microscope. The same is tru for the papillomaviruses which, for decades, were thought only to cause harmless warts. However, it has now been known for some time that these minute organisms can also cause cancer of the skin and of the mucous membranes. The handling of these pathogens, which of course are invisible to the naked eye, thus demands special protective measures; these were strictly observed in the construction of the building which houses the Research Program "Applied Tumor Virology".

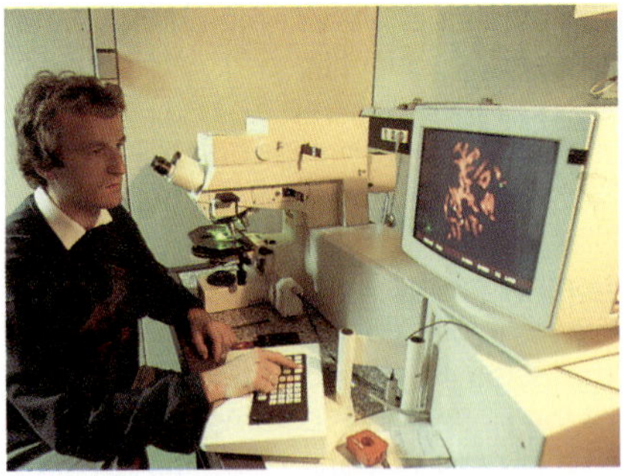

Fig. 84
Dr. Peter Lichter, head of the new division "Organization of Complex Genomes", at work on the computer

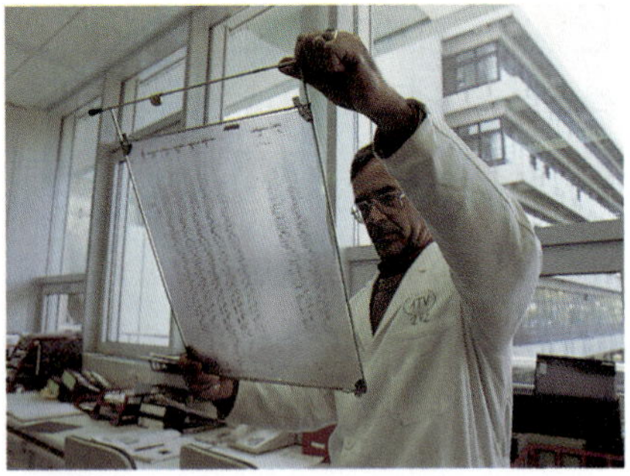

Fig. 85
The head of the new division "Virus-Host Interactions", Prof. Dr. Claus Hobe Schröder, in the laboratory

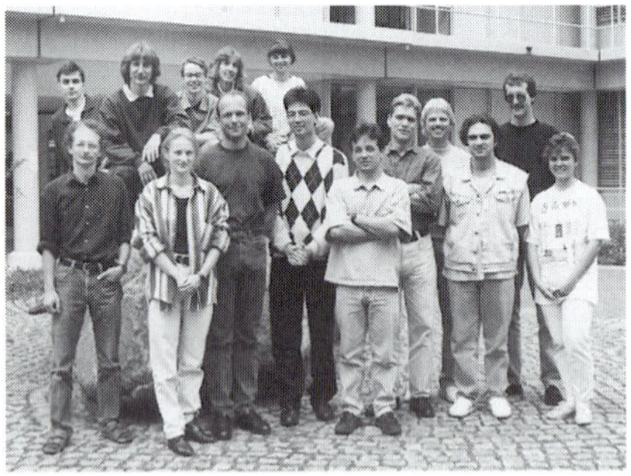

Fig. 86
Staff of the new division "Tumor Virus Immunology" with their divisional head Prof. Dr. Hans-Georg Rammensee (front row, far left)

Most virus diseases are harmless. After the infection, however, a few viruses leave behind parts of their hereditary material in the affected somatic cells. This, too, is usually of no great consequence. But in a small minority of patients the foreign genetic material becomes actively involved in the instructions for generating new cells, and this can cause tumors to develop. Two subvarieties of the wart viruses or papillomaviruses with which Ethel-Michele de Villiers works can induce cervical can-cer – but only one in 30 infected women are affected. How, when, and, most importantly, for whom this mechanism takes effect are questions that are still being researched. An essential aspect of the work is the international search for new types of virus in human tumor tissue. To collect and collate this information de Villiers' division incorporates the "Reference center for human-pathogenic papillomaviruses," which plays a world-wide, essential role in the identification and characterization of new types of virus belonging to this group.

The division "Molecular Pharmacology" began its work in early 1992 under the leadership of Priv. Doz. Dr. Peter Gierschik. This medical researcher and his staff are concerned with the regulation of cell growth a process that is frequently disrupted in cases of cancer and their aim is to develop new pharmacological approaches to tumor therapy. At the forefront of their efforts is the wish to better understand the process of signal transduction at the cell membrane and the G-proteins involved in this process. In October, 1993, Peter Gierschik took over as head of the Department of Pharmacology and Toxicology at the University of Ulm. Thus, after a period of transition, the work of his research group will be continued at the University of Ulm.

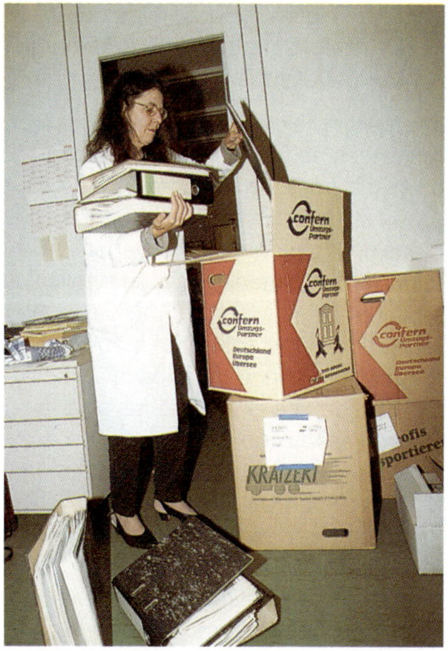

Fig. 87
The new division "Tumor Progression and Tumor Defense" is moving into refurbished premises. Seen here is the divisional head Prof. Dr. Margot Zöller

The division "Tumor-Virus Immunology" has been headed, since the middle of 1993, by Prof. Dr. Hans-Georg Rammensee. His subject area, the so-called MHC proteins, are cell-surface molecules that play an important role in the regulation of immune defense. The task of these molecules is to bind to peptide fragments from the cellular metabolism, and to present these at the cell surface to a particular group of white blood corpuscles, the cytotoxic T-cells. The latter can distinguish between foreign and non-foreign complexes and can thus selectively fight against and destroy cells that are infected with foreign material, for example, a virus. Hans-Georg Rammensee and his staff have developed a procedure with which the protein fragments displayed by the MHC proteins can be isolated and detected directly. They thereby succeeded in deciphering the rules according to which the peptides are bound to the MHC molecules. A future aim is to establish where and how the peptides arise and which of the cell's own proteins are presented in particular infectious, tumor, and autoimmune diseases. In the long term the results of this research could be useful in the development of vaccines and methods of immune therapy.

The new division "Toxicology and Cancer Risk Factors" tackles questions posed by the still young subject of molecular epidemiology. Here, scientists from the two former divisions "Environmental Carcinogens" and "Carcinogenesis and Chemotherapy" work together under the leadership of Prof. Dr. Helmut Bartsch. Their top priority is to analyze the "genetic fingerprints" of human tumor cells produced by the effects of cancer-causing substances. Such results allow conclusions to be drawn about the type of cancer-causing factors, and one can also judge the extent to which the data gathered in animal experiments can be usefully related to humans. It should thereby become possible to assess cancer risks more accurately. Using highly sensitive measurement techniques it should also be feasible to detect changes to the human DNA produced by exposure to carcinogenic substances and thus to identify groups of people who are particularly at risk. Contributions to the interdisciplinary research field of molecular epidemiology come from experimental scientists, clinicians, and epidemiologists, who endeavor through their joint efforts to further our knowledge of the causes and prevention of cancer.

The main research emphasis of the new division "Immune Suppression by Viruses" headed by Priv. Doz. Dr. Hans-Georg Kräusslich is the molecular-biological characterization of the processes occurring in the late stages of the replication cycle of viruses. A further goal of this division is to study in detail the early phases of viral infection including the replication of the genome. Among other things, this will facilitate a better understanding of the effect of antiviral substances. Particularly interesting systems that are being studied as part of this project include the medically important retroviruses, for example, the HIV type 1 virus. A final and no less important aspect of the division's work is the development of antiviral agents on the basis of chemotherapeutic and gene-therapeutic concepts.

"Molecular Embryology" is the name of another new division, headed by Dr. Christof Niehrs. The processes involved in embryonic development have many parallels to those that occur in cancer. Similar to metastatic spread – the process by which tumor cells migrate to distant organs – embryonic cells, too, wander through foreign tissue. Another common feature is the active and rapid replication of both types of cell. Finally, under certain conditions, embryonic cells are able to develop a so-called teratocarcinoma, a tumor of the testis that can occur in young men. Christof Niehrs has focused his attention on the control of migration and differentiation of mesodermal cells in the clawed frog – the traditional research object in embryology. He is particularly interested in the regulator protein goosecoid which obviously serves as a kind of "main safety switch" for the embryonic development program.

The new division "Biophysics of Macromolecules" led by Prof. Dr. Jörg Langowski is seeking and studying the physical laws determining the three-dimensional structure of the genetic material. Three-dimensional superhelical structures play an important role in the regulation of the activity of many genes, for example during the growth and differentiation of a cell, and thus also in the processes constituting cancer. As model systems the scientists make use of ring-shaped DNA molecules which are intertwined within themselves. They introduce into these rings sequences that lead to a local curvature, or bind proteins to the DNA molecules which cause them to bend. The structural changes in the molecules are then investigated using methods of dynamical light scattering. From the scattering of the laser light, Langowski and his colleagues can extract information about the internal motion of the DNA molecule. Further important results for their work stem from measurements of the neutron and low-angle x-ray scattering performed at the neutron reactor and the European synchrotron in Grenoble.

In a second, theoretical, approach the scientists in this new division attempted to work out the structure and dynamics of superhelical DNA on the basis of model calculations. They succeeded in quantitatively describing the internal motion of rings comprising between 900 and 3000 base pairs. Through the comparison of such results with experimental data it is also possible to adjust and optimize the computer model used.

The division "Classical and Molecular Cytogenetics" led by Prof. Dr. Manfred Schwab – previously the project group "Cytogenetics" – is concerned with discovering the ways in which genetic modifications contribute to the development of human cancers. Here attention is focused on the neuroblastoma, a cancer affecting nerve cells in children, and on a hereditary form of colon cancer. To deduce the mechanisms of cancer causation and in order to perform genome analysis of human cancer cells, a variety of experimental approaches from cytogenetics, molecular genetics, and protein chemistry are combined.

The division "Molecular Biology of Mitosis," led by Prof. Dr. Herwig Ponstingl, has been created from the project group of the same name. Its research concerns cell division, which is studied with a view to revealing the causes of the unchecked replication of cancer cells.

At the end of 1992 the project group "Human Retroviruses" became the division "Retroviral Gene Expression". The researches group headed by Prof. Dr. Rolf Flügel investigates the interaction of the spumaretrovirus with its host cells and the role of this virus in certain diseases.

The project group "Tolerance and Immune Response" of Priv. Doz. Dr. Margot Zöller has become the division "Tumor Progression and Immune Defense". Together with her co-workers, Dr. Zöller studies cell-surface molecules that change during the course of metastasis, or are even newly created. In the winter semester 1993/1994 she was appointed to the chair of Applied Genetics at the University of Karlsruhe. A special arrangement between the University of Karlsruhe and the Deutsches Krebsforschungszentrum will ensure that she can continue her research work at the Deutsches Krebsforschungszentrum.

Distinctions and Appointments

From 1991 to 1993, as in the past, scientists at the Deutsches Krebsforschungszentrum once more received numerous prizes and honors.

1990 Prize of the Heidelberg Association for Natural History and Medicine for the best PhD thesis in medicine at the university (Dr. Jenny Chang-Claude)

1991 Falcon Prize (Dr. Petra Boukamp and Dr. Rudolf Leube); Natural Sciences Prize of the Fritz Winter Foundation (Prof. Dr. Ingrid Grummt); 1991 Kind Philipp Prize for Pediatric-Oncological Research (Prof. Dr. Peter Krammer, together with an external clinician); 1991 Karl Freudenberg Prize (Dr. Peter Lichter); INSTAND Sponsorship Prize of the Institute for Standardization and Documentation and 1991 Ernst Krokowski Prize (Priv.-Doz. Dr. Dr. Ulrich Abel, Tumor Center Heidelberg/Mannheim); 1991 Ludolf Krehl Prize of the Society for Internal Medicine of Southwest Germany (Dr. Thomas Efferth); Sponsorship Prize of the Bavarian Gastroenterological Society (Dr. Martin Volkmann, shared equally with two other external scientists); 1991 Philips Prize of the German Society for Medical Physics (Dr. Gunnar Brix)

1992 Aronson Prize (Prof. Dr. Stefan C. Meuer); 1992 German Cancer Prize for Experimental Research (Prof. Dr. Rudolf Preußmann and Prof. Dr. Manfred Schwab); 1992 Farmitalia Carlo Erba Prize (Prof. Dr. Walter Jens Zeller, together with three external scientists); 1992 Ernst Derra Prize of the German Society for Thoracic, Cardiac, and Vascular Surgery (Priv.-Doz. Dr. Hans-Peter Meinzer, together with an external clinician); 1992 Scientific Prize of the German Society for Human Genetics (Dr. Peter Lichter); 1992 Sponsorship Prizes of the Society for the Promotion of Molecular-Biological Research (Dr. Jan Michael Peters and Dr. Thomas Höger); 1992 Ruprecht Karls Prize of the University of Heidelberg (Dr. Jenny Chang-Claude); 1992 Premio Sebetia Ter Prize of the Sebetia Ter Center for Art and Culture and Beijerinck Virology Medal of the Royal Dutch Academy of Arts (Prof. Dr. Harald zur Hausen); 1st Ludolf Krehl Prize of the Society for Internal Medicine (Dr. Wilfried Hefter); Dr. Alfredo Jacob Prize of the Argentinean Society for the Pathology of the Genitals and Colposcopy (Dr. Thomas Kahn, together with Argentinean colleagues)

1993 Clinical Research Award of the Federation of European Cancer Societies (Prof. Dr. Harald zur Hausen); 1993 Philips Prize for Medical Physics and Sponsorship Prize of the German Ultrasound Society (Dr. Dr. Jürgen Debus); 1993 Robert Koch Prize (Prof. Dr. Hans-Georg Rammensee, one half); Olympus Prize of the Olympus Europe Foundation "Science for Life" (Priv.-Doz. Hans-Peter Meinzer); 1993 Varian Poster Prize of the German Society for Medical Physics (Knut Jöchle); 1993 Scientific Sponsorship Prize of the Heidelberg Association for Natural History and Medicine (Dr. Markus Freyaldenhoven); Scientific Prize for Medical Research of the Smith Kline Beecham Foundation (Priv.-Doz. Dr. Peter Gierschik); 1993 Friedrich Weygand Prize (Dr. Stefan Stevanovic); 1993 Amersham Buchler Prize (Dr. Dirk Bosse meyer); 1993 Poster Prize of the German X-Ray Society (Dr. Peter Peschke and Dr. Frederik Wenz)

In 1991, Prof. Dr. Harald zur Hausen was awarded an honorary doctorate by the Northern Swedish University of Umeå. In the same year, he was elected Vice President of the biomedical section of the Academia Europaea and made an honorary member of the Scientific Medical Society of Virology in Sofia, Bulgaria. In 1992, the Hungarian Cancer Society made Prof. zur Hausen an honorary member. He was also admitted as an honorary member to what was then the Czechoslovakian Microbiological Society. In 1993, Prof. zur Hausen was elected President of the European Organization of Cancer Institutes (OECI). Furthermore, in 1993, he was made a corresponding member of the Academia Nacional de Medicina in Caracas, Venezuela.

In 1991, Prof. Dr. Stefan C. Meuer was appointed to the organizing committee of the "Center for Molecular Medicine" in Berlin-Buch and to the advisory board "Oncology" of the State of Baden-Württemberg. In 1992, he was elected spokesman of the Heidelberg Transplantation Center.

Prof. Dr. Günther Schütz was admitted as a member of the Academia Europaea in 1991.

In 1991, Prof. Dr. Jürgen Wahrendorf was appointed to the organizing committee of the Institute for Nutrition in Potsdam-Rehbrücke. In 1993, he was appointed a member of the Bremen Institute for Prevention Research and Social Medicine.

In 1991, Priv.-Doz. Dr. Martin Berger was made an honorary member of the Brazilian Society for Hematology and Hemotherapy.

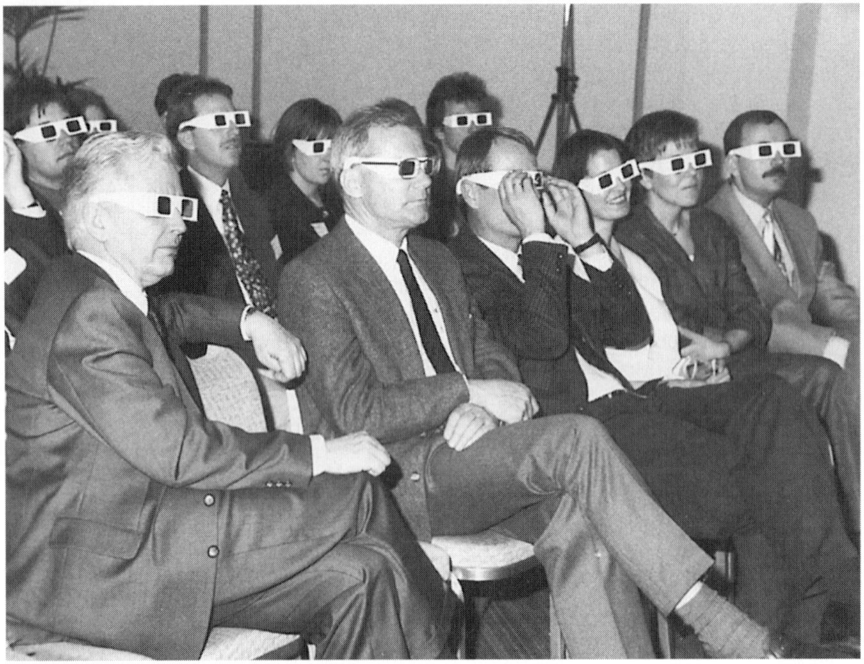

Fig. 88
The spatial structure of protein kinases, the research area of Dr. Dirk Bossemeyer, can be made visible with the help of 3-D glasses. Dr. Bossemeyer was awarded the 1993 Amersham Buchler Prize and is seen here giving his talk on the occasion of the presentation of the prize

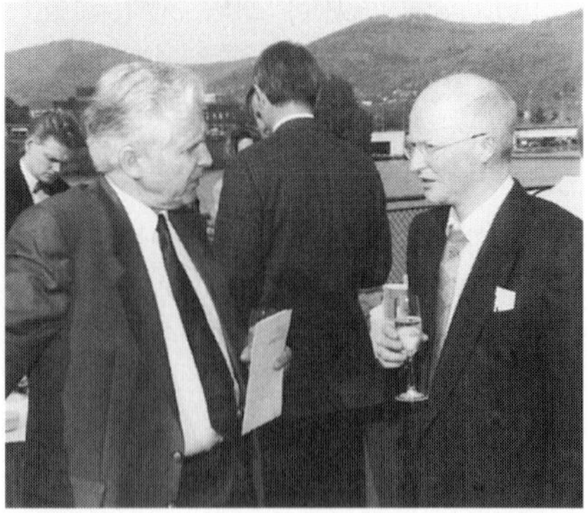

Fig. 89
Prof. Dr. Harald zur Hausen, Scientific Member of the Management Board of the Deutsches Krebsforschungszentrum, talking to the prize-winner after the presentation (on the right)

In 1991, Prof. Dr. Norbert Fusenig was elected Chairman of the Society for Cell and Tissue Culture for a 3-year term.

Prof. Dr. Volker Schirrmacher was elected President of the Metastasis Research Society in 1991. In 1993, he joined the editorial board of the International Journal of Oncology.

In 1991, Dr. Lutz Edler was elected Scientific Secretary of the International Association for Statistical Computing (IASC).

Priv.-Doz. Dr. Regine Heilbronn received a Heisenberg grant from the German Research Association (DFG) in 1992.

In 1993, Prof. Dr. Klaus Frieder Munk was awarded the Order of Merit of the Federal Republic of Germany.

Prof. Dr. Wolfgang Schlegel was appointed an honorary member of the Hungarian Radiotherapy Society in 1993.

Prof. Dr. Gustav Wagner was named an honorary member of the German Medical Specialist and Professional Press Association in 1993.

Dr. Maria Blettner was elected a member of the advisory board of the German International Biometrical Society and appointed representative of the Biometrical Society for the German work group "Epidemiology".

Prof. Dr. Lutz Gissmann was admitted as a corresponding member to the Mexican Academy of Sciences.

Former divisional heads

Between 1991 and 1993, a number of division heads of the Deutsches Krebsforschungszentrum retired or were given emeritus status. Nearly all members of the generation which has represented the Center since it was founded in 1964 and which laid the basis for and continuously developed its research program over many years will have retired by the year 2000. In the past few years this applied to Prof. Dr. Ernst Weber, Division of Biostatistics within the former Institute for Documentation, Informatics, and Statistics (1990), Prof. Dr. Klaus Munk, Division of Human Tumor Viruses, former director of the Institute for Viral Research (1993), Prof. Dr. Hans Osswald, Division of Experimental Chemotherapy, former Institute for Toxicology and Chemotherapy, Prof. Dr. Klaus Goerttler, Division of Pathomorphology, former director of the Institute for Experimental Pathology, and Prof. Dr. Rudolf Preussmann, Division of Environmental Carcinogens within the former Institute for Toxicology and Chemotherapy (all 1993). In 1994, Prof. Petre Tautu, Division of Mathematical Models, previously within the Institute for Documentation, Informatics, and Statistics, retired.

The aims and tasks of the divisions were redefined. In the case of several divisions it has already been possible to appoint new heads (cf. "Evaluation of results and research focuses, new divisions and project groups").

Two new division heads have received invitations to accept a professorship elsewhere: Priv.-Doz. Dr. Peter Gierschik, head of the new Division of Molecular Pharmacology, has accepted a professorship at Ulm University; Dr. Heinz D. Osiewacz, head of the Division of Molecular Biology of Aging has taken on a new task at the University of Frankfurt. Prof. Dr. Margot Zöller, head of the Division of Tumor Progression and Immune Defense has accepted a professorship at Karlsruhe Technical University; however, she will continue her research work at the Deutsches Krebsforschungszentrum.

Prizes awarded by the Deutsches Krebsforschungszentrum

Three prizes for exceptional achievements in the field of cancer research or early detection of cancer are awarded in cooperation with the Deutsches Krebsforschungszentrum.

Since, 1981, the Wilhelm and Maria Meyenburg Foundation has awarded the Meyenburg Prize for outstanding accomplishments in cancer research. The prize is endowed with DM 30000. In addition, the board of the foundation supports research visits by scientists from Germany and abroad to the Deutsches Krebsforschungszentrum as well as research projects of scientists from the Deutsches Krebsforschungszentrum and the facilities cooperating with them.

In 1992, the Meyenburg Prize was awarded to Prof. Dr. Walter Birchmeier, professor for molecular cell biology at the university hospitals in Essen. He was awarded the prize for research that led to a better understanding of the molecular mechanisms of metastasis. Among other things, Birchmeier and his group succeeded in characterizing a molecule called E-cadherin, which is responsible for the adhesion of tumor cells to one another. If this molecule is missing, tumor cells are capable of leaving the cell aggregate and forming metastases elsewhere in the body. On the basis of this knowledge new therapies can be developed with the aim, for example, of using viruses to insert the blueprints of E-cadherin into tumor cells so as to prevent metastasis.

In 1993, Dr. Johannes Gerdes from the Institute for Experimental Biology of the Bostel Research Institute was awarded the Meyenburg Prize for his outstanding work on the molecular basis of cell division. Johannes Gerdes and his coworkers have discovered a monoclonal antibody, Ki-67, which reacts exclusively with the cell nuclei of dividing cells. A knowledge of the proportion of cells that are dividing at a given moment is of enormous importance for the treatment of cancer. Without any inconvenience to the patients it is thus possible to gain medically valuable additional information which helps to improve therapy planning.

The Walther and Christine Richtzenhain Prize is awarded annually by the Deutsches Krebsforschungszentrum for contributions to the field of experimental cancer research. It is awarded alternately to PhD students from research facilities in Heidelberg and to scientists from all over Germany. It is endowed with up to DM 15000 and is financed from the estate of Walther and Christine Richtzenhain.

The winner of the 1991 prize was the Mexican guest scientist Vianney Ortiz-Navarrete, who is working in the Division of Somatic Genetics at the Deutsches Krebsforschungszentrum. In cooperation with Prof. Dr. Peter Klötzel from the Molecular Biology Center of Heidelberg University (Zentrum für Molekulare Biologie, ZMBH), he discovered the genes responsible for "cutting through" exogenous proteins. This process is of central importance for triggering immune reactions in the body. The results open up a new dimension in the search for the causes of genetically determined immunological diseases in humans.

Dr. Thomas Metz of the European Molecular Biology Laboratory was the winner of the Richtzenhain Prize in 1993.

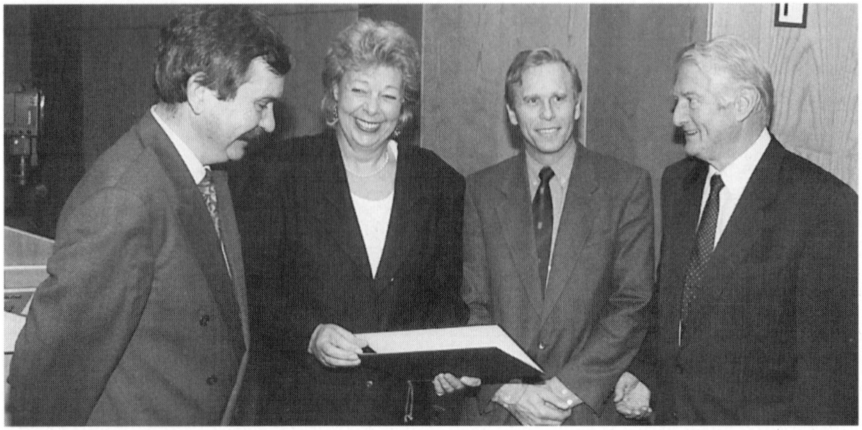

Fig. 90
Presentation of the 1993 Meyenburg Prize to Priv.-Doz. Dr. Johannes Gerdes (left) by Dr. Marion Meyenburg. On the right is Prof. Dr. Klaus Munk, long-standing member of the board of the Meyenburg Foundation. The laudation was made by Prof. Dr. Harald Stein of the Pathological Institute of the Steglitz University Hospitals (second from the right)

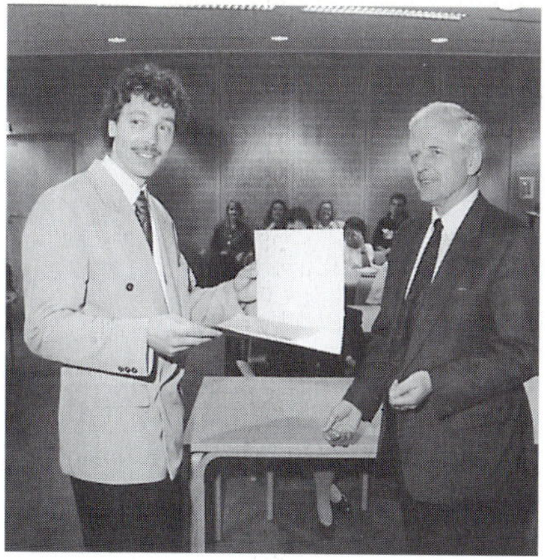

Fig. 91
Dr. Thomas Metz of the European Molecular Biology Laboratory was awarded the Richtzenhain Prize in 1993 by Prof. Dr. Harald zur Hausen

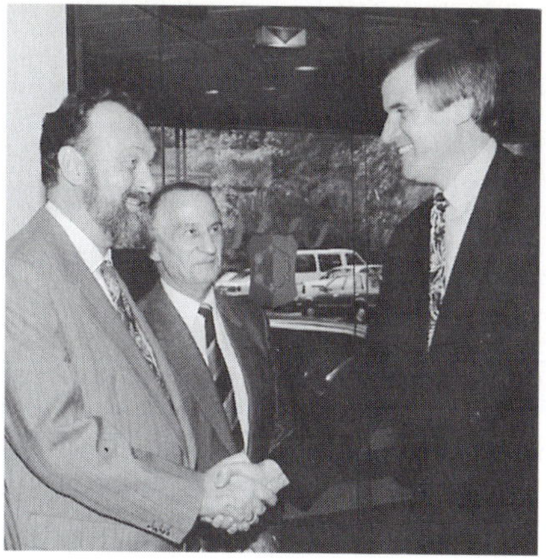

Fig. 92 a
The German Minister of Health Horst Seehofer congratulating the winners of the 1992 Ernst von Leyden prize for early cancer detection: Dr. Joachim Geiling (left) and Prof. Dr. Günter Möbius (center) from Schwerin

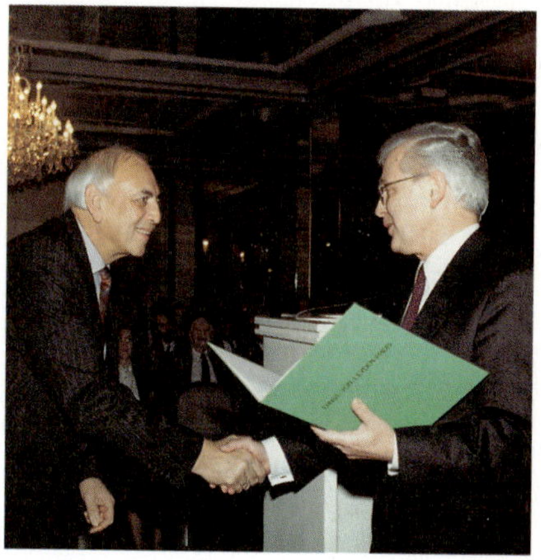

Fig. 92 b
Prof. Dr. Harald zur Hausen congratulating the medical journalist Dr. h. c. Hans Mohl on winning the Ernst von Leyden Price in 1994

He received the prize for his PhD thesis, in which he examined the interactions between various cancer-causing genes (oncogenes).

Since 1990, the Deutsches Krebsforschungszentrum has awarded the Ernst von Leyden Prize every two years as an encouragement and a reward for outstanding activities in the field of early cancer detection. The prize, which is donated by the company Procter & Gamble Pharmaceuticals Germany GmbH, formerly Röhm Pharma GmbH, is endowed with DM 20 000. Its presentation is supervised by the Press and Public Relations Department of the Deutsches Krebsforschungszentrum.

The 1992 prize was shared equally by Prof. Dr. Günter Möbius, director of the Pathological Institute of Schwerin Clinics until 1991, and to Dr. Joachim Geiling, head of the Department for Gynecological Cytodiagnostics of the Pathological Institute in Schwerin. Under the most difficult circumstances and thanks to a strong personal commitment, the two pathologists managed to raise the rate of women participating in cytological early detection examinations in what is today Mecklenburg-Vorpommern from 1.5 percent in 1965 to 53 percent in 1989 (of females aged 20 and above). Thanks to the intensified examination of cytosmears about 90 000 preparations were checked by the Pathological Institute every year, the number of invasive cervical tumors has decreased from 130 in 1968 to 56 in 1988. While in 1968, 39 women in 100 000 developed a late stage of this cancer, in 1988 there were only 18 such cases.

The prize is named after the physician Ernst von Leyden (1832–1919), who was for many years chairman of the German Central Committee for Cancer Research and director of the 1st Clinic for Internal Medicine of the Charité in Berlin. He is regarded as a pioneer of cancer research in Germany.

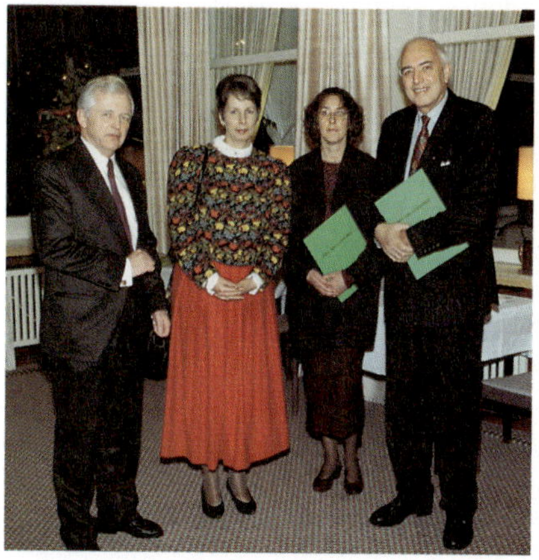

Fig. 92 c
The winners of the 1994 Ernst von Leyden Prize: Hans Mohl and Helga Ebel (second from the right), together with Dr. Sabine Bergmann-Pohl, Parliamentary Secretary of the German Ministry of Health, and Prof. Dr. Harald zur Hausen

Publications

The results of the scientific work of the Deutsches Krebsforschungszentrum are published on a regular basis in the listing "Veröffentlichungen aus dem Deutschen Krebsforschungszentrum". By the end of 1993, the Center's scientists had published a total of 11 342 scientific articles. Out of these, 7 238 were published in scientific journals, 1 121 were diploma theses, dissertations and habilitations, and 510 were books and articles in handbooks that appeared in 1990, 1991, 1992, and 1993.

These publications are supplemented by thousands of lectures held at scientific congresses and for the interested general public.

The listing is published every year and can be ordered by any interested party.

It is the task of the Center's Departement of Press and Public Relations to make the results of the research known to the general public and to explain its significance in the prevention, the early detection, and the therapy of cancer. The Department maintains permanent contacts with all media and with interested citizens (see the article on Press and Public Relations).

Detailed information on the research activities is provided by the "Research Report" of the Deutsches Krebsforschungszentrum. The current issue 1992/93 was published in 1994.

International and National Collaboration

The integration of the research activities of the Deutsches Krebsforschungszentrum into international research concepts is documented by the high percentage (approx. 50%) of joint publications with scientists from other research institutes in Germany and abroad. The research program of the Deutsches Krebsforschungszentrum comprises cooperation with researchers from a total of 29 countries. On the national level there is cooperation with more than 30 universities and 70 other research institutes. The cooperation with the University of Heidelberg is centered around the joint clinical-experimental projects within the Heidelberg/Mannheim Tumor Center. By 1994, this cooperation could look back on 14 years of history. Of special interest in the field of fundamental research is the collaboration within the special research programs of the Deutsche Forschungsgemeinschaft, namely, the special research program Nr. 229 “Molecular mechanisms of gene expression and differentiation”.

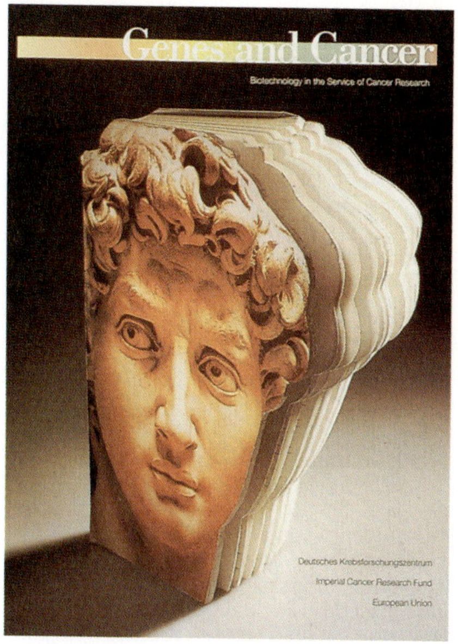

Fig. 93
Cover page of the special issue of the journal “einblick” entitled “Genes and Cancer”, which was published in cooperation with the Imperial Cancer Research Fund, London, in 1994

The excellent international standing of the Center is confirmed by the frequency of citations from publications of the Deutsches Krebsforschungszentrum in international specialist journals and by reports on the Center in the American, French, and Italian specialist press. Evenin the journalistic area it was possible to realize a cooperation with financial support of the European Union: a joint edition of the Center's journal “einblick” with the Imperial Cancer Research Fund (ICRF) in London (einblick 4/93), which also appeared as a brochure both in German (“Gene und Krebs”) and English (“Genes and Cancer”).

The long-standing cooperations with scientists in the United States, Japan, Israel, France, and many other countries were intensified. The establishment of a work unit of the French research organization INSERM (Institut de la Santé et de la Recherche Médicale) at the Center in 1993 bears witness to the increasing attraction of the Center for international cooperations (cf. “New divisions and project groups”). Further support for this claim is provided by the large number of guest scientists visiting the Center for a prolonged stay (168 reseacrhers in 1993).

On the national level the founding of the “Association for Clinical-Biomedical Research” (“Verbund Klinisch-Biomedizinische Forschung”) has marked an important step in strenghthening clinically oriented research efforts in research insitutions outside the universities.

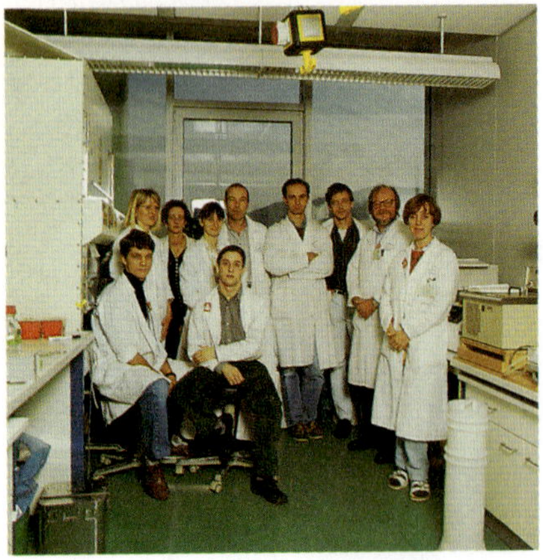

Fig. 94
The working group of the French research organization INSERM at the Deutsches Krebsforschungszentrum. In the center (fifth from the right), its head Prof. Dr. Jean Rommelaere

Collaboration on the basis of bilateral agreements with other countries has been continued and intensified as well. The cooperation with the United States is based on the "Memorandum of Understanding" with the American National Cancer Institute (NCI) in Bethesda, Maryland. The agreement concluded with the National Council of Research and Development (NCRD) in Israel has secured 12 years of highly successful scientific cooperation with scientists in various Israeli research institutions, including the Ben Gurion University, Tel Aviv University, the Hebrew University of Jerusalem, the Weizmann Institute of Science, the Technicon in Haifa and the Hadassah University Medical Hospital in Jerusalem. Close contacts have also been established in the field of administration, in particular with the Weizmann Institute, which has lead to the dispatch of delegations from Israel and from Germany, as well as to an intensive exchange of administrative solutions, which is continually carried on.

The research program agreed upon with the Tanzania Tumor Centre in Dar es Salam comprises projects in molecular biology, epidemiology, and clinical research. On the organizational, technical, and humanitarian levels this cooperation is supported by the society "Tanzania Tumor Support" whose members are scientists from the Deutsches Krebsforschungszentrum and other citizens of Heidelberg. The society provides help for the Tanzania Tumour Centre in the form of regular donations of scientific and medical instruments, by providing technical equipment and staff training at the Deutsches Krebsforschungszentrum, as well as by collecting clothes and money.

Direct contacts between scientists from different nations continue to be a characteristic feature of the research work. Official agreements are particularly supportive when there is a question of the use of special funds.

International Scientific Exchange

Science needs the exchange of ideas and it profits substantially from the discussion with guest scientists. This is true particularly for cancer research which is concerned with nearly all fields of medicine and most fields of natural science.

On the one hand, the research stays for a limited time give the guests an insight into certain lines of research and enables them to learn techniques in which scientists of the Deutsches Krebsforschungszentrum are preeminent. On the other hand, they serve to recruit scientists with specific know-how, with which they can rationally complement the scientific work at the Deutsches Krebsforschungszentrum.

A further objective of international collaboration is the development and implementation of joint projects and programs in the field of cancer research.

The figures of recent years impressively show the intensity of international and national collaboration in the Deutsches Krebsforschungszentrum:

In 1991, 1992, and 1993, a total of 489 guest scientists from 40 different countries worked at the Deutsches Krebsforschungszentrum.

In addition to internal grants and scholarship programs the guest scientists were supported by the following organizations:

German Academic Exchange Service (DAAD)

Humboldt Foundation

German Research Association (DFG)

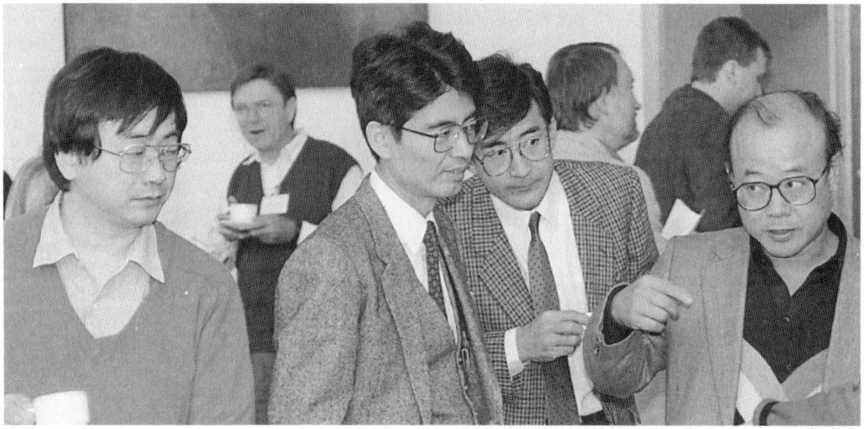

Fig. 95
Scientists from Japan at one of the regular German-Japanese workshops

Study Foundation of the German Nation

Meyenburg Foundation

European Molecular Biology Organization

NATO

Council of Europe

Catholic Academic Exchange Service

Konrad Adenauer Foundation.

Furthermore, there is an active international and national collaboration.

In the guest houses of the Center in Heidelberg, 41 completely fitted residential units (one-room to three-room apartments) are available for the guest scientists.

In view of the intensive international research contacts the guest houses are still completely used to capacity. Thus, they still cover their costs.

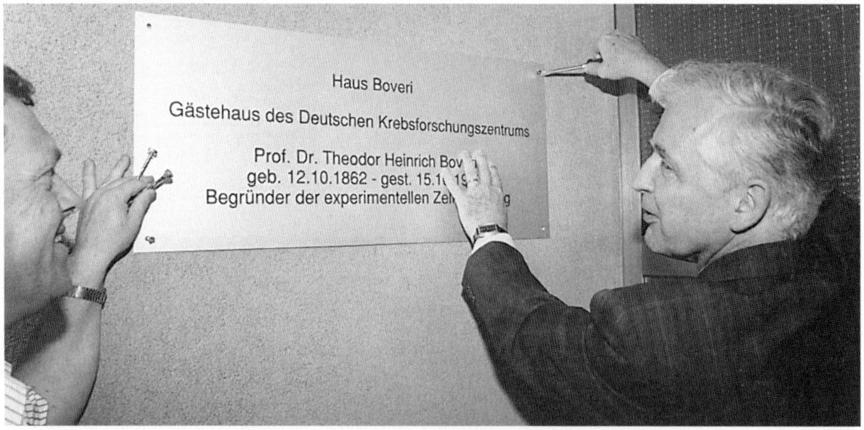

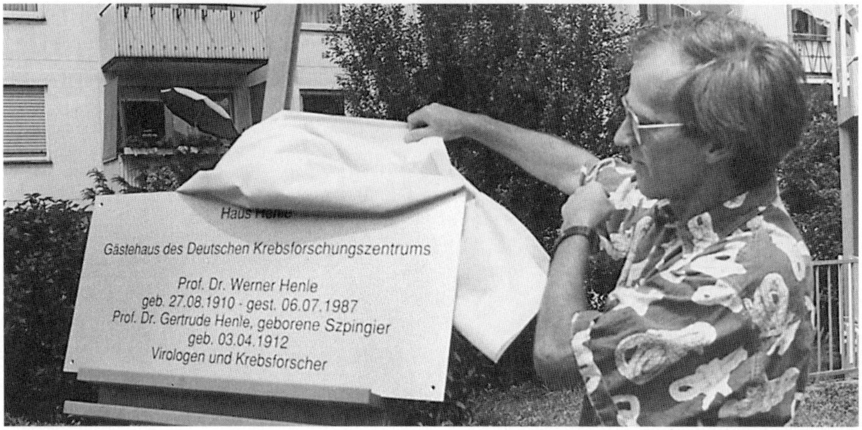

Fig. 96, 97
The apartment houses for guests of the Deutsches Krebsforschungszentrum, "Haus Boveri" and "Haus Henle," were named after prominent scientists. Prof. Dr. Harald zur Hausen affixes the name plaque to the wall of "Haus Boveri"; Prof. Dr. Günter Hämmerling, chairman of the committee for guest scientists' affairs unveils the plaque for "Haus Henle" (below)

Twenty Years of Successfull German-Israeli Cooperation in Cancer Research

Collaboration in cancer research between the Deutsches Krebsforschungszentrum and research establishments in Israel was initiated in 1976. It covers many different aspects of cancer and is based upon a treaty between the Deutsches Krebsforschungszentrum and the National Council for Research and Development (NCRD) in Israel as the immediate partner organizations. During the past nearly 20 years this treaty was transposed successfully from its paper form into vivid scientific reality. The scientific program is verified by common projects, usually composed of one Israeli subproject and one subproject from the Krebsforschungszentrum. They have cooperated actively for three years. If desired thematically, in singular cases also a competent partner from the University of Heidelberg or from another German university may join in. So far nine Israeli research establishments of excellence in medical research and in science were engaged in the cooperational program, each by a number of subprojects: Ben-Gurion University, Beer-Sheva; The Hebrew University of Jerusalem; Technion, Haifa; Tel-Aviv University; The Weizmann Institut of Science, Rehovot; Hadassah Medical Center, Jerusalem; Ichilov Hospital, Tel-Aviv; Kaplan Hospital, Rehovot; Sheba Medical Center, Tel-Hashomer.

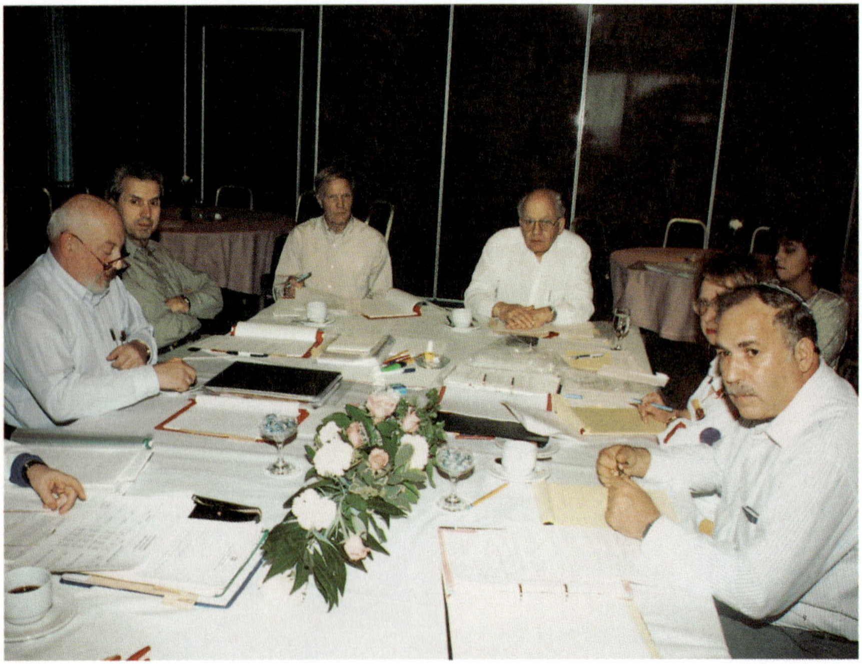

Fig. 98
Scientists from Israel and Germany at a joint workshop in Tel Aviv in 1994

The cooperational program is advised and evaluated in detail by a Scientific Program Committee. It consists of eight members, namely six independent scientists and a Program Coordinator from each of the partner organizations. Of the scientific members three are appointed by the NCRD from Israel and three by the Deutsches Krebsforschungszentrum from among the international scientific community. The committee operates along the outlines of its "Temporary procedures to generate common projects". These summarize important and proven rules to be of assistance in the development of common projects, from the announcement of Priority Topics up to approval and conclusion of a project. Several thematically related projects constitute a project group under a common priority topic. The latter are proposed by the Krebsforschungszentrum, discussed and approved by the Program Committee, and advertised in Israel and in the Center.

Out of the presently running 13 projects six belong to the priority topics below which are considered basic research:

1 "Role of growth factors, hormones and signaling cascades in cell-specific gene regulation"
2 "Gene control of cell proliferation, differentiation and tumorigenesis."

Previous project groups dealt with patient-related priority topics:

1 "Epidemiology (Case-control-studies, cancer registries, biochemical epidemiology)"
2 "Recurrence and progression of adenomatous polyps: an epidemiological model for prevention of colorectal cancer."

The Program Committee meets annually, alternatively in Israel and Germany, and makes site visits and evaluations of ongoing subprojects in the partner country. These activities are fortified by the annual and concluding reports of the projects. Also during Program Committee Meetings, numerous applications for new projects, preselected after external scientific evaluation, are analyzed and discussed. Out of them, actual projects are selected and approved according to their scientific merit.

Preferentially, the cooperational program lives from and by the personal contacts between the participating Israeli and German scientists. They are verified under the roof of the project by common bench work and by exchange of experience and knowledge during mutual visits in Israel and in Germany. Moreover, every third year a common Workshop ("Status-seminar") takes place to report to the plenum (of the members of the program committee and of the scientists of the projects) current results of all ongoing projects and to discuss and evaluate them critically. The 6th Workshop of the cooperational program in combination with the 17th Program Committee Meeting took place in 1994 in Tel Aviv, Israel.

At the beginning of this cooperational program a certain "fear of contact" was prevalent among the participating Israeli and German scientists. With increasing time and numbers of projects the individual contacts became more intimate; today they often lead to lasting friendships between scientists from the two countries. Simultaneously, also the scientific quality of the common projects increased steadily with the years. Altogether the cooperational program has so far granted 62 common projects. Forty-nine of them have concluded and 13 projects are currently underway. By the end of 1991, 266 publications had resulted out of common projects. Many of them were co-authored by the Israeli and German partners and were accepted for publication by scientific journals of worldwide prestige, such as, e.g., Cancer Research, Carcinogenesis, Cell, European Journal of Immunology, The EMBO Journal (European Molecular Biology Organization), Journal of Cancer, Journal of Biological Chemistry, and Journal of Immunology.

In various areas of cancer research remarkable achievements were made, specifically in investigations of the molecular-genetic basis of cancerogenesis, in immunobiology of cancer, in the role of growth factors, of oncogenes and tumor suppressor genes. Also, important insights were gained into the interaction of cancer cells with their surrounding matrix and into their motility. As one of the highlights resulting from the cooperational program a phenomenon may be mentioned which proved to become particularly important: it is the induction of so-called "gene amplification" by chemical risk factors of cancer of the tumor initiator type, but not by such risk factors of the tumor promoter type. A comparable induction of gene amplification was shown to take place also by virus of the herpes group, vaccina- and adenovirus. This phenomenon was worked out in a particularly impressive way during the period 1986–1988 within the common project of Dr. Sara Lavi and co-workers from University of Tel Aviv and Dr. Jörg R. Schlehofer and co-workers from Deutsches Krebsforschungszentrum, Heidelberg. In addition to investigations of the mechanism of DNA amplification also the inhibition of cancerogen- and virus-induced gene amplification by (tumor inhibitory) adeno-associated Parvovirus were integrated in the studies. The results of the project have contributed enormously to stimulate wordwide new investigational approaches to study cancerogenesis induced by chemical and viral risk factors by means of techniques of molecular biology. They permit to experimentally challenge for the first time the fundamental so-called "somatic gene mutation hypothesis of cancerogenesis" postulated about 60 years ago. This may eventually allow to develop the theory further and to specify it in mechanistic terms.

The success of this cooperational program has demonstrated clearly that the mutual stimulation of ideas, the exchange of novel technologies as well as of freshly developed methodologies, together with common manual work on the spot by national talents can expand the capabilities of the individual scientific partners to achieve high-ranking goals: truly, one plus one can equal more than two.

Prof. Dr. Erich Hecker
Coordinator of the German-Israeli Cooperation and deputy chairman of the Program Committee

Tumor Center Heidelberg/Mannheim

The Tumor Center Heidelberg/Mannheim was founded in 1979 with the aim of bringing together the large hospitals and research centers in the Heidelberg area to form an interdisciplinary cooperative association.

Even earlier, in 1966, an Oncological Working Group was founded in Heidelberg, and this was followed, in 1973, by the initiation of a similar enterprise in Mannheim.

Both cancer therapy and cancer research have a long tradition in Heidelberg. As early as the turn of this century, the surgeon Vincenz Czerny introduced intraoperative radiation therapy, and, in 1906, Heidelberg was the location of the first international cancer congress, also organized by Czerny. He also founded the interdisciplinary cancer research institute, inspired by the similar institutes already existing in Moscow (Morosow Institute) and in Buffalo/USA (Roswell Park Memorial Institute). Finally, K.H. Bauer, director of the Heidelberg University Surgical Hospital from 1941 to 1964, took the initiative in creating the Deutsches Krebsforschungszentrum, a public foundation of the State of Baden-Württemberg, and later a National and State Research Center.

The Tumor Center Heidelberg/Mannheim is a collaboration between the University Hospitals in Heidelberg, the Thorax Clinic in Heidelberg-Rohrbach, the medical faculty of Heidelberg University in the Mannheim City Hospital, and the Deutsches Krebsforschungszentrum. In addition to its main concern of ensuring the best possible treatment and care of tumor patients in the hospitals and in the region, the Tumor Center has taken up the challenge of translating the research results achieved at the Deutsches Krebsforschungszentrum into clinical practice. This aim is served by interdisciplinary clinical/fundamental-scientific research projects. Cooperations with other tumor centers and special oncological institutions in Baden-Württemberg are also being increasingly developed. A basis for this was provided by the Cancer Association of Baden-Württemberg, which, with its annual conferences (Association of Tumor Centers and Specialist Oncological Institutions, Baden-Württemberg – ATO) offered an additional opportunity for the exchange of experience and information.

The running of the Tumor Center Heidelberg/Mannheim is in the hands of the Steering Committee. This consists of 14 members who represent the contractual partners, i.e., the University Hospitals of Heidelberg and Mannheim, the Thorax Clinic Heidelberg-Rohrbach, and the Deutsches Krebsforschungszentrum, along with practicing doctors, and the chairpersons of the two Oncological Working Groups Heidelberg and Mannheim. The Steering Committee decides upon the main areas of activity of the Tumor Center. It is supported by an advisory council comprising doctors and scientists along with representatives from industry and public affairs. The chairman of the Steering Committee is Prof. Christian Herfarth, who also heads the coordination and administrative office.

The main emphases of the work of the Tumor Center are in the following areas:

1. Clinical Oncology:

1.1 Coordination and regulation of the care of cancer patients (in part via the Oncological Working Groups)

1.2 Planning and coordination of continuing and further education

1.3 Organization of the hospitals' internal cancer registers

2. Planning and organization of collaborative research projects

1. Clinical Oncology

Within the domain of caring for patients with malignant diseases, the Oncological Working Groups play a decisive role. They form a common forum for the interdisciplinary discussion and collaboration in clinical oncology. They draw up recommendations for the diagnosis and therapy of individual tumors. These are published as guidelines of the Tumor Center. To date, 22 such guidelines dealing with particular tumor forms and general cancer care have appeared within the series of brochures known as the "grüne Reihe" (green series). New editions ensure that the information contained in these works remains up to date. Within the Tumor Center Heidelberg/Mannheim, the recommendations are regarded as binding, although their practical application in individual cases remains the responsibility of the doctor concerned.

The publications which have so far appeared in this series are:

1. "Das Bronchialkarzinom" (The Bronchial Carcinoma), 1st edition 1979 – now replaced by issue No. 8
2. "Gastrointestinale Tumoren" (Gastro-intestinal Tumors), 1st edition Jan. 1981 – replaced by issue Nos. 9, 12, 15, and 17
3. "Malignes Melanom" (Malignant Melanoma), 4th completely revised edition Sept. 1991
4. "Weichteilsarkome im Erwachsenalter" (Soft Tissue Sarcomas in Adults), 4th edition, April 1992

5. "Morbus Hodgkin", 3rd revised edition Dec. 1993
6. "Das Mammakarzinom" (The Mammary Carcinoma), 4th completely revised edition Jan. 1993
7. "Non-Hodgkin-Lymphome" (Non-Hodgkin Lymphomas), 2nd edition July 1985
8. "Die bösartigen Tumoren von Lunge, Pleura und Thymus" (Malignant Tumors of Lung, Pleura, and Thymus), 2nd revised edition Sept. 1991 – new edition of brochure No. 1
9. "Das Pankreaskarzinom" (The Pancreatic Carcinoma), 1st edition Jan. 1986
10. "Das Nierenzellkarzinom" (The Renal Cell Carcinoma), 2nd revised edition June 1991
11. "Das Schilddrüsenkarzinom" (The Thyroid Carcinoma), 2nd revised edition May 1993
12. "Das kolorektale Karzinom" (The Colorectal Carcinoma), 1st edition Jan. 1987
13. "Das Sozialrecht in der medizinischen und sozialen Rehabilitation von Krebskranken" (Social Legislation in the Medical and Social Rehabilitation of Cancer Patients), 3rd revised edition April 1993
14. "Diagnostik und Therapie des Tumorschmerzes" (Diagnosis and Therapy of Tumor-Induced Pain), 2nd revised edition Jan. 1993
15. "Das Magenkarzinom" (The Stomach Carcinoma), 1st edition Jan. 1990
16. "Die bösartigen Tumoren der ableitenden Harnwege" (Malignant Tumors of the Efferent Urinary Tract), 1st edition Dec. 1990
17. "Das Oesophaguskarzinom" (The Esophagus Carcinoma), 1st edition Jan. 1991
18. "Die bösartigen Tumoren der männlichen Geschlechtsorgane" (Malignant Tumors of the Male Genitals), 1st edition June 1991
19. "Hausärztliche Mit- und Nachsorge von Tumorpatienten" (Care and Aftercare of Tumor Patients by the Family Doctor), 1st edition Jan. 1992
20. "Die bösartigen Tumoren der Kopfspeicheldrüsen" (Malignant Tumors of the Salivary Glands), 1st edition July 1992
21. "Das Prostatakarzinom" (The Prostate Carcinoma), 1st edition Nov. 1992
22. "Der geriatrische Tumorpatient" (The Geriatric Cancer Patient), 1st edition March 1993

Brochures in preparation will deal with gynecological and with hypophysial tumors. The brochure on non-Hodgkin lymphomas is presently being revised. These brochures are made available to all cooperating and other interested doctors as a source of diagnostic and therapeutic recommendations. One copy of each brochure can be obtained free of charge from the coordination and administrative office of the Tumor Center Heidelberg/Mannheim, Im Neuenheimer Feld 105/110, D-69120 Heidelberg, Germany, Telephone ++6221/472645, 566558, 566559, FAX ++6221/563094.

Special oncological units at the hospitals of the Tumor Center form certain crystallization points for particular oncological, diagnostic, and therapeutic problems. These units are also responsible for a part of the clinical/fundamental-scientific research coordination. They include:

- the Section for Surgical Oncology at the University Surgical Hospital Heidelberg
- the Department of Internal Medicine V of the Medical Hospital and Out-Patient Clinic of the University of Heidelberg
- the Oncology-Hematology Section of the University Pediatric Hospital Heidelberg
- the Orthopedic-Oncology Section of the Foundation Orthopedic Hospital of the University of Heidelberg
- the Section for Special Oncology of the III Medical Clinic, Oncological Center at Mannheim University Hospitals, and
- the Oncological Department of the Thorax Clinic Heidelberg-Rohrbach of the State Insurance Institution, Baden.

At the clinic for radiation therapy of the Radiological University Hospital the patients almost exclusively comprise cancer sufferers. Other clinical institutions which are also concerned with the treatment of cancer patients cooperate via the Oncological Working Groups and through interdisciplinary discussions.

In 1984, the Psychosocial Aftercare Facility at the Heidelberg University Surgical Hospital was taken over by the State of Baden-Württemberg. It contributes to the aftercare of cancer patients at the University Surgical Hospital, the Universiaty Gynecological Hospital, and the Out-Patient Clinic.

The organization of continuing and further education at the Tumor Center Heidelberg/Mannheim takes place at several different levels:

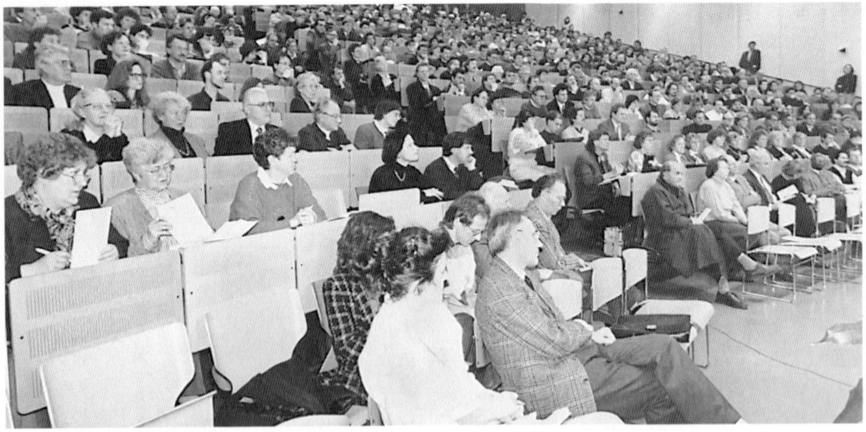

Fig. 99
A continuing education seminar for general practitioners on the topic of breast cancer, organized by the Oncological Working Group of the Tumor Center Heidelberg/Mannheim

The first regular vocational seminars were held by the Psychosocial Aftercare Facility at the University Surgical Hospital in Heidelberg. Doctors, psychologists, nursing staff, and social workers form the target group for this course, which, for the most part, is also supported by the Federal Health Ministry and the Social-Welfare Ministry of Baden-Württemberg.

Continuing and further education for nursing has been offered since the 1980s. With the support of the Federal Health Ministry and the Social-Welfare Ministry of Baden-Württemberg, vocational training courses in oncology were developed for practicing nursing staff. The main topics dealt with are the special demands encountered in nursing care of cancer patients and the psychosocial aspects of this task. A remarkable success achieved by this initiative in 1992 was the recognition of the course by the State of Baden-Württemberg as an approved further education measure. Present efforts are particularly directed towards establishing the specially trained oncological nursing staff as a professional group with corresponding salary scales.

Among the aims specified in the statutes of the Tumor Center is the continued and further education of doctors in oncology. The Tumor Center holds regular advanced training events which are held by the Oncological Working Groups Heidelberg and Mannheim in collaboration with the Academy for Advanced Medical Training of the District Medical Chamber of North Baden. These training events complement the above-mentioned volumes of the "grüne Reihe". They treat particular malignant diseases and organ tumors or topics such as paraneoplastic syndrome, microcarcinoma, special questions relating to chemotherapy, and nutritional problems. The advanced training events have gained wide acceptance from doctors. The topics dealt with most recently were:

Oncological Working Group Heidelberg:

1994 (02.05.): Tumors of the urogenital tract – the state of the art of therapy

1993 (02.06.): Breast cancer – new developments in diagnostics and therapy

1992 (02.01.): Paraneoplastic symptoms and syndromes

Oncological Working Group Mannheim:

1994 (10.15.): Malignant tumors of the hepatobiliary system

1993 (10.16.): New approaches in surgical tumor therapy

1992 (10.17.): Curative chemotherapy

Every 2 years, special advanced courses for family doctors are held in Heidelberg. They address "Oncology for the family doctor – topics relating to prevention, treatment, and aftercare". The last two such events were held on 12.05.92 and 12.03.94.

The tumor documentation at the Tumor Center Heidelberg/Mannheim takes the form of a clinical cancer register, kept separately for each of the three clinical partners. Data protection concerns prevent the maintenance of a central cancer register for the Tumor Center as a whole.

Cooperative Research Projects

In the 1980s the cooperative research projects were oriented towards investigations of individual organ tumors. Since 1992 the main research focus has been on methodological questions. The research projects are organized analogously to a Special Research Program ("Sonderforschungsbereich") and are each headed by two coordinators. One is a representative from clinical science and the other from basic research. In detail, the present research projects are the following:

I. Immunologiocal and molecular-biological approaches in tumor diagnostics

(Coordinators: Prof. Peter Möller, Pathology Institute, University of Heidelberg, and Dr. Gerhard Moldenhauer, Deutsches Krebsforschungszentrum)

Subprojects:

1. Detection of numerical and structural chromosomal aberrations in chronic lymphatic neoplasms by means of classical cytogenetic analysis and non-radioactive in-situ hybridization (Project leaders: Dr. Hartmut Döhner, Department of Internal Medicine V of the Heidelberg University Hospital, and Dr. Peter Lichter, Deutsches Krebsforschungszentrum)

2. Normal and aberrant p-53 gene expression in hepatocellular carcinoma and chronic liver disease in relation to the hepatitis B virus status (Project leaders: Dr. Peter Galle, Department of Internal Medicine IV of the Heidelberg University Hospital and Dr. Martin Volkmann, Deutsches Krebsforschungszentrum)

3. Proliferation- and apoptosis-mediating cell surface molecules in brain tumors (Project leaders: Prof. Marika Kiessling, Pathology Institute, University of Heidelberg, and Prof. H. Peter Krammer, Deutsches Krebsforschungszentrum)

4. Structure and function of adhesion and differentiation molecules on leukemia and lymphoma cells of the B-cell type (Project leaders: Dr. Karin Koretz, Pathology Institute, University of Heidelberg, and Dr. Reinhard Schwartz-Albiez, Deutsches Krebsforschungszentrum)

5. Influence of homing receptor expression on the dissemination of B-cell type lymphomas and the interaction of the intratumoral T cells with the lymphoma cells (Project leaders: Prof. Peter Möller, Pathology Institute, University of Heidelberg, and Prof. Volker Schirrmacher, Deutsches Krebsforschungszentrum)

6. Extrafollicular B lymphocytes and B-cell lymphomas (Project leaders: Prof. Peter Möller, Pathology Institute, University of Heidelberg, and Dr. Peter Lichter, Deutsches Krebsforschungszentrum)

7. Antibody labeling with heavy-metal nuclides: In-vivo labeling with bispecific antibodies / new ligands for immune therapy (Project leaders: Priv.-Doz. Dr. Sepp Kaul, University Gynecological Hospital, Heidelberg, and Dr. Jochen Schuhmacher, Deutsches Krebsforschungszentrum)

II. Biological response modifiers and molecular therapies (Coordinators: Dr. Klaus-Michael Debatin, University Pediatric Hospital, Heidelberg, and Prof. Stefan C. Meuer, Deutsches Krebsforschungszentrum)

Subprojects:

1. Induction of apoptosis in pre-B- and pre-T-cell leukemias in vitro and in vivo (Project leaders: Dr. Klaus-Michael Debatin, University Pediatric Hospital, Heidelberg, and Prof. Peter H. Krammer, Deutsches Krebsforschungszentrum)

2. Molecular basis of abnormal growth control in malignant T lymphocytes (Project leaders: Prof. Stefan Meuer, Deutsches Krebsforschungszentrum, and Priv.-Doz. Dr. Sepp Kaul, University Gynecological Hospital, Heidelberg)

3. Immune response to tumor-associated mucin in breast cancer (Project leaders: Priv.-Doz. Dr. Sepp Kaul, University Gynecological Hospital, Heidelberg, and Prof. Stefan C. Meuer, Deutsches Krebsforschungszentrum)

4. Bispecific hybrid antibodies for the therapy of human lymphatic leukemias and malignant lymphomas of the B-cell type (Project leader: Dr. Gerhard Moldenhauer, Deutsches Krebsforschungszentrum)

5. Biological basis of the action of rHu-TNF-alpha in malignant ascites (Project leaders: Prof. Daniela Männel, University of Regensburg, and Priv.-Doz. Dr. Ulrich Räth, Department of Internal Medicine IV of the Heidelberg University Hospital)

6. Immune therapy of brain tumors (Project leaders: Prof. Stefan Kunze and Dr. Hans-Herbert Steiner, University Neuro-Surgical Hospital, Heidelberg)

7. Effectiveness of active specific immunization (Project leaders: Prof. Peter Schlag, University Surgical Hospital, Heidelberg, and Max-Delbrück Center, Berlin, and Prof. Volker Schirrmacher, Deutsches Krebsforschungszentrum)

III. Loco-regional tumor therapy – research on radiation therapy, including diagnostics (Coordinators: Priv.-Doz. Dr. Rita Engenhart, University Radiological Hospital, Heidelberg, and Prof. Gerhard van Kaick, Deutsches Krebsforschungszentrum)

Subprojects:

1. Photon conformation radiotherapy (Project leaders: Priv.-Doz. Dr. Rita Engenhart, University Radiological Hospital, Heidelberg, and Prof. Wolfgang Schlegel, Deutsches Krebsforschungszentrum)

2. Developments in the field of neutron therapy (Project leaders: Dr. Karl-Heinz Höver, Deutsches Krebsforschungszentrum, and Priv.-Doz. Dr. Rita Engenhart, University Radiological Hospital, Heidelberg)

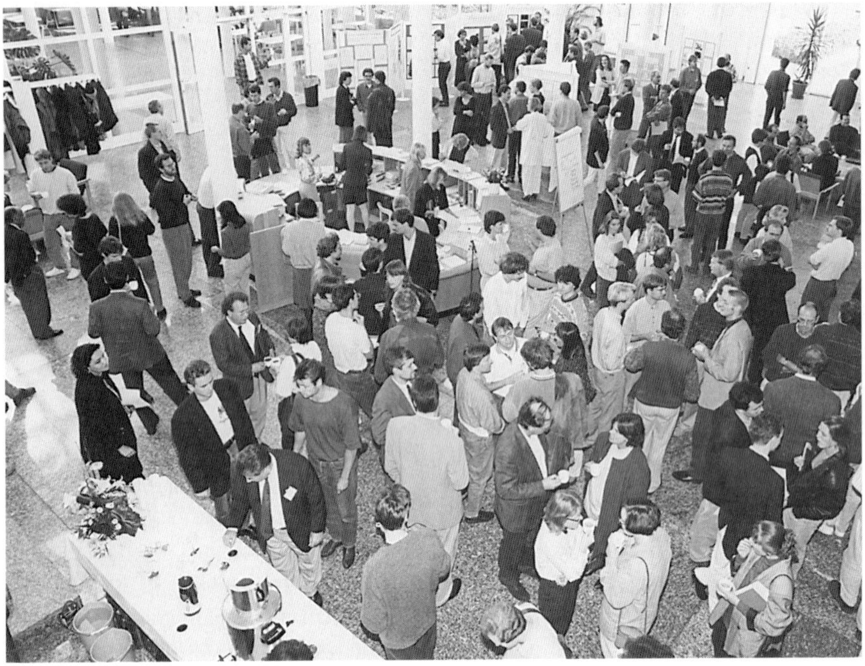

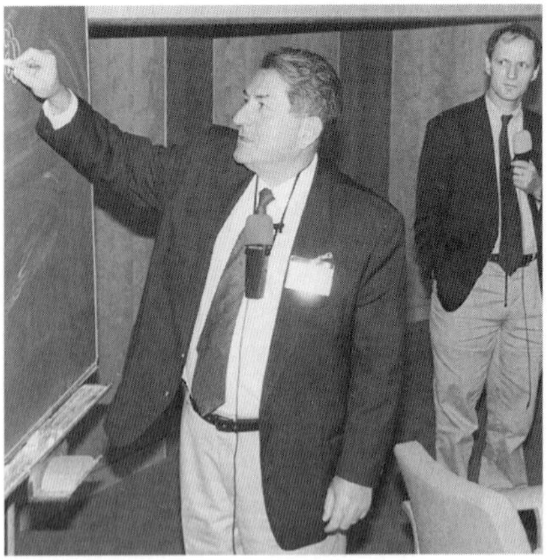

Fig. 100, 101
Symposium of the Association for Clinical-Biomedical Research on the topic of gene diagnosis and gene therapy in 1993 in Heidelberg. The picture shows Prof. Dr. Max Birnstiel of the Research Institute for Molecular Pathology in Vienna during his lecture

3. Carrier-mediated local chemotherapy of malignant brain tumors (Project leaders: Dr. Birgit Eifert, University Neuro-Surgical Hospital, Heidelberg, and Prof. Jens Zeller, Deutsches Krebsforschungszentrum)

4. Functional tumor diagnostics with MRS and MRT (Project leaders: Priv.-Doz. Dr. Rita Engenhart, University Radiological Hospital, Heidelberg, and Dr. Michael Knopp, Deutsches Krebsforschungszentrum)

5. Functional tumor diagnostics with PET (Project leaders Dr. Egbert Hagmüller, Surgical Clinic of the Mannheim City Hospital, and Dr. Uwe Haberkorn, Deutsches Krebsforschungszentrum)

6. The use of lasers in diagnostics and therapy – LIFD and PDT (Project leaders: Prof. Christian Herfarth, University Surgical Hospital, Heidelberg, and Dr. Wolfgang Maier-Borst, Deutsches Krebsforschungszentrum)

IV. Tumor cell heterogeneity, metatasis, and resistance (Coordinators: Prof. Werner Franke, Deutsches Krebsforschungszentrum, and Priv.-Doz. Dr. Thomas Lehnert, University Surgical Hospital, Heidelberg)

Subprojects:

1. Recognition, monitoring, and biological and clinical relevance of cell-type heterogeneity for selected tumors (Project leaders: Prof. Werner Franke, Deutsches Krebsforschungszentrum, and Priv.-Doz. Dr. Ingrid Moll, Skin Clinic of the Mannheim City Hospital)

2. Genetic modifications as markers for heterogeneity, growth behavior, metastasis, and genetic susceptibility of human tumors (Project leader: Dr. Manfred Schwab, Deutsches Krebsforschungszentrum)

3. Growth behavior of chemosensitive and chemoresistant cells in carcinomas that respond to chemotherapy (Project leaders: Prof. Peter Drings, Thorax Hospital, Heidelberg-Rohrbach, and Priv.-Doz. Dr. Christoph Granzow, Deutsches Krebsforschungszentrum)

4. Aromatase expression and tumor growth (Project leader: Prof. Walter Pyerin, Deutsches Krebsforschungszentrum)

5. Molecular-biological investigations of the heterogeneity of gene expression in epithelial tumors and dysplastic lesions (Project leader: Dr. Franz Bosch, Ear,

Nose, and Throat Hospital of the University of Heidelberg)

6. Significance of parathyroid-hormone-related protein as plasma and cell marker in hypercalcemia-inducing tumors (Project leaders: Prof. Werner Franke, Deutsches Krebsforschungszentrum, and Prof. Friedhelm Raue, Department of Internal Medicine I of the Heidelberg University Hospital)

7. Metastasis-specific membrane proteins: Function and diagnostic/therapeutic usefulness (Project leaders: Priv.-Doz. Dr. Wolfgang Tilgen, University Skin Clinic, Heidelberg, and Prof. Margot Zöller, Deutsches Krebsforschungszentrum)

8. Adhesion and glycosylation of metastasizing tumor cells from human biopsy material (Project leader: Priv.-Doz. Dr. Wolfgang Kemmner, Institute of Biochemistry II, University of Heidelberg)

9. Disequilibrium of cathepsins and their inhibitors (Project leaders: Dr. Stefan Riedl, University Surgical Hospital, Prof. Werner Ebert, Thorax Hospital Heidelberg-Rohrbach, and Prof. Eberhard Spiess, Deutsches Krebsforschungszentrum)

The research activities of the Tumor Center decribed here are also partly supplemented by studies that are carried out in collaboration with other tumor centers and research institutes. These include the European Organisation for Research on Treatment of Cancer (EORTC), the Swiss Institute for Applied Cancer Research (SIAK), and the oncological working groups of the German Cancer Society.

Clinical oncology is financed from the budgets of the participating hospitals; prospective oncological research projects are supported by external funding; and the programs of continuing education have, for the last 2 years, been financed by the State of Baden-Württemberg.

The funding of the research activities of the Tumor Center is based on external assessment and is provided for by the budget of the Deutsches Krebsforschungszentrum, supplied in turn by the Federal Ministry for Education, Science, Research and Technology (90%) and the State of Baden-Württemberg (10%).

The running of the coordination and administrative office and its activities is financed by the four contractual partners. The constant up-dating and extension of the book series is made possible in part by donations.

The Association for Clinical-Biomedical Research

The Association for Clinical-Biomedical Research Verbund Klinisch-Biomedizinische Forschung (KBF) was founded in 1992 by five members of the Association of National Research Centers Arbeitsgemeinschaft der Großforschungs-einrichtungen (AGF) engaged in research related to health. The founder members in alphabetical order are:

DKFZ – Stiftung Deutsches Krebsforschungszentrum, Heidelberg

GBF – Gesellschaft für Biotechnologische Forschung mbH, Braunschweig

GSF – GSF-Forschungszentrum für Umwelt und Gesundheit GmbH, München

KFA – Forschungszentrum Jülich GmbH, Jülich

MDC – Stiftung Max-Delbrück-Centrum für Molekulare Medizin, Berlin-Buch

Two more AGF members, the Kerforschungszentrum Karlsruhe (KfK) and the Gesellschaft für Schwerionenforschung mbH Darmstadt (GSI), were admitted in Spring 1993 and in February 1994, respectively. In Fall 1993, the Zentralinstitut für Seelische Gesundheit in Mannheim became an associate member. Thus, the Association now encompasses eight research institutes.

The aim of the Association is to contribute to the improvement of clinically oriented biomedical research by optimizing the quality of relevant research endeavors and specifically supporting joint projects with clinical partners.

The Association has two organs, the Board and the Coordinating Committee, which control its work in close co-operation with each other. The Board consists of the scientific directors of the participating institutes and two members from business. The Coordinating Committee is appointed by the Board and consists of prominent scientific representatives of the respective institutes. Their number depends on the proportion of health-related research in the overall scientific activities of the institute. Currently, the Coordinating Committee consists of 13 members. The Board and the Coordinating Committee usually meet jointly to discuss questions relating to the organization and subject matter of the Association.

Quality optimization is sought mainly by an appropriate appointment policy and an evaluation of the research performed at the member facilities.

The participating research institutes have agreed to admit to their appointment commissions two external members named by the Association. It is thereby hoped that, on the basis of a broad expertise, the candidates best qualified for leading positions will be chosen.

The members of the Association attach great importance to the regular evaluation of their research work by internal and external as a rule internationally staffed expert commissions. The Association endeavors to harmonize the appraisal procedures in the member institutes and to ensure that the best scientists in a particular research area comment on the work done or, if required, give recommendations concerning a reorientation of the work. These evaluations can have a profound influence on the structure and orientation of existing focuses of research. Representatives of the Association always take part in inspections of the member facilities.

Furthermore, the Association tries to undertake a certain coordination of future research efforts, aiming, in particular, to prevent large overlap of the scientific activities.

In addition to the above-mentioned organizational measures aimed at quality optimization, the Association wants to make a contribution to clinical research by specifically supporting cooperation projects between groups from the member facilities and clinical partners preferably university hospitals and by providing funds for working visits of scientifically active clinicians to member facilities. For the duration of their research activity at member institutes, it is planned to compensate the hospitals for the loss of their medical skills.

The Association reports on the work done in annual meetings which are connected with a scientific symposium. The first such symposium was held in Fall 1993 at the Deutsches Krebsforschungszentrum in Heidelberg on the topic “Gene Diagnosis and Gene Therapy”.

Sixteen leading scientists from Europe and the USA gave talks and presented their latest results on the topics “Gene Diagnosis and Identification,” “Gene Delivery Systems,” “Gene Targeting,” and “Gene Therapy.” Research Minister Dr. Paul Krüger was present on the first day. The high attendance more than 300 participants from Europe and overseas bore witness to the great interest in this topic.

In 1994, the symposium, this time on the topic “Genetic Instability and Cancer,” will take place at the GSF-Forschungszentrum für Umwelt und Gesundheit in Neuherberg near Munich.

Organs of the Foundation

As provided by § 7 of its Statutes and Articles, the Foundation has the following organs:

- the Board of Trustees with the Scientific Committee,
- the Management Board, and
- the Scientific Council.

The Board of Trustees

As provided by § 8 of the Statutes and Articles of the Foundation, the Board of Trustees supervises the legality, expediency, and economy of the conduct of the Foundation's transactions. It decides on the aims of research and important research policy and financial affairs of the Foundation. In addition, it determines the principles of management and those governing efficiency control, and it sets up long-term financial plans including programs for development and investment. Normally, the Board of Trustees convenes twice a year.

In the period 1991–1993, the Board of Trustees dealt with the following issues:

- Approval of the new structure of the Deutsches Krebsforschungszentrum.
- Approval of the establishment of the new Research Programs and the nomination of their Coordinators.

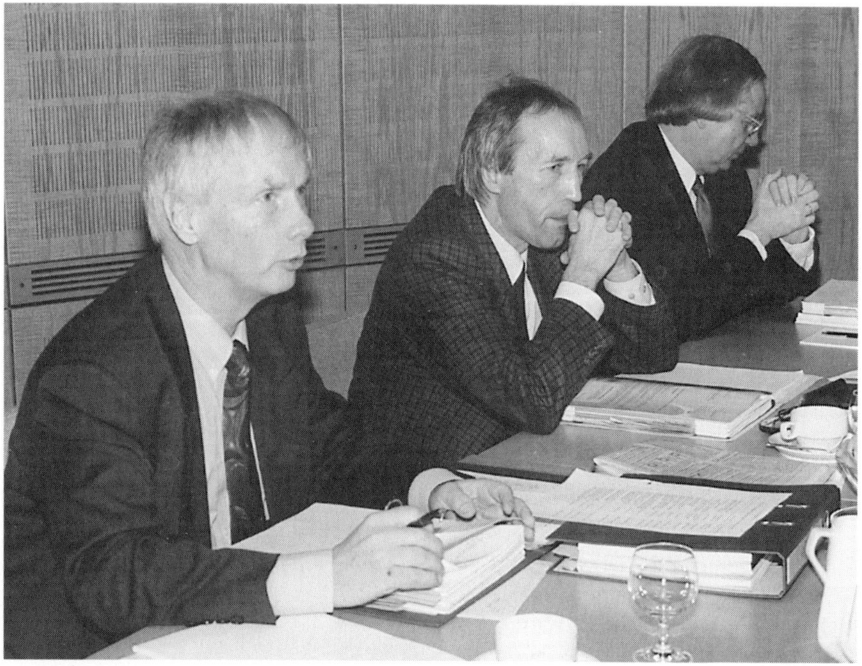

Fig. 102
Meeting of the Board of Trustees and the Scientific Committee of the Deutsches Krebsforschungszentrum. From left to right: MinDirig. Dr. Knut Bauer, Chairman, MinDirig. Dr. Heribert Knorr, Vice Chairman, Dr. Werner Schmidt, Finance Ministry of Baden-Württemberg

- Approval of the establishment of clinical cooperation units on the basis of a general agreement.
- Approval of the foundation of the Association for Clinical-Biomedical Research (Verbund Klinisch-Biomedizinische Forschung, KBF).
- Approval of the report by the Management Board on the present state of affairs and prospects for the future.
- Approval of the establishment of the clinical cooperation unit "Molecular Oncology/Hematology".
- Appointment of Dr. Peter Lichter as head of the division "Organization of Complex Genomes".
- Appointment of Prof. Dr. Hans-Georg Rammensee as head of the division "Tumor-Virus Immunology".
- Appointment of Prof. Dr. Helmut Bartsch as head of the division "Toxicology and Cancer Risk Factors".
- Appointment of Priv.-Doz. Dr. Sandor Suhai as head of the division "Molecular Biophysics I".
- Appointment of Prof. Dr. Herwig Ponstingl as head of the division "Molecular Biology of Mitosis".
- Appointment of Prof. Dr. Thomas Boehm as head of the division "Experimental Therapy".
- Nomination of the Scientific Member and Chairman of the Management Board, Prof. Dr. Dres. h. c. Harald zur Hausen, for another 5-year term.
- Nomination of the Administrative Member of the Management Board, Dr. Reinhard Grunwald, for another 5-year term.
- Nomination of Prof. Dr. Jean Rommelaere as Coordinator of the Research Program "Applied Tumor Virology".

- Conversion of the project "Gene Expression and Cytopathogenicity of the Human Spumaretrovirus" into the division "Retroviral Gene Expression" and appointment of Prof. Dr. Rolf Flügel as its head.
- Conversion of the project "Tolerance and Immune Response" into the division "Tumor Progression and Immune Response" and appointment of Prof. Dr. Margot Zöller as its head.
- Approval of the establishment of the divisions "Virus-Host Interactions" and "Tumor-Virus Characterization" and appointment of Prof. Dr. Claus Hobe Schröder as provisional head of the division "Virus-Host Interactions" and of Priv.-Doz. Dr. Ethel-Michele de Villiers as provisional head of the division "Tumor-Virus Characterization".
- Discussion of the results of the external assessments of
  - the Institute of Biochemistry
  - the Institute of Immunology and Genetics
  - the Division of Applied Tumor Virology
  - the project "Tolerance and Immune Response"
  - the project "Cytogenetics" (second assessment)
  - the Division of Cell Biology (second assessment)
- Approval of the establishment of the division "Molecular Pharmacology" and appointment of Priv.-Doz. Dr. Peter Gierschik as its head.
- Approval of the establishment of the division "Cytogenetics".
- Approval of the establishment of the division "Molecular Biophysics II" and appointment of Prof. Dr. Jörg Langowski as its head.
- Approval of the establishment of the division "Immune Suppression by Viruses" and appointment of Priv.-Doz. Dr. Hans-Georg Kräusslich as its head.
- Approval of the establishment of the division "Molecular Embryology" and appointment of Dr. Christof Niehrs as its head.
- Disbandment of the division "Genetics of Tumor Viruses".
- Disbandment of the division "Mathematical Models".

As provided by § 10 of the Statutes and Articles of the Foundation, the Scientific Committee prepares the decisions of the Board of Trustees in all scientific matters. In particular, it is responsible for the continuous evaluation of the results of the research work by scientific expertise. Aside from elaborating the basis for decisions for the Board of Trustees, the Scientific Committee appoints consultative commissions, composed of leading international scientists, for external evaluations.

The Management Board

As provided by § 14.1 of the Statutes and Articles, the Management Board directs the Foundation. It consists of at least one scientific and one administrative member (§ 15.1). The Board of Trustees appoints the members of the Management Board after consultation with the Scientific Council (§ 15.2).

Since May 1, 1983, Prof. Dr. med. Dres. h.c. Harald zur Hausen has directed the Management Board as its chairman and as its scientific member. In May 1988 and in May 1993, he was re-appointed for an additional five-year terms. Since July 1, 1984, Dr. jur. Reinhard Grunwald has been the administrative member of the Management Board. In 1994, he was re-appointed for five-year terms.

In a multi-disciplinary, complex and necessarily decentralized research institution the traditional management functions of planning, decision making, and supervision, are less hierarchically structured. Scientific management is primarily based on encouraging and promoting ideas, coordinating processes, and balancing multiple interests.

Thus, when defining the scientific program of the Deutsches Krebsforschungszentrum, the Management Board focuses on considering how to initiate and to terminate Research Programs, how to distribute the Center's resources depending on performance, and how to further improve organizational processes. The collaboration with the Foundation's committees and its sponsors and the cooperation with scientific partners in Germany and abroad are important aspects of the work of the Management Board. The experiences and the results of the analyses of the work completed so far have been integrated into a restructuring plan which is to give the Center the flexibility that it needs for continued success. An important instrument is the internal evaluation of all scientific divisions. The Chairman and Scientific Member is supported in his task by the scientific consultants of the Management Board.

The work of the Management Board is considerably supported by advisory committees. In the past, the Management Board has delegated the following tasks to permanent commissions: selection of scientists for awards, bonuses, upgrading, and tenure, assessment of all applications for the use of laboratory animals in the Center according to the German Law on Animal Protection, and examination of all applications and supervision of all work and installations subject to the German Gene Technology Law.

Other tasks are delegated to ad hoc committees. The Management Board is supported in its work by staff departments and by the administration.

The Scientific Council

The task of the Scientific Council is to advise the Board of Trustees and the Management Board on all relevant scientific issues. In a number of particularly important matters, decisions of the Management Board require the consent of the Scientific Council.

The Scientific Council deals with research projects and programs, appointments, the utilization of research results, recording of achievements, the advancement of scientific information exchange, the collaboration with universities and other research facilities, budget planning and investment programs.

The Scientific Council consists of 16 members, comprising the coordinators of the eight Research Programs and an equal number of elected representatives of the scientific staff.

Members of the Scientific Council (as of March 1994)

Prof. Dr. Werner Wilhelm Franke (Chairman)
Dr. Jürgen Kartenbeck
Research Program Cell Differentiation and Carcinogenesis

Prof. Dr. Norbert Fusening
Prof. Dr. Friedrich Marks
Research Program Tumor Cell Regulation

Dr. Norbert Frank
Prof. Dr. Jürgen Wahrendorf
Research Program Cancer Risk Factors and Prevention

Prof. Dr. Stefan Meuer
Dr. Klaus Wayß (Deputy Chairman)
Research Program Diagnostics and Experimental Therapy

Prof. Dr. Walter Lorenz
Prof. Dr. Wolfgang Schlegel
Research Program Radiological Diagnostics and Therapy

Prof. Dr. Jean Rommelaere
Dr. Elisabeth Schwarz
Research Program Applied Tumor Virology

Prof. Dr. Peter H. Krammer
Dr. Gerhard Moldenhauer
Research Program Tumor Immunology

Dr. Sándor Suhai
Prof. Dr. Claus O. Köhler
Research Program Bioinformatics

Dipl.-Math. Siegfried Herz
Secretary of the Scientific Council

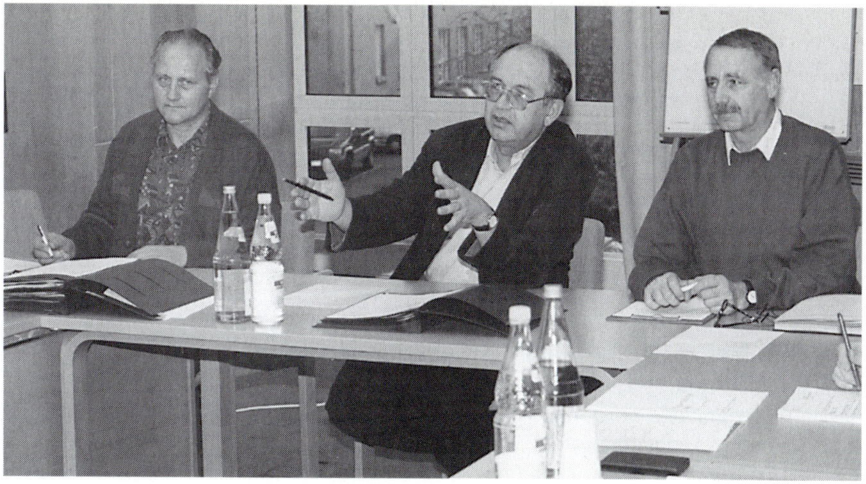

Fig. 103
the Scientific Council convenes once a month. In the center, its Chairman Professor Dr. Werner W. Franke and the former Deputy Chairman, Priv.-Doz. Dr. Klaus Wayß (right). On the left, the secretary of the Scientific Council, Dipl.-Math. Siegfried Herz

As a rule, the Scientific Council holds 12 meetings a year. A number of expert commissions and a permanently staffed office support the Council in its work and in the preparation of decisions.

The current 3-year term of office started in February 1992, after the early election of a new Council according to the new Statutes of the Foundation.

Members of the Scientific Council (as of February 1995)

Prof. Dr. Werner Wilhelm Franke (Chairman)
Dr. Jürgen Kartenbeck
Research Program Cell Differentiation and Carcinogenesis

Prof. Dr. Friedrich Marks
Dr. Petra Boucamp
Research Program Tumor Cell Regulation

Prof. Dr. Helmut Bartsch
Dr. Nikolaus Becker
Research Program Cancer Risk Factors and Prevention

Prof. Dr. Stefan Meuer
Prof. Dr. Melvyn Little
Research Program Diagnostics and Experimental Therapy

Prof. Dr. Walter Lorenz
Prof. Dr. Wolfgang Schlegel
Research Program Radiological Diagnostics and Therapy

Prof. Dr. Jean Rommelaere
Priv.-Doz. Dr. Elisabeth Schwarz (Deputy Chairperson)
Research Program Applied Tumor Virology

Prof. Dr. Peter Krammer
Dr. Gerhard Moldenhauer
Research Program Tumor Immunology

Prof. Dr. Claus O. Köhler
Priv.-Doz. Dr. Sándor Suhai
Research Program Bioinformatics

Dipl.-Math. Siegfried Herz
Secretary of the Scientific Council

Staff Council

The rights and duties of the Staff Council are laid down in the Staff Representation Law of the State of Baden-Württemberg.

Considering that, of the total staff of about 1600, only about 40 percent are employed under permanent contracts, it is easy to anticipate the problems which arise: short-term contracts, high fluctuation, and a lack of continuity in the entire staffing structure.

This, in turn, means that staff can easily lose a sense of responsibility for their work, and that lack of care can jeopardize the observation of safety regulations.

The research and science policy at the Deutsches Krebsforschungszentrum is based on the idea that outstanding scientific results can best be obtained during the course of research projects that run for a limited time and from staff who are employed only temporarily. The Staff Council believes that this also contributes to an increase in pressure and stress, as well as fear of unemployment-factors which burden the employees and have negative effects on their work.

The introduction of new research activities goes hand in hand with the breaking up of existing working units and the establishment of new research groups. This leads to a mobility of staff which certainly has some benefits, but also means that when a short-term contract runs out, there may be no further position available. The consequences are unemployment and reduced financial and social status.

The Staff Council has recently addressed the following topics:

– the drafting of rules to ensure the protection of data privacy in recording and dealing with personal data and other information about individuals;

– support of the cooperation with the women's initiative that has been founded at the Center. This includes involvement in the discussion about a women's representative for all women working at the Center, and the drawing up of specifications for the function and qualifications of the women's representative;

– fulfilling the requirements contained in the legal regulations on working place, safety at work, radiation protection, and others. On the basis of the existing legal regulations the commercial inspectorate has demanded the introduction of certain measures as prerequisites for granting permission for the use of open radioactive substances in the laboratories.

Members of the Staff Council (Status: December 1994)

Hanspeter Götz
Siegfried Herz
Brigitte Hobrecker, chair
Annekathrin Kollenda
Ingeborg Kühni
Heinz Löhrke
Jutta Müller-Osterholt
Hartmut Richter
Heinrich Schmitt, vice chairman
Rolf Schmitt, member of the board
Annemarie Schrödersecker
Ingeborg Vogt, member of the board
Heinz Wiesner, deputy vice chairman

The Administration of the Deutsches Krebsforschungszentrum

In the past few years, administrative work was dominated by the growth and changing tasks of the Center and by the reorganization of its research structure.

Central activities included the administrative involvement in:

– the reorganization of the research structure of the Deutsches Krebsforschungszentrum. In this context the following activities deserve special mention: participation in the researchers' discussions on the new statutes and on the changes

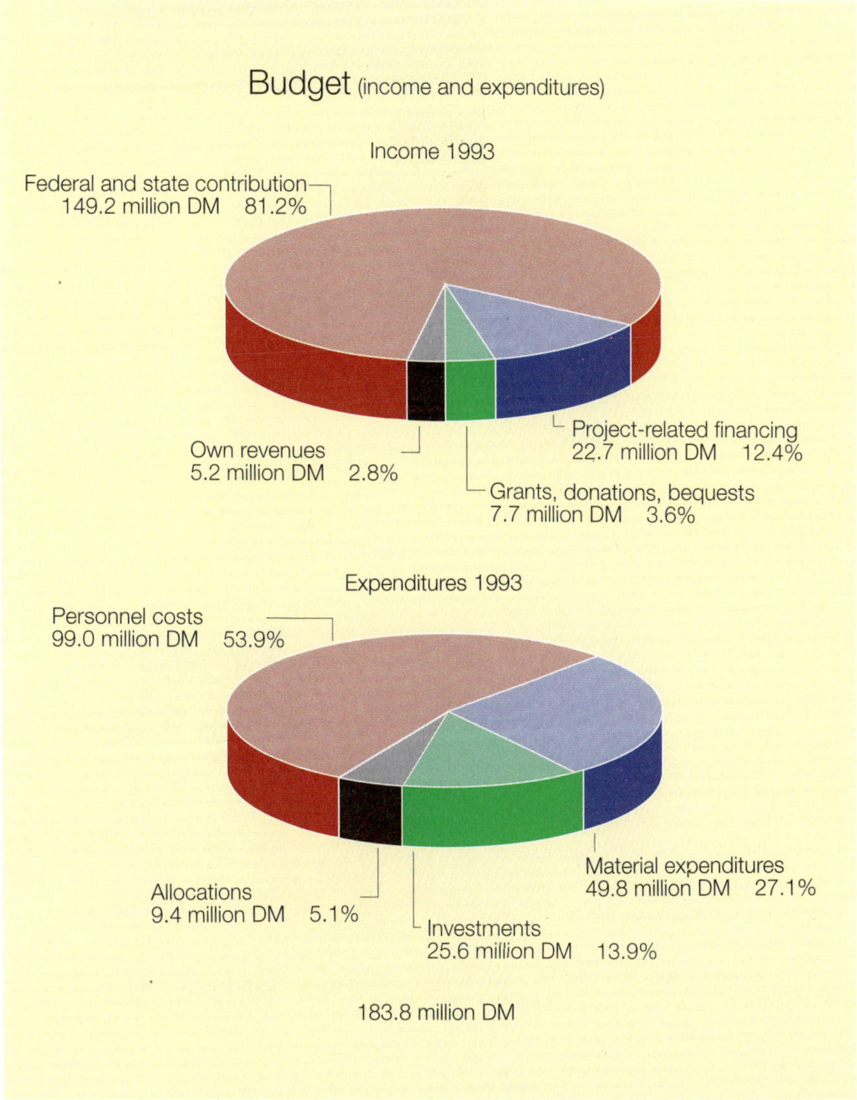

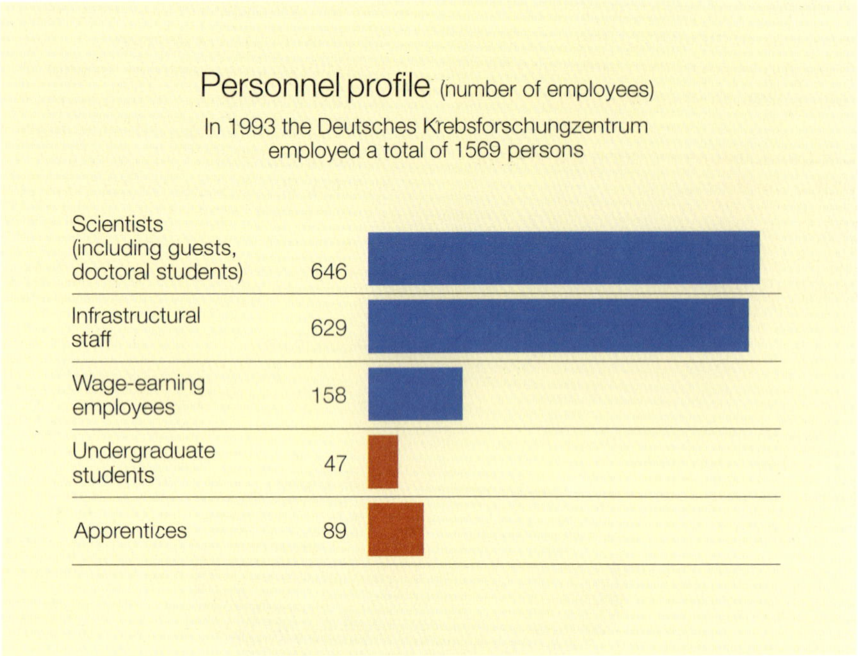

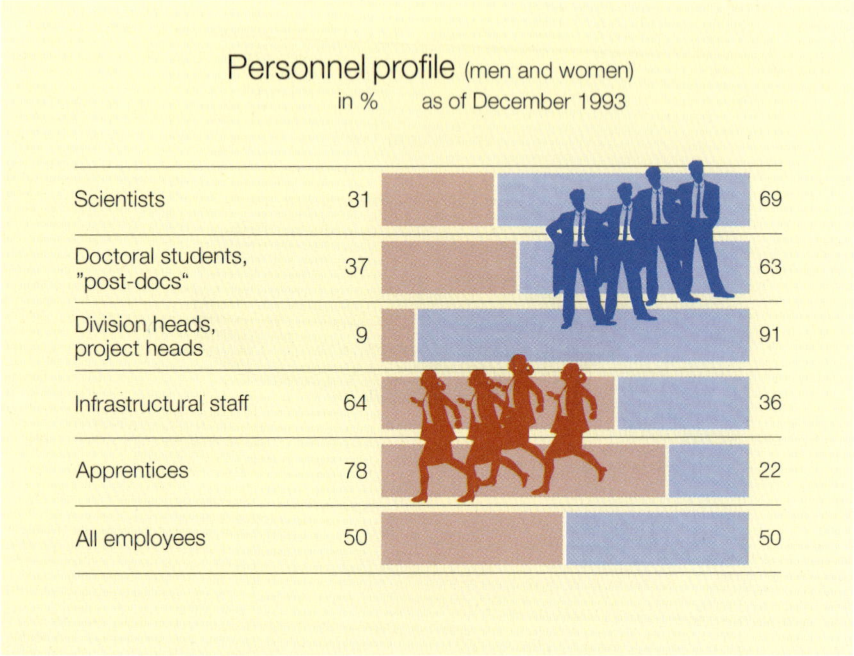

in the existing rules and regulations emanating from the new structure; the discussions in the subcommittees of the Scientific Council on the implementation of the changes and their consequences for individual divisions, projects, and working groups;

- the establishment of new divisions and projects, the reorganization of existing ones and the associated measures concerning staff, funding, and buildings;
- the closure and disbandment of divisions and projects including, above all, the related personnel measures;
- the planning and realization of central renovation measures such as the disposal of asbestos and the creation of safety areas according to the stipulations issued by the trade inspectorate.

Alongside these activities, staff members of the administration of the Deutsches Krebsforschungszentrum were involved in measures to support research institutions in the former East Germany and in activities within the framework of the Association of National Research Centers (Arbeitsgemeinschaft der Großforschungseinrichtungen, AGF). They took a major part in the work of the AGF's committees and subcommittees.

Meetings of administrators from Heidelberg research institutions with administrators from Israeli research institutions, which took place alternately in Heidelberg and in Rehovot, Israel, constituted further highlights. These meetings provided the opportunity of a transnational exchange of experiences. Mutual visits of administrative staff from the Deutsches Krebsforschungszentrum at Is-

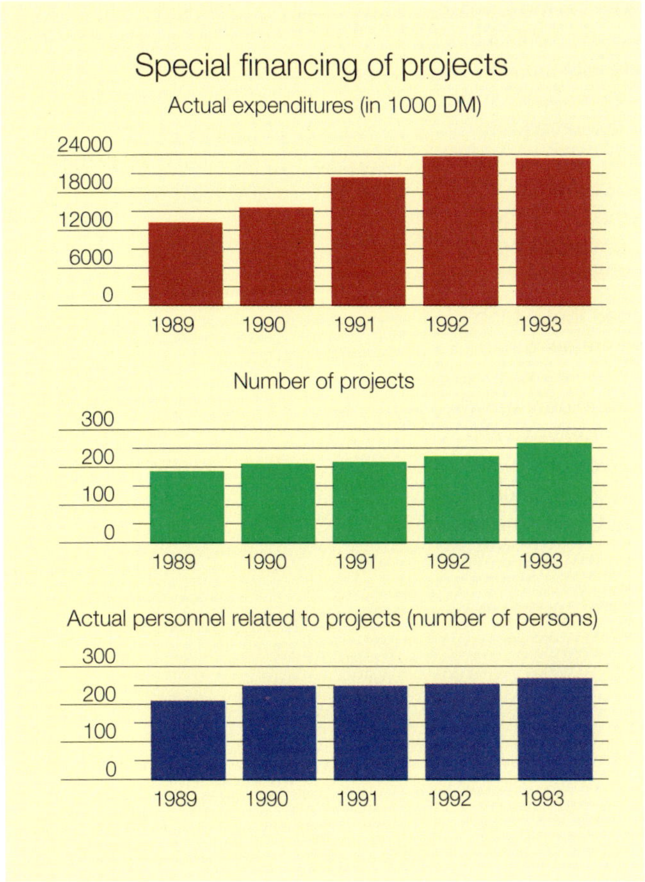

raeli research centers and vice versa supplemented the exchange of experience, providing immediate insights into the structure of a research institution abroad.

Furthermore, the administration has implemented an administrative data processing system that meets today's standards, thereby improving the tools necessary for the planning, realization, and control of administrative tasks. Following an analysis of the internal work flows, suggestions for streamlining them were worked out and implemented in agreement with the employees concerned.

The administration of the Deutsches Krebsforschungszentrum takes into account that strictly hierarchical and centralized structures, characterizing the traditional administrative image of many government agencies and other public services to the present day, cannot or only partly be applied to the administration of a research center. The Center's administration is convinced that the "decentralization and segmentation of administrative services in accordance with customer and market requirements," a principle which plays a major role in considerations concerning a reform of public administration, is better suited to meet the demands of a research administration. The issue of "customer focus," related, in particular, to the researchers as the main consumers of administrative services, will in future gain even more importance in all areas of administration.

A decentralization of administrative processes at the Deutsches Krebsforschungszentrum can provide the individual scientist with a broader scope of action when managing his or her administrative requests. However, it is important that the responsibility for administrative actions is clearly defined and that scientists do not take over immediate administrative tasks except to improve the conditions for research work. The example of decentralized procurement of small capital goods and non-cash resources may serve to illustrate this point. A researcher who makes use of the possibility of directly ordering assets in accordance with the Center's procurement regulations is responsible for managing and documenting the procurement process according to the public stipulations on the allocation of goods. Often it will be difficult to tell what benefits the scientist more: a decentralized procurement process with quicker ordering and supply or a centralized one where the scientist benefits from the administrative services offered and is relieved from the administrative activities and duties associated with procurement. Therefore, the administration concentrates its efforts primarily on offering qualified services when required, thereby leaving it to the scientists to choose the best mode of action in the individual situation.

Professional Categories in the Technical Department

Electrical engineering

- Electrical power engineering
- Automation engineering
- Communications engineering

Scientific apparatus engineering

- Light engineering
- Glass blowing

General maintenance and mechanical engineering

- Refrigeration engineering
- Ventilation engineering
- Heat engineering
- Sanitary engineering
- Fitter's shop

General services

- CAD construction
- Materials handling technology
- Painting and decorating
- Joiner's shop

Considerations on technology transfer are gaining new importance for administrative work. Even in aresearch institution like the Deutsches Krebsforschungszentrum, which focuses primarily on basic research, models for the commercial exploitation of research results are worth discussing. It is particularly important to transfer results from government-funded research as quickly as possible into practical applications, thereby making them available for the public. Moreover, the intensification of technology transfer provides the Center and its scientists with new possibilities of establishing contacts with industry. These contacts can substantially facilitate the acquisition of resources from industry. In addition, they offer a chance of improving the job prospects of young scientists from the Deutsches Krebsforschungszentrum following the professional orientation phase.

In the future, it is planned that a technology broker shall help make out inventions, prepare them for industrial exploitation on the basis of expert knowledge, establish contacts between scientists and representatives of industry, and speed up the process of making research results available for commercial exploitation.

Dr. Wolfgang Henkel
Head of Administration

Teaching, Professional Training, and Refresher Courses for Employees

Teaching

The scienties of the Deutsches Krebsforschungszentrum offer a wide range of seminars, colloquia, lectures, and laboratory courses for advenced students. All together, they teach more than 100 courses at the University of Heidelberg and, to a lesser degree, at the Universities of Karlsruhe, Tübingen, and Kaiserslautern, as well as at various professional colleges. From 1991 through 1993, 760 doctoral and diploma students participated in research work at the Center. During this period, they submitted 285 diploma, doctorial, and postdoctorial theses. The Center also organizes postgraduate training courses, refresher courses for staff members, and special courses for physicans, which are mainly held by scientists of the Research Program Radiological Diagnostics and Therapy. Courses in ultrasound are offered regularly at three levels – introductory, intermediate, and advanced.

In order to promote highly qualified young researchers, five posts for young scientists and 10–15 posts within team-oriented project proposals are sponsored per year by the Center's special fund, i.e., by donations given to the Center. Within the framework af projects competitively proposed by the Center's scientists, young researchers are thus offered the possibility to do research work for up to 3 years. A trainee program is also devoted to the promotion of young scientists. Students of the Study Foundation of the German People (Studienstiftung des Deutschen Volkes) and of Stanford University (Krupp Foundation), U.S.A., are offered 8-week practicals.

The winners of the competition "Researching Youth" (Jugend forscht), held by the German States, are regularly invited to the Krebsforschungszentrum and may work for up to 2 weeks in a division of their choice.

In addition, international courses for the introduction of scientists to new techniques and methods of research are organized by the Center on a regular basis.

The Center's collodquia are organized as an instrument for introducing new scientific ideas and for stimulating scientific discussion among researchers of the Center and of other institutions. From 1991 through 1993, scientists from more than 28 countries held more than 550 lectures. The Center's colloquia program is part of of the program "bio-scientific lectures" of the University of Heidelberg, the Max Planck Institutes in Heidelberg, and the European Molecular Biology Laboratory. The lecture announcements of all of the abovementioned institutions are compiled monthly by the Center's Department of Public Relations and mailed upon request.

Professional Training

Since 1976, the Deutsches Krebsforschungszentrum has offered professional training as specified in the Professional Training Law and, since 1985, this has been carried out in collaboration with the professional colleges of Baden-Württemberg. The initial emphasis was to offer young people the opportunity to train for a profession in the laboratories. This professional training has become an established part of the Center's activities and is highly regarded by the industrial companies of the Rhein-Neckar region.

In recent years the range of careers for which professional training is offered has grown, and now encompasses:

Laboratory professions:

- medical assistant
- biology laboratory assistant
- chemistry laboratory assistant
- radiation protection engineer (diploma of the professional college)
- animal keeper (specializing in the care of domestic and experimental animals)

Technical professions:

- precision engineer
- mechanical engineer
- joiner

Managerial professions:

- business management (diploma of the professional college, specializing in State-run institutions)
- commercial clerk in office communication

The Deutsches Krebsforschungszentrum takes on many young people from the local region far more than are actually needed for later employment at the Center in order to provide as many school-graduates as possible with a useful and modern professional training.

By the end of 1993, over 580 apprentices had successfully qualified, whereby the high level of competence demanded by the training was maintained throughout. Despite the fact that the Center is unable to offer positions to many of the qualified apprentices, these young workers generally find good positions either in the region or further afield. Professional training at the Deutsches Krebsforschungszentrum is clearly an attractive option, as demonstrated by the relatively large number of applicants.

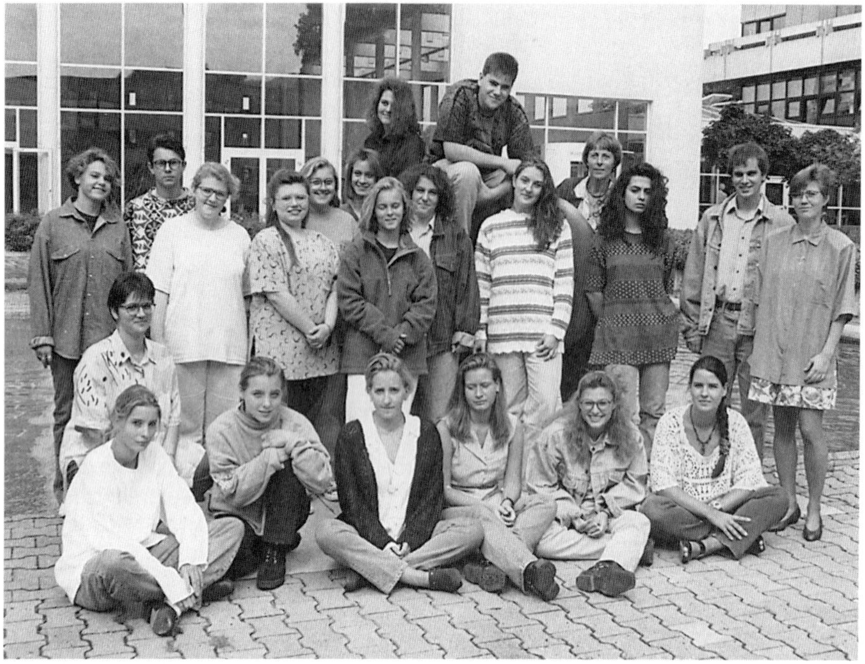

Fig. 109
Apprentices from the Center with the head of training Dr. Nesta Ehler (back row, fourth from the right)

The low birthrate years have influenced the number of applications received: In 1990, 452 school-graduates applied for 25 apprenticeships at the Center; in 1991, the number fell to 309 applicants, but in 1993, it had risen once more to 380. In the future the demands placed on the professional training will continue to increase. Today, the young people working in the various departments, regardless of whether they are being trained in laboratory or managerial skills, are already learning sophisticated modern techniques that will prepare them for the challenges of the future. During their training the apprentices spend periods in several of the different Research Programs in order to get to know the broad and continually changing spectrum of activities of a research institute.

The practical training in the laboratories is complemented by regular practical and theoretical instruction in the training laboratory, leading to an appropriate synthesis of theoretical knowledge and practical skills.

The content of the Center's training program goes well beyond statutory requirements. This is evidenced by the high proportion of apprentices who qualify early – almost 50% – and by their excellent examination results. It is a frequent occurrence for an apprentice biology laboratory assistant from the Deutsches Krebsforschungzentrum to obtain the best results awarded by the professional association.

The professional training offered at the Deutsches Krebsforschungszentrum is the responsibility of three full-time staff members. Their expertise has also gained recognition outside the Center.

Trainees

In addition to school classes visiting the Center to learn about the main areas of research in the scientific laboratories, in the years 1991–1993 more than 120 high-school students have attended practical vocational training courses in our specialist laboratories. Individual wishes of the students are taken into account as much as possible in selecting the specialist field which they encounter. The time spent on the practical course – which ranges from a few days to several months – gives the students important guidance in choosing their professions.

Last year, more than 50 students from technical colleges studying biotechnology, computer science, electronic engineering, and chemistry spent their practical semester working at the Center.

Students of biology and medicine are applying in increasing numbers for the opportunity to do practical work at the Center during their university vacations. The most popular areas are molecular biology, biochemistry, immunology, and genetics.

The large number of trainees who undertake unpaid practical work at the Center demonstrates the high expectations placed on the professional experience gained in the research laboratories.

Continuing Education for Employees

For the staff of the Deutsches Krebsforschungszentrum, continuing education is essential, since skills and knowledge are being overtaken by new advances faster than ever before. The spectrum of scientific endeavors and their aims has changed significantly in recent years. The ever increasing complexity of the tasks of the research center place great demands on its staff members. But the success of the Center depends strongly on the people who work there. Learning is itself a form of work, and the willingness of individuals to learn is an expression of their commitment to the Deutsches Krebsforschungszentrum. The systematic program of continuing education is thus an investment which, in the long term, is as valuable to the staff as it is to the Center.

On the basis of a service agreement, the staff of the Deutsches Krebsforschungszentrum is offered a wide-ranging continuing education program,

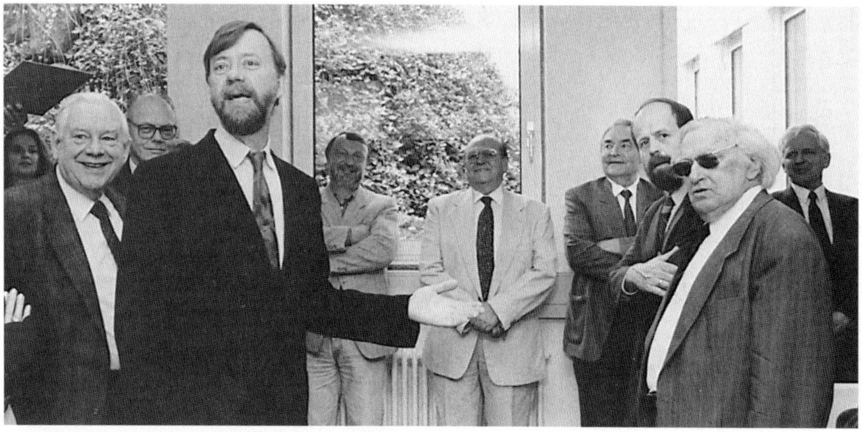

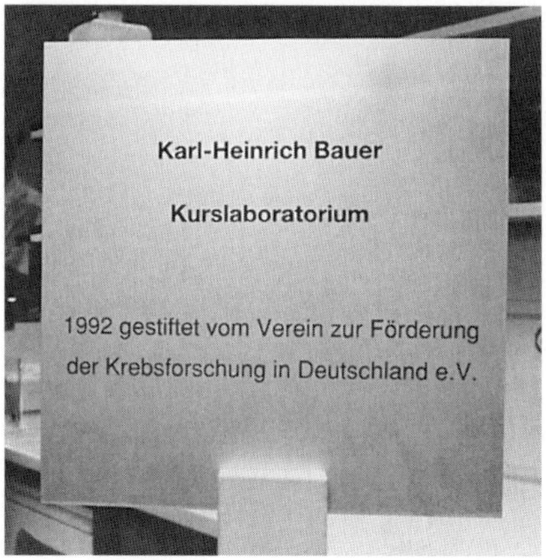

Fig. 110, 111
In 1993, the Karl Heinrich Bauer Course Laboratory was established at the Center for teaching purposes. Priv.-Doz. Dr. Jürgen Kartenbeck, who is responsible for the course laboratory, presents its rooms at the inauguration. In the foreground on the right is Dr. Ernst Grieser, member of the board of the Association for the Furtherance of Cancer Research in Germany, which provided significant financial support for the extension. The course laboratory was named after the founder of the Deutsches Krebsforschungszentrum, Prof. Dr. Karl Heinrich Bauer

which has so far been extended every year. It contains, on the one hand, the proven courses of previous years, and, on the other, it takes into account the changing needs and wishes of the staff by including, at the suggestion of the various organizational units, both subjects of general interest and specialist courses.

These aspects are reflected in the annually appearing program of continuing education and in the decisions about releasing staff from their duties in order that they can attend courses. The Center's continuing education activities include:

- specific measures to provide the staff with knowledge tailored to their individual needs,
- measures to provide groups from various organizational units with the necessary training for coping with the constantly changing demands,
- events aimed at improving cooperation and communication.

During the past 2 years, participants in the continuing education program each spent an average of nearly 3 days involved in training activities. This, it should be noted, does not include time spent at scientific lectures or meetings of the various research divisions or project groups.

The Continuing Education Department is also intensifying its program of instruction for the 250 doctoral and diploma students, since their knowledge and skills play a decisive role in the overall performance and success of the Center.

The interdisciplinary seminars that form part of the graduate support program, offering for example an introduction to the subject of laboratory animals including practical work, or on biostatistics, are very well attended by the young scientists, as are the more general topics such as the preparation of scientific manuscripts or presentation techniques.

Support of young scientists

The Scientific Member of the Management Board of the Deutsches Krebsforschungszentrum had the idea of establishing a grant program designed to reinforce infection research – especially AIDS research – in Germany. In 1989, with the support of the German Research Association (DFG), the Deutsches Krebsforschungszentrum was entrusted with the administrative management of the program. It is financed by the Federal Ministry of Research and Technology.

The research projects submitted are assessed by an independent board of scientists. Following a personal interview with the applicants, the board decides on the award of the grants.

The first phase of the grant consists of a 2-year stay abroad, which is designed to acquaint young scientists with the top international standards in AIDS research. This is followed by a 3-year stay at a German research institute. So far, grants have been awarded to medics and natural scientists who had performed outstanding work during their post-doctoral or even their doctoral research. In a first stage, the grant-holders work at internationally renowned research centers for 2 years in order to develop their own projects. The Dana-Farber Cancer Institute in Boston, the Scripps Clinic La Jolla, and the National Institute of Health in Bethesda, all in the U.S.A., are but a few examples of the first-class laboratories which have provided recipients with a working place.

Following an evaluation of the stay abroad, the recipients return to continue their work at an appropriate research institute in Germany. Their positions are financed for a period of 3 years. The first reports after 2 years' work in Germany are now available and serve to confirm that top-class research is being conducted within the program.

What is more, on returning to Germany all recipients can choose from several offers of where to continue their research work. In the years up to 1993 more than 60 5-year grants were awarded. Altogether, the program, which runs from 1989 until the end of 2002, will make available more than DM 45 million as grants supporting infection research.

Graduate Student Adviser

About 300 PhD and diploma students are on the staff of the Deutsches Krebsforschungszentrum at any time. Most of them are students from Heidelberg University, but they also come increasingly from numerous other German and foreign universities. Even though they are employed only on a temporary basis, they contribute substantially to the Center's scientific work.

The Center considers the support and encouragement of these young scientists to be a very important task. To this end, a special program for the benefit of graduates was started in 1990. In the last 3 years the activities of this program have been focused on continuing scientific education, presentation techniques, and neighboring areas of our immediate scientific sphere of interest. Continuing scientific education is offered in the form of short courses in which certain technical skills are taught and insights provided into new or particularly complicated scientific research methods; they are held mainly by experienced in-house colleagues. The courses in presentation techniques, which are held by trained specialists, are designed to develop the students' ability to present themselves and their scientific work in an adequate form. One highlight of these activities is the yearly poster exhibition where PhD students and diploma students can present their work to the in-house public, not least in the hope of gaining inspiration from this circle and making new contacts. In the third focus of the program, the PhD students' own initiatives come to fruition. Three different work groups have dealt with topics such as contacts to industry, insights into matters of business administration, and ethical questions in science. Results of this work are a brochure on recruitment methods of German industrial enterprises and visits to such companies, in the course of which opportunities for applicants and the situation of young scientists were discussed. In response to the interest in matters of business administration two seminars entitled "Introduction to Business Administration" were organized in cooperation with Mannheim University; both seminars lasted several days. A particularly strong impression was made by the discussion forum "Ethical questions of genetic engineering," where PhD students and academics from the disciplines of ethics in natural sciences, theology, and medicine, discussed this topic in front of a large audience.

Encouraged by the positive response to all these events, we have decided to make them permanent elements of the continuing education program of the Deutsches Krebsforschungszentrum.

Graduate student adviser:
Prof. Dr. Eberhard Spiess

Current Topics

Biological Safety

The German Law on the Regulation of Genetic Engineering has now been in force for 3 years. A first amendment to this law was introduced with the intention of relaxing certain excessively strict stipulations, but this applies less to the field of basic research. The law and its regulations control the handling and use of genetically modified organisms, also providing a definition of what an organism is. Accordingly, cells of animal origin that are grown in vessels in the laboratory are also to be regarded as organisms. The great majority of the genetic engineering projects undertaken at the Deutsches Krebsforschungszentrum involve work with – or the creation of – sublines of cells that have been selectively modified via the introduction of foreign genetic material, i.e., cells that have become genetically modified organisms.

The four safety levels

Level 1 applies to genetic engineering work involving nonpathogenic organisms which, according to our present knowledge, can be considered without risk to man and environment. Laboratories undertaking such work require a single initial registration which includes the first planned experiments. Follow-up work needs only to be documented.

Facilities and initial experiments in the levels 2, 3, and 4 require authorization, and follow-up experiments must be registered. In the application procedure the applicant must always await the decision of the authorities.

Level 2 relates to work with pathogenic organisms which, however, pose only a low risk to man or environment. The transfer of oncogenes, for example, generally falls into this category. At the Deutsches Krebsforschungszentrum almost two dozen laboratories presently have to observe the regulations associated with safety level 2. This level also applies to all new laboratory zones dedicated to Applied Tumor Virology. Access to these areas, which must be marked with the warning "biological hazard," is granted only to authorized persons wearing protective overalls.

Level 3 comprises work with pathogenic organisms that are associated with a moderate risk for man and environment. At the Deutsches Krebsforschungszentrum the corresponding safety measures are required for investigations of the AIDS HI viruses and experiments with a transfer system that stems from smallpox viruses. These experiments are carried out in a screened and monitored security laboratory.

Level 4 applies where there is reason to believe that the work involves a high risk, for example, genetic engineering experiments with the infectious anthrax bacillus or with the agent that causes foot-and-mouth disease. At the Deutsches Krebsforschungszentrum no experiments at safety level 4 are carried out.

The number of individuals and groups that can carry responsibility is strictly controlled by the legislation and is limited to managers of a genetic engineering establishment, in this case the Management Board, to the manager's appointed project leaders, and to the biological safety officers. The commission for biological safety is a legal prerequisite.

There were intitially two aspects which caused some difficulties: 1) The level of information about the law and its stipulations needed by the scientists concerned and 2) the willingness to accept the regulations. These problems were overcome firstly through the advice made available by the biological safety officers, and secondly by means of courses which dealt with the general legal requirements, and particularly with the evaluation of risks and the safety measures necessary in genetic engineering work. The overall aim is to give as many staff as possible the formal basis and knowledge that would enable them to take on the tasks of a project leader.

Longer-term, or at least continuing difficulties concern the procedures for acquiring authorization; these typically begin with the filling out of numerous forms. The lists kept by the Central Commission for Biological Safety in Berlin (ZKBS) do allow a certain reduction in the sea of paper: They comprise a group of organisms, including some that are genetically modified, for which special forms are no longer needed since the organisms are known to the authorizing body. The ZKBS plans to continually update these lists. There has also been a certain reduction of pressure within the Center since new genetic engineering projects that are relatively low-risk (safety level S2) can now increasingly be affiliated to existing projects, or under the latest laws can be more quickly approved because they are comparable to projects elsewhere that have already been approved. Projects of safety level S2 at the Deutsches Krebsforschungszentrum are mainly concerned with oncogene DNA, which can be the cause of malignant transformations of cell growth, and with human and animal pathogens for which there are effective treatments or vaccines. Work on the AIDS virus is classified in higher safety level S3 because neither of these safeguards is presently available.

The supervision of genetic engineering projects and of their project leaders by specialist colleagues – at present numbering 12 at the Center – has proved to be a fundamentally sound idea and provides an alternative to the assignment of full-time safety officers. A prerequisite for this scheme is the support of the Management Board.

Regular inspections of individual sections of the Center by staff of the regional board in Tübingen not only served as a control, but also facilitated communication between the various levels of responsibility. The emphasis placed by the representatives of the authorities make evident the competition and overlap between the stipulations in the various safety areas (genetic engineering, human pathogens, animal pathogens, radiation protection, general laboratory safety). In this situation the responsible officer finds himself playing the role of a contact person for the authorities and for the project leader. In addition, the cooperation with the Center's Safety Division is particularly important in ensuring a fruitful interaction with the regional board. It becomes clear from the examples quoted that the biological safety officers, alongwith their official task, also have another central aspect to their work, namely the supervision of matters of general laboratory safety.

The continual increase in the amount of laboratory space that is part of a genetic engineering facility bears witness to the growing importance of this subject in both basic and applied research. Assuming that this growth will continue, it is desirable that this should be achieved not by an increase in the number of genetic engineering facilities but rather by an expansion of the existing ones. This facilitates the internal communication and also the transport of genetically modified organisms.

Prof. Dr. Claus Hobe Schröder

Chairman of the Biological Safety Commission

Safety in Research Work

Staff involved in modern biochemical and medical research have to deal with a broad spectrum of chemical, biological, infectious, and radioactive substances. In the laboratories high technology devices and automation systems are employed. And today, the methods of genetic engineering have largely replaced classical laboratory techniques. This demands corresponding safety measures, which must be continually adjusted to new developments in order to protect the workers from exposure.

For the realization of the necessary protective measures, safety engineers and medical officers were hired, as required by the law on safety at work, together with officers responsible for radiation protection and biological safety, in accordance with the respective regulations on radiation protection and genetic engineering. All these persons have well-defined functions in their particular areas. They advise the scientists and the Management Board on questions of safety. The control measures stipulated by the various safety laws provide a means of ensuring that the relevant safety rules are properly observed. One such control measure is the regular performance of safety audits. These are inspections of the work place which, through a combined effort of all parties, allow an effective identification of shortcomings.

Partly as a result of the harmonization of laws within the European Union, the rule book (incorporating laws, ordinances, accident-prevention regulations, guidelines, norms, etc.) is becoming ever longer and more complex. An important response has been the construction of an internal set of guidelines. These help the laboratory staff to deal with safety questions, and also serve to complete the range of measures relat-

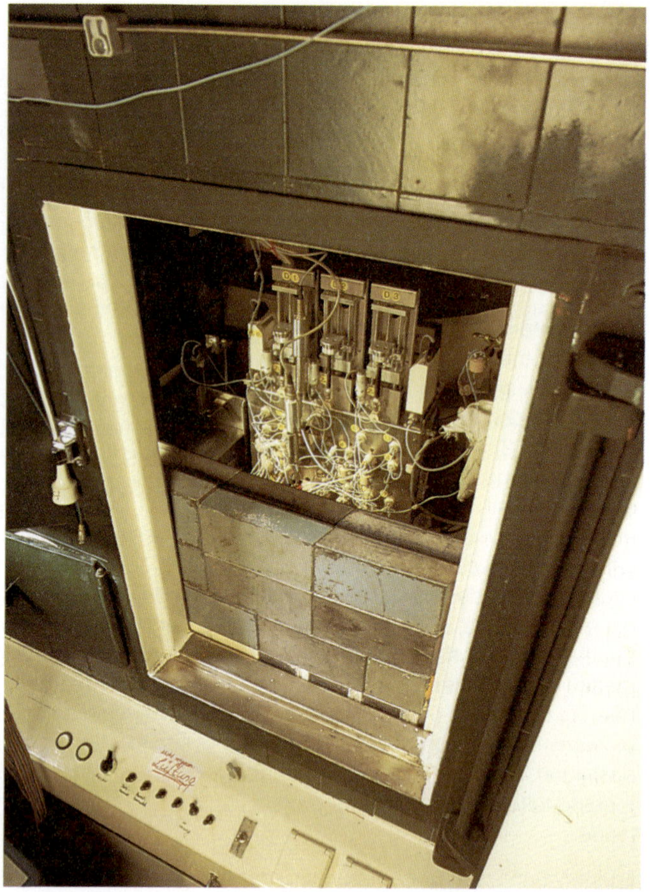

Fig. 113
Apparatus for synthesizing radiopharmaceuticals. To protect staff against radiation and contamination while dealing with open radioactivity, the apparatus is surrounded by a lead screen and is controlled by an external process computer

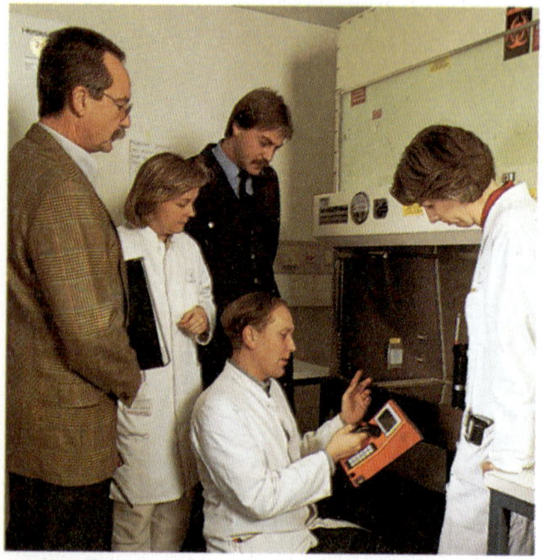

Fig. 112
Safety inspection in a laboratory. Participating are members of the fire brigade, the officers responsible for radiation protection and safety at work, and representatives from the Technical Services Department. As a rule, the staff doctor also takes part

ing to protection at work. A large number of implementation instructions – both for dangerous substances and for procedures – is needed, as is evident when one remembers that several thousand different chemicals and reagents may be employed in a typical research institute. The availability of databases providing the staff with rapid access to information about safety parameters is to be recommended.

Depending on the particular field and the scale of the research, it may be necessary to take on additional officers. The law on waste materials specifies that every scientific institute should have an officer responsible for waste management. He or she has both advisory and control functions and, in particular, provides support for the department specializing in waste disposal. The internal waste guidelines drawn up at the Deutsches Krebsforschungszentrum, which contain a listing of the individual types of waste, have proven to be very valuable. Special officers responsible for the protection of water resources or those stipulated by the federal law on emissions are only necessary when the corresponding plants or installations are present. Effluent and emission control are normally taken care of by the usual safety staff.

In order to avoid putting pregnant women at risk in the research environment, an early and comprehensive counseling is necessary, together with an inspection of the working place. The handling of dangerous substances can usually be reduced to an acceptable level by transfering the woman concerned to a less hazardous work place.

The honorary safety officers of the departments play a joint advisory role as members of the committee for safety at work. This committee meets several times a year. Any safety problems that have arisen are discussed here and measures are adopted for solving them.

According to its size, an institution may be well advised to maintain its own volunteer fire-fighting service. This is the case at the Deutsches Krebsforschungszentrum. This ancillary force is called upon in the case of accidents and emergencies which the laboratory personnel cannot deal with alone, for example, incidents requiring breathing apparatus. These fire-fighters should stay in close contact with the professional fire-brigade.

An essential activity facilitating information exchange and mutual aid is participation on external boards and committees, for example, those of the Association of National Research Centers (AGF), the insurance associations, the Association of German Safety Engineers (VDSI), and international organizations.

Of course all safety specialists, medical and other officers interact closely among themselves and with the Staff Council. This is the only way to ensure that staff are protected from danger and exposure. The low numbers of accidents and work-related illnesses at the Deutsches Krebsforschungszentrum confirm the effectiveness of the efforts made.

Dipl.-Ing. Edgar Heuss
Head of the Safety Division

Animal Protection at the Deutsches Krebsforschungszentrum

Experiments on animals form an indispensable element in the range of methods used in cancer research. At the Deutsches Krebsforschungszentrum they are performed in order to develop cancer models which can help to elucidate how cancer arises and also to study and facilitate new therapeutic and diagnostic strategies. In this type of research, it is essential to consider questions concerning professionalism, appropriateness, and ethical justification.

As long as animal experiments remain irreplaceable, the best means of realizing a practical protection of the animals is to keep them under optimum conditions including the best possible standards of hygiene. The better the animals are kept, the lower the number of experiments that need to be performed in order to attain a particular scientific goal. A comprehensive and routine examination of the animals' state of health by veterinarians and their staff from the Central Animal Laboratory guarantees a high standard of hygiene of the animals used for experiments (in cancer research mainly mice and rats).

Animal experiments may only be carried out following approval of an application by the responsible authority (regional council Karlsruhe). The Animal Protection Law of 1986 and the regulations which it imposes provide the relevant basis. The observation of the legal rules and regulations is the responsibility not only of the project leaders, but also of six animal welfare officers employed at the Center to cope with this arduous task. Their duties include advising the researchers and commenting on each

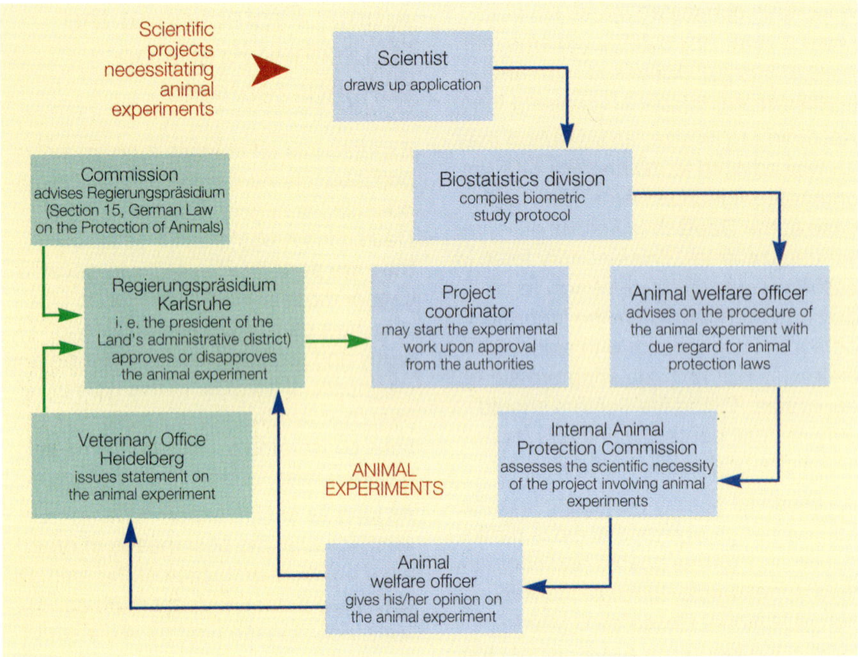

Scientific projects necessitating animal experiments
Scientist
draws up application
Biostatistics division
compiles biometric study protocol
Commission
advises Regierungspräsidium (Section 15, German Law on the Protection of Animals)
Regierungspräsidium Karlsruhe
i. e. the president of the Land's administrative district) approves or disapproves the animal experiment
Project coordinator
may start the experimental work upon approval from the authorities
Animal welfare officer
advises on the procedure of the animal experiment with due regard for animal protection laws
Veterinary Office Heidelberg
issues statement on the animal experiment
ANIMAL EXPERIMENTS
Internal Animal Protection Commission
assesses the scientific necessity of the project involving animal experiments
Animal welfare officer
gives his/her opinion on the animal experiment

application to perform animal experiments. The animal welfare officers are the contact persons for the supervisory body (Veterinary Authority Heidelberg), which also monitors the research through visits to confirm that the legal stipulations are being observed. A further control body, which goes beyond the legal requirements, is the Internal Animal Protection Commission, founded 10 years ago by the management of the Deutsches Krebsforschungszentrum. This commission comprises several scientists and one layperson. Its task is to judge all proposed animal experiments prior to submission of an official application in terms of their scientific necessity, and to determine whether they conform to present scientific standards.

Thanks to the cooperation of the three groups concerned with animal protection and the appropriate sensitivity of the researchers, animal experiments at the Center are limited to the necessary minimum. Thus, almost all applications made in recent years to the regional council in Karlsruhe were deemed worthy of approval. The entire application procedure takes from 2 to 3 months. Science lives, of course, from spontaneous ideas and their immediate realization. In the manner described above, a compromise has been found between the scientists' desire to carry out experiments as soon as possible and society's concern that their ethical justification be assessed through an independent evaluation.

Dr. Bernd Arnold
Chairman of the Internal Animal Protection Commission

The Waste Concept – Refuse Reduction and Disposal

One of major problems of environmental protection in Germany is the question of how to dispose of waste material without harming the environment. According to the law on waste materials of 27 August 1986, each person is obliged to avoid the creation of refuse wherever possible. If this is impossible, the amount of refuse should be reduced, the amount of toxic substances in waste products be minimized, and waste materials be utilized.

Up until 1990, the Deutsches Krebsforschungszentrum produced approximately 2000 cubic meters of refuse annually – enough to fill to the brim two swimming pools 25 meters long, ten meters wide and four meters deep. More than 60% of this refuse was domestic waste. About 500 cubic meters – i.e., a quarter of the total waste – was sent for recycling; this was mainly waste paper, glass, and scrap metal from discarded equipment. Then there was a further 280 tons of waste needing special surveillance (special waste). Of this, 214 tons were composed of soiled litter from animal houses, and the rest was special waste from laboratory work.

In view of the growing importance of treating wastes without harming the environment, a new full-time position was assigned to the House Services Department. This made it possible to better fulfill the legal waste-materials requirements and, above all, the task of advising the other staff in matters relating to waste avoidance and reduction. In cooperation with the scientific divisions and the Safety Division, a strategy was developed to refine the internal refuse guidelines, which stem from 1989 and deal with the avoidance, reduction, utilization, and environmentally safe disposal of waste materials. At the same time, all types of waste occurring in the different departments were recorded systematically and analyzed as to their potential for recycling.

The next step was to establish stations for the collection of reusable materials throughout the Center on all floor levels, and staff were required to separate glass, waste paper, aluminum, polystyrene, metal, batteries, and plastics. For the common rooms, library, and office areas, additional containers for compostable waste materials were provided. The daily collection of all these materials is guaranteed by the House Services Department.

In the years since 1990, the amount of paper recycled increased from 26 to 59 tons in 1991, and from 59 to 108 tons in 1992.

Another problem was the treatment of the huge quantities of special waste produced. One measure to reduce the quantity of special waste is the register of dangerous substances that was compiled for all laboratories by the Center's Safety Division. This register enabled dangerous substances to be replaced by safer and perhaps even environmentally harmless alternatives. Thus, for example, the dangerous and environmentally problematic chromium sulphuric acid, used to remove fats from glassware, was replaced by harmless, degradable detergents that are equally effective. No further mercury-containing thermometers were bought; instead those based on alcohol were employed. For dealing with special fluid waste created in the laboratories, seven containers were installed. These fluids are now disposed of separately according to the categories: non-halogenated solvents; halogenated solvents; cell culture media containing dangerous substances; acids; leaches; aqueous noncombustible wastes; and other chemicals that do not fit into one of these categories or react with substances in the other categories. In addition, special containers are distributed to the laboratories for collecting fluid waste that can be recycled. These measures are presented in the second edition of the Center's waste guidelines, a brief A to Z of waste materials entitled „Das kleine Abfall-Lexikon von A wie Abluftfilter bis Z wie Zytostatika," which appeared in February 1992.

However, despite the huge progress that has been made in the field of waste disposal, it remains true that to avoid the creation of waste is the best protection of the environment. The obvious place to start was the canteen. Why use disposable items when reusable ones are so much better for the environment? Alternatives were presented for plastic cups, drinks in cans, individual milk portions in plastic containers, etc. In December 1992 an automatic cup dispenser was installed next to the coffee vending machine. Staff who do not bring their own coffee mugs can now buy paper cups, previously provided free of charge, for 20 pfennigs each. Very soon a noticeable decline in the quantity of waste cups became apparent. The switching from canned drinks to those in reusable deposit bottles reinforced this development.

Encouraged by these experiences, which have shown that the consumers are willing to give up old habits for the sake of environmental protection, the

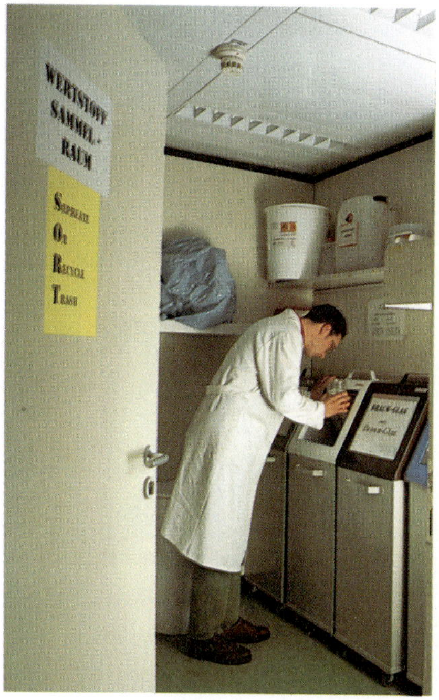

Fig. 115
One of the collecting points for recyclable waste products. Here the waste can be separated, for example, into glass, paper, aluminum, polystyrene, metal, and plastics

Center has also pursued new neans of packaging and wrapping – one of the main culprits in the growth of the rubbish mountains. Products in transport packaging, contained in a further packaging, often padded out with polystyrene chips or the environmentally harmful polyurethane foam are no longer accepted by the Department for Procurement and Material Management following a modification of the delivery conditions for all new products. Today, products are delivered in environmentally friendly bio-degradable packaging, or special contracts ensure the right to return the discarded goods, e. g., batteries and equipment.

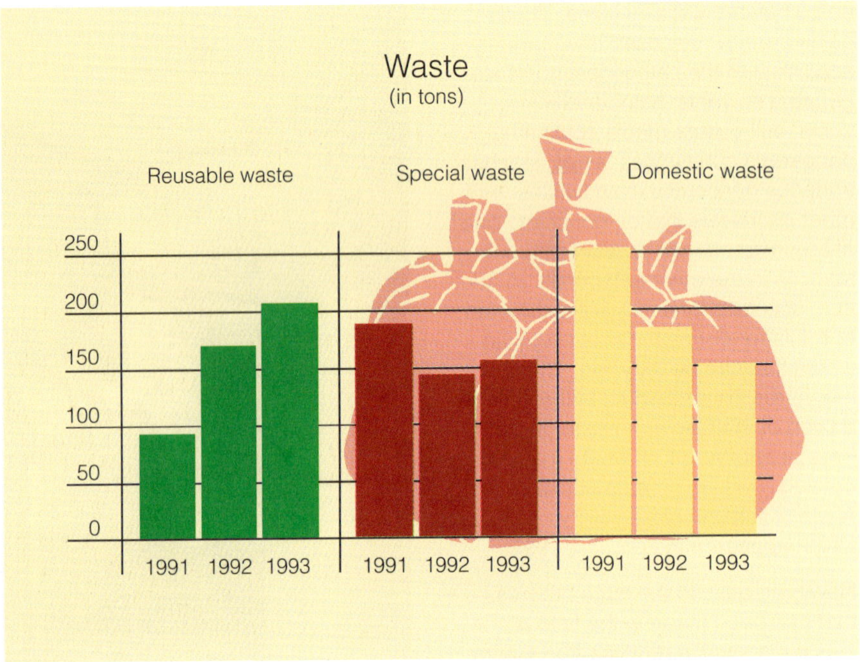

On 31 March 1993 the federal cabinet brought before the German Bundestag a bill for a new law on waste materials. The aim of this law is the further development of waste management into a recycling economy. According to this law, all refuse arising in a company has to be recorded. For the management of the refuse the law stipulates the following order of priorities: avoidance – recycling – incineration – waste treatment and waste disposal. Everything which, according to the law on recycling, can be re-utilized is a secondary raw material. Waste materials are then only those refuse products whose nature and properties prevent them from being utilized as secondary raw materials. This bill initiated a further critical revision of the Center's waste guidelines. The result of this revision, the third edition of the waste guidelines of the Deutsches Krebsforschungszentrum, appeared in January 1994. The central points of the expected recycling law were thereby already incorporated in advance. In addition, the waste guidelines were augmented by a hygiene plan and a list of incompatible chemicals. Along with waste avoidance, reduction, and disposal, matters of safety at work and environmental protection are also essential points.

By taking these measures, the Deutsches Krebsforschungszentrum has contributed to the shrinking of the refuse mountains. A computer-aided recording system ensures that the present 45 different types of waste find their way into the correct disposal and recycling channels. The success is measurable: The quantity of unusable residual waste was reduced from 280 tons in 1990 to 149 tons in 1993. At the same time, the quantity of reusable waste materials rose from 45 tons in 1990 to 206 tons in 1993. The special fluid waste fell from 64 tons in 1990 to 36 tons in 1993. The Deutsches Krebsforschungszentrum regards these successes as an encouragement to continue to make every effort to further reduce its waste production in the future.

Hans-Joachim Buchholz
Hazardous Goods Officer

Press and Public Relations

The media

The years 1991, 1992, and 1993 were marked by a sustained interest of the general public in questions related to cancer research. Cooperation with the media reached a quantitative peak which was difficult to manage with the existing capacities. The topic of genetic engineering in cancer research has attracted ever more interest and today dominates media coverage. European Cooperation is beginning to become visible in this area, too. Contacts to journalists abroad have been extended and intensified in the past few years. A reflection of this international development was a symposium attended by science journalists from all over Europe, which took place in early December 1993 at CERN in Geneva. Its aim was to exchange problems of scientific research coverage and to seek joint European solutions. As early as 1992, the Deutsches Krebsforschungszentrum took up the ideas concerning a European orientation of the media coverage of cancer research by organizing a European workshop for journalists entitled "New Aspects in Cancer Research – A Network of European Cooperation in Science". The event was sponsored by the Commission of the European Union and took place within the framework of the program "Europe Against Cancer". From November 29 to December 1, 1992, research projects involving cooperation with European partners or forming part of European programs were presented. The aim of the workshop was to reveal the European interconnections in cancer research and the fact that even national projects are integrated into the European scientific discussion. It was intended that every journalist should emphasize a national aspect as a starting point for his or her reporting. The workshop, which was held in English, was divided into the topics: "The roots of cancer," "What does cancer live on?" "Seeing, before there is anything to see," "Fighting cancer – The body's own arms," "The run-of-the-mill method is out," "New forms of cooperation between cancer research and clinical practice," and "Cancer care as social prevention". The talks were given by scientists from the Deutsches Krebsforschungszentrum, from university hospitals, other National Research Centers, the World Health Organization (WHO), and foreign research institutions. Of the 50 participating journalists about one third came from abroad. The language barriers within Europe, particularly in relation to journalistic coverage, will in future make it necessary to make use of simultaneous interpreters.

Fig. 117
European workshop for journalists on "New Aspects in Cancer Research" in November 1992. Prof. Dr. Richard Peto, ICRF Cancer Studies Unit, Oxford, England, on the left; on the right Dr. Anthony Michaelis, "Interdisciplinary Science Reviews," London, England

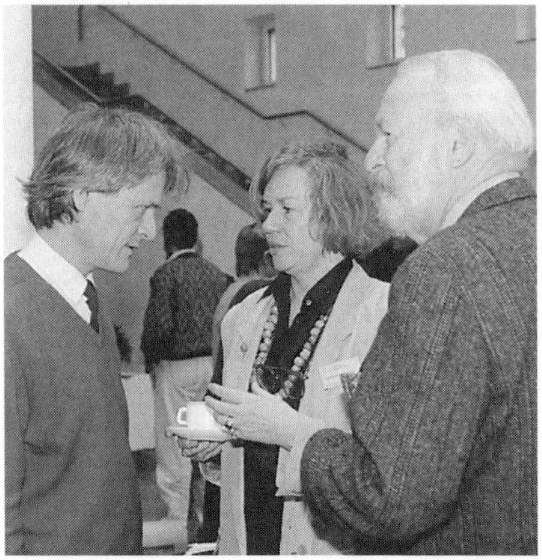

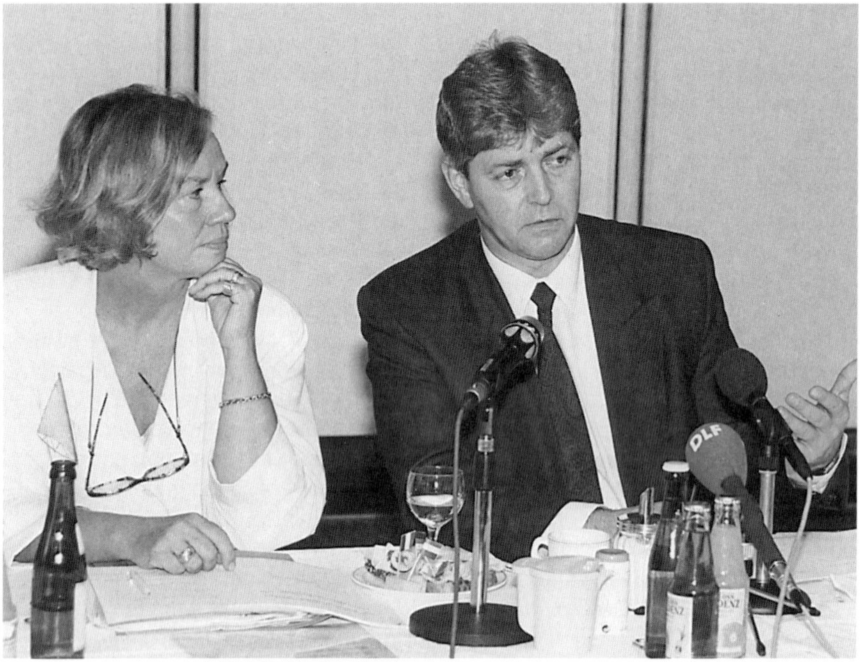

Fig. 118
Press conference of the German Minister for Research and Technology Dr. Paul Krüger on October 5, 1993 on the topic of the Federal Government's involvement in genetic engineering

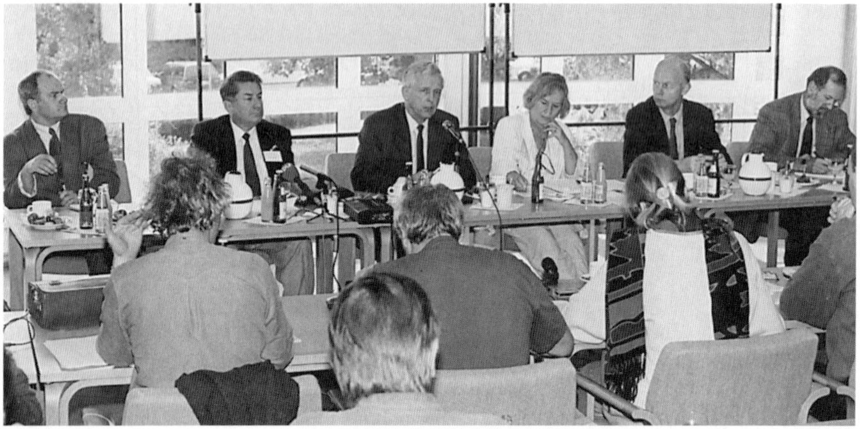

Fig. 119
Press conference on the occasion of the symposium on gene diagnosis and gene therapy of the Association for Clinical-Biomedical Research (Verbund Klinisch-Biomedizinische Forschung, KBF) in Heidelberg on October 5, 1993. From left to right: Prof. Dr. Ernst Böhnlein, Vienna International Research Cooperation Center, Vienna, Prof. Dr. Max Birnstiel, Research Institute for Molecular Pathology, Vienna, Prof. Dr. Harald zur Hausen, Scientific Member of the Management Board of the Deutsches Krebsforschungszentrum and President of the KBF, Hilke Stamatiadis-Smidt, head of the Division of Press and Public Relations of the Deutsches Krebsforschungszentrum, Prof. Dr. Detlev Ganten, Scientific Member of the Management Board of the Max Delbrück Center for Molecular Medicine, Berlin-Buch, Prof. Dr. Anton Berns, Netherlands Cancer Institute, Amsterdam

The symposium helped to establish many contacts and also laid a base for further focal events of this kind.

The following figures bear witness to the intensive cooperation with the media. From 1991 to 1993, more than 80 film reports were produced in the Deutsches Krebsforschungszentrum. Almost 300 interviews with scientists and about 140 background talks took place. In addition, the staff of the Press and Public Relations Division dealt with about 600 inquiries from journalists concerning information, interview partners, statistical material, etc. every year. This flood of inquiries is partly due to the press releases which are regularly published – more than 100 in the above period.

Along with the European workshop, other events were organized with the aim of presenting information specifically for journalists. These included a press talk on June 27, 1991 on the future orientation of the Deutsches Krebsforschungszentrum and the establishment of clinical cooperation units, an invitation by the Associaton of the German Medical Specialist and Professional Press on September 26, 1992, and two press conferences on the occasion of the conference of the Association of Clinical-Biomedical Research (Verbund Klinisch-Biomedizinische Forschung, KBF) entitled "Gene Diagnosis and Gene Therapy" from 4 to 7 October 1993. At this symposium, at a press conference held on 4 October with the participation of the Federal Research Minister, Dr. Paul Krüger, and at a press conference on October 5, more than 50 science and medical journalists learned about current developments in gene-therapeutic and gene-diagnostic research and the state of the debate on genetic engineering in the political context. Press talks were organized and carried out for the Association for Experimental Cancer Research of the German Cancer Society in 1991 and 1993; for the AGF symposium on June 5, 1992 on early cancer detection (AGF = Arbeitsgemeinschaft der Großforschungseinrichtungen, Association of National Research Centers) which was organized by the Coordination Committee for Cancer Research (Koordinierungsausschuß Krebsforschung) in Heidelberg; for the annual conference of the Tumor Centers of Baden-Württemberg in 1991; and for the continuing education seminar on "Breast Cancer – New Developments in Diagnostics and Therapy" offered by the Tumor Center Heidelberg/Mannheim on February 2, 1993. Twenty-two journalists from Germany and abroad were present at the press conference that was organized by the Center's Press and Public Relations Division on the occasion of the annual meeting of the Academia Europaea on September 18, 1991.

If scientific symposia, which are usually held in English, are considered to be of interest for German journalists too, the press office sends out the programs and draws attention to the possibility of participating. The same applies to conferences of the University Hospitals, in particular of the Tumor Center. In addition, press releases concerning individual activities of the Tumor Center are issued.

In 1993, the Deutsches Krebsforschungszentrum established the Wolfgang Rieger Grant intended to support a sound media coverage of scientific issues and at the same time to provide further training for science and medical journalists. Recipients visit the Center's laboratories for a period of 1 to 4 weeks and are given a chance to acquire a knowledge of molecular-biological techniques and methods, to get to know the basics of new scientific developments and thus encounter new issues and problems, and, in close contact with scientists and technical staff, to become acquainted with the practical research work. This grant is awarded within the framework of the "European Initiative for Communicators of Science (EICOS)," a program of the Max Planck Society. The Rieger Grant extends this initiative to German journalists. In addition, the Center awards two further grants to European science and medical journalists who are also named by the panel of experts of the EICOS program. The Wolfgang Rieger Grant was awarded for the first time in 1993 to Lilo Berg, a science editor at the Süddeutsche Zeitung. The grants will contribute to the evolution of a European perspective on research in the media and also enhance the professionalism of journalists.

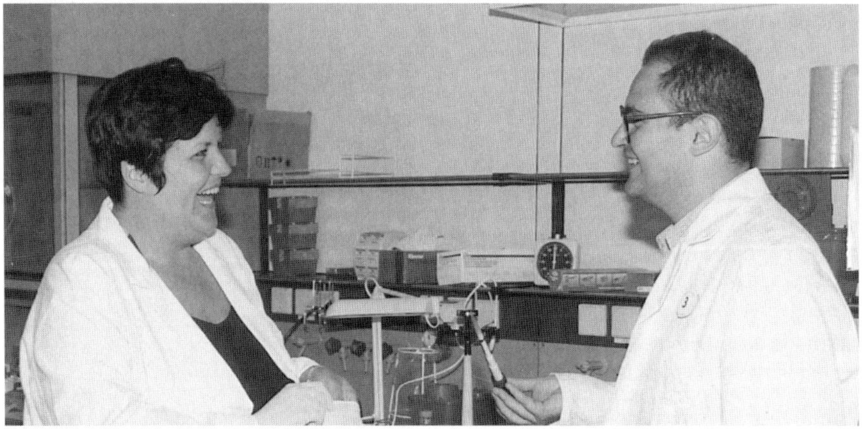

Fig. 120
The first two foreign journalists who received the Wolfgang Rieger grant of the Deutsches Krebsforschungszentrum. During their three-week visits at the Center, they were acquainted with the work of several different divisions. On the left, Tünde Tuscher from Hungary; on the right, Oscar Menéndez from Spain

The journal "einblick"

The Deutsches Krebsforschungszentrum and the Imperial Cancer Research Fund in London have shown that this European perspective can be put into practice in a joint project, even if this demands a strong commitment. They agreed to carry out a joint project: a special issue of the journal "einblick" in German and English. The result of these efforts is a double issue of the journal which is devoted exclusively to the topic of genetic engineering in cancer research ("Gene und Krebs," German issue; "Genes and Cancer"; English issue). The project was supported within the framework of the Biotechnology Program of the European Union following an application by the Center that was approved in 1992. The articles, which, for the most part, were written by German and English science journalists, provide short but typical insights into the scientific revolution in genetic engineering over the past few years. In a manner that can be understood by the layman, the journal's 64 pages describe the possibilities emanating from this new approach to fighting the causes of cancer. The double issue of "einblick 3/4 1993" can be obtained free of charge from the press office, as can the current issue of the journal. The English issue is designed to disseminate information to the wider European audience which aims at helping to judge the real pros and cons of genetic engineering, especially in cancer research.

Texts that can readily be understood, vivid illustrations, and an appealing layout – these are the tools that "einblick" uses to inform the public about cancer research. The journal, which was started in 1987, appears three to four times

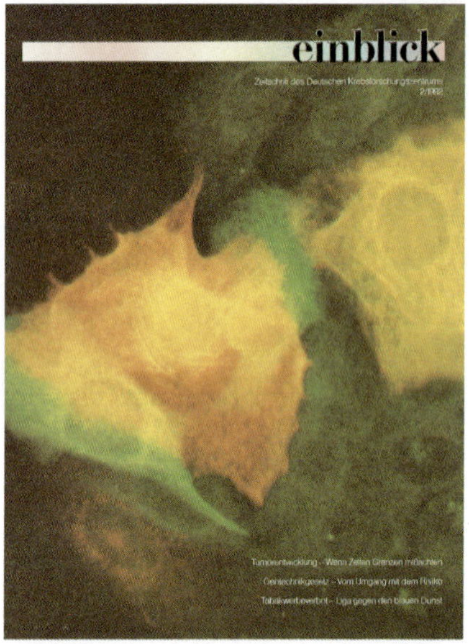

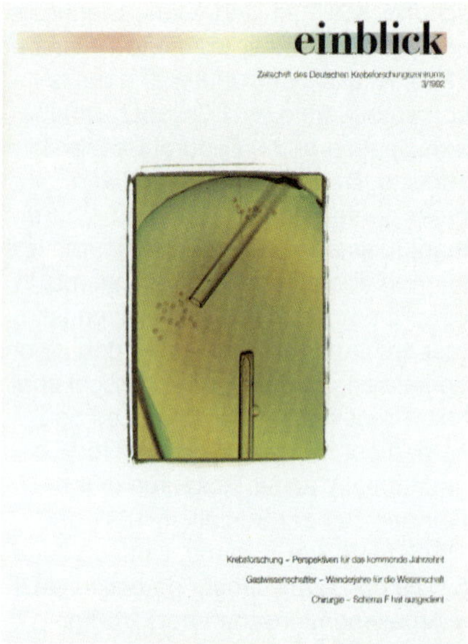

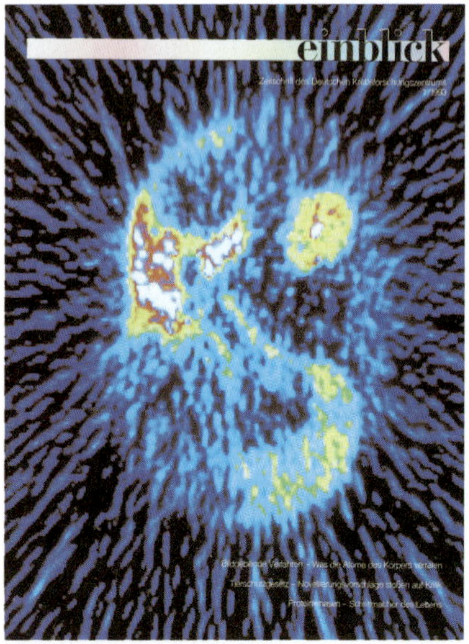

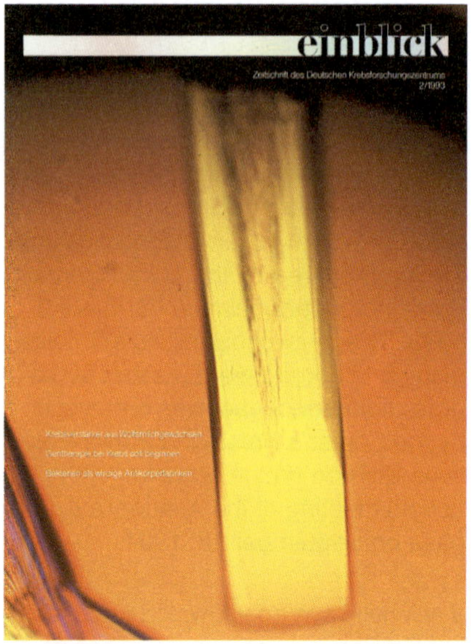

Fig. 121, 122, 123, 124
Covers of the journal "einblick"

Fig. 125
"The ten rules for fighting cancer and their scientific background," an information brochure for the general public

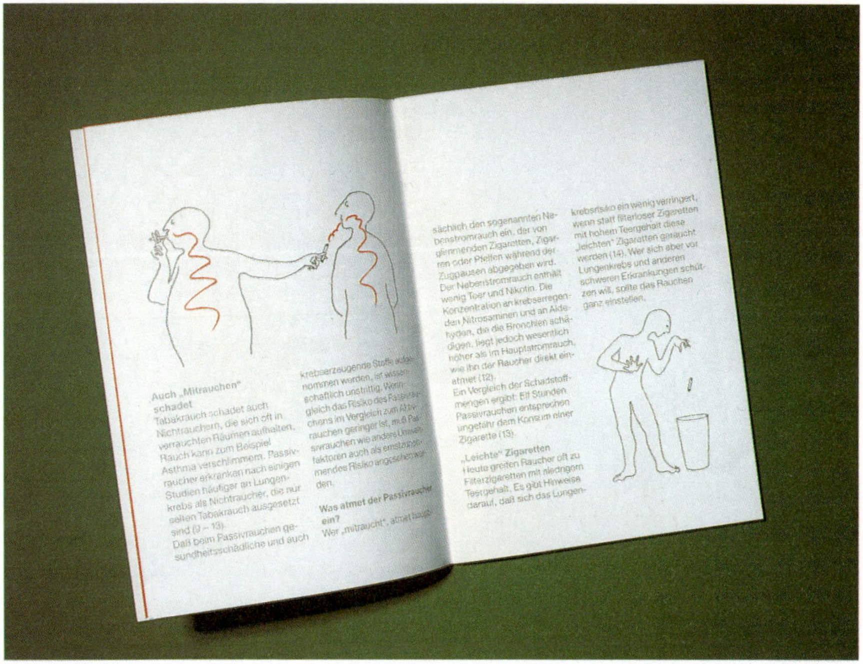

a year. The reader is given insights into the various disciplines in which scientists are working to solve the cancer problem. Freelance journalists who cooperate with the inhouse editors ensure a critical view "from the outside". The journal addresses the general public and can be obtained on a regular basis free of charge from the press office.

Publications

Besides the journal "einblick" and the publications "Krebsforschung heute," and "Current Cancer Research," the press office also published a reprint of the brochure "Die zehn Regeln zur Bekämpfung des Krebses und ihre wissenschaftlichen Grundlagen" (The ten rules for fighting cancer and their scientific background) with further financial support from the European Union, since the first edition of 20 000 copies was out of print after 1 year (reprint: another 20 000 copies). In 1991, a brochure entitled "Neues aus der Krebsforschung" (News from cancer research) appeared. Its 100 pages contain survey articles on new findings in the areas of carcinogenesis and cancer prevention, diagnostics and therapy research. In 1993, with a subsidy from the European Union, the brochure "Krebs – Krebsprävention mit dem Schwerpunkt der Verhinderung aller auf das Zigarettenrauchen zurückführbaren Krebsformen" (Cancer – cancer prevention focusing on all forms of cancer that can be ascribed to cigarette smoking) appeared. It provides information for teachers and was written by Prof. Dr. Volker Kinzel. Furthermore, a new detailed self-portrait of the Center has been published in German and English, a short version of which is also in preparation. In addition, work has started on a brochure about means of making donations to the Deutsches Krebsforschungszentrum, and on a publication for new staff members, which is designed to serve as a "guide" to the Center's services, duties, and internal agreements.

Information booths

The Press and Public Relations Division endeavors to present the activities of the Deutsches Krebsforschungszentrum "on the spot" by organizing information booths at selected conferences. In 1991, the Center was represented at the second Conference of German Physicians in Dresden, and in 1992 at the Conference "Computer Assisted Radiology" (CAR) in Berlin, at the German Cancer Conference, and at the Hanover Fair, where the developments in the radiotherapy of cancer were presented. In 1993, the state of the art in the use of fast neutrons to treat cancer was documented at the Hanover Fair, and 1994 "Genetic Engineering". At the 1993 CAR Conference in Berlin the radiotherapy planning method developed at the Deutsches Krebsforschungszentrum was demonstrated. In addition, the Cancer Information Service (KID: Krebsinformationsdienst) organized information booths at 12 events in various places including Dresden, Bremen, Bremerhaven, Heidelberg, Berlin, Erfurt, Weimar, and Munich (1991–1993).

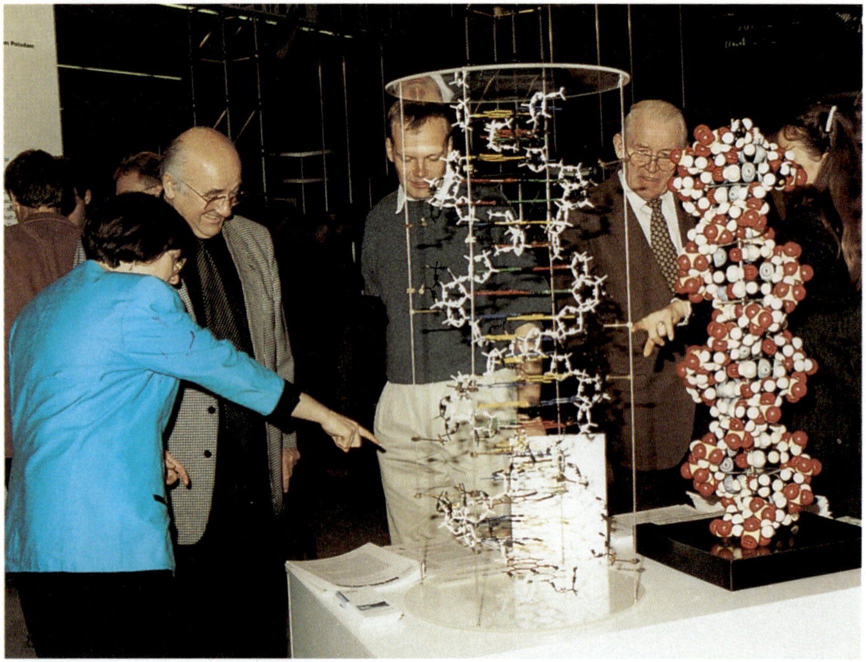

Visitors' service

The visitors' service within the Press and Public Relations Division endeavours to offer interested groups a continuous spectrum of visiting programs tailored to their particular profile. In 1991, 1992, and 1993, a total of 199 groups of visitors comprising almost 5500 people learned about current developments in cancer research, their fundamentals and problems, both in lectures and at first hand in the laboratories of the Deutsches Krebsforschungszentrum.

A new concept for visitors was conceived in 1992 and put into practice in 1993. Since the number of interested citizens had been increasing continuously over the years, the individual supervision of single groups began to exceed the existing capacities. This problem was solved by concentrating on events aimed at only one target group at a time. Within this new concept, the first Pupils' Forum of the Deutsches Krebsforschungszentrum took place on

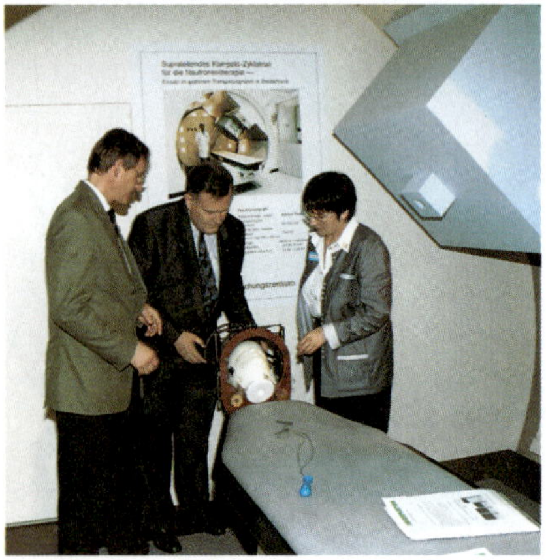

Fig. 126 a, b
Presentation of the Deutsches Krebsforschungszentrum at the Hanover Fair in 1993 and 1994; a) Topic "Genetic Engineering". On the left, Dr. Martina Pötschke-Langer, Division of Press and Public Relations; b) Topic "Neutron Therapy". In the center, Erwin Teufel, Chief Minister of the State of Baden-Württemberg, in conversation with Priv.-Doz. Dr. Günther Gademann, Division of Oncological Diagnostics and Therapy, and Dr. Martina Pötschke-Langer

Fig. 127
A work of Angelika Dirscherl

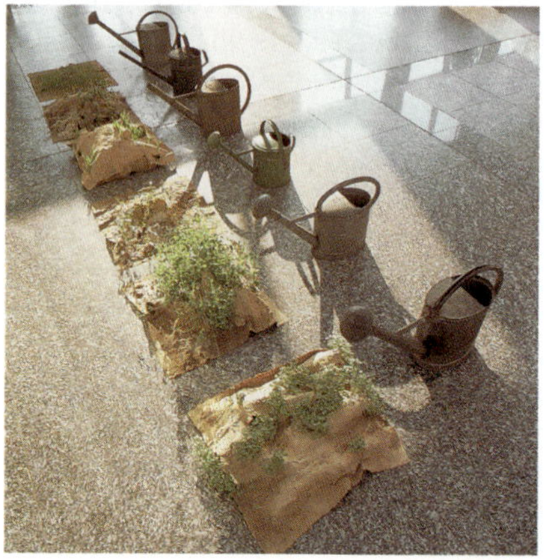

Art exhibitions

The art exhibitions, which form part of the internal communication and have been initiated and organized by the press office since 1981, have been continued. Thirteen exhibitions took place. They are aimed at furthering contacts between citizens of Heidelberg and staff members of the Deutsches Krebsforschungszentrum and at enlivening the "social climate".

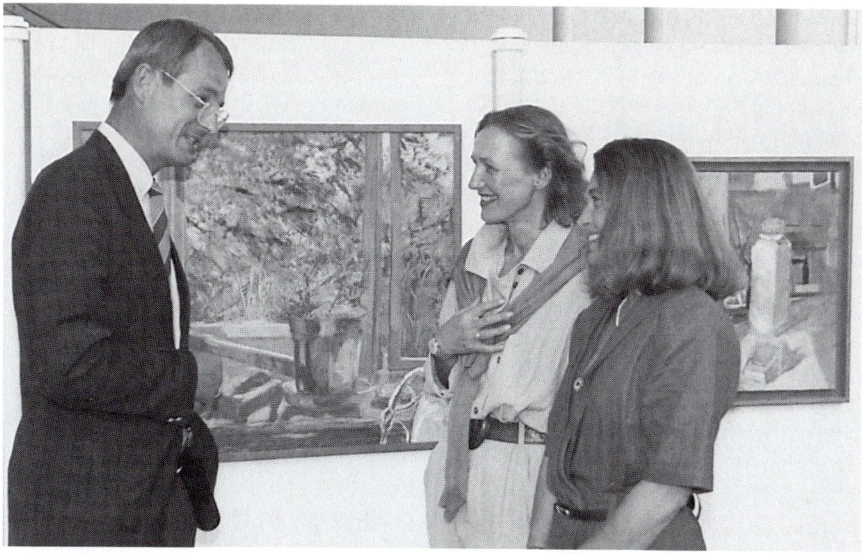

Fig. 128

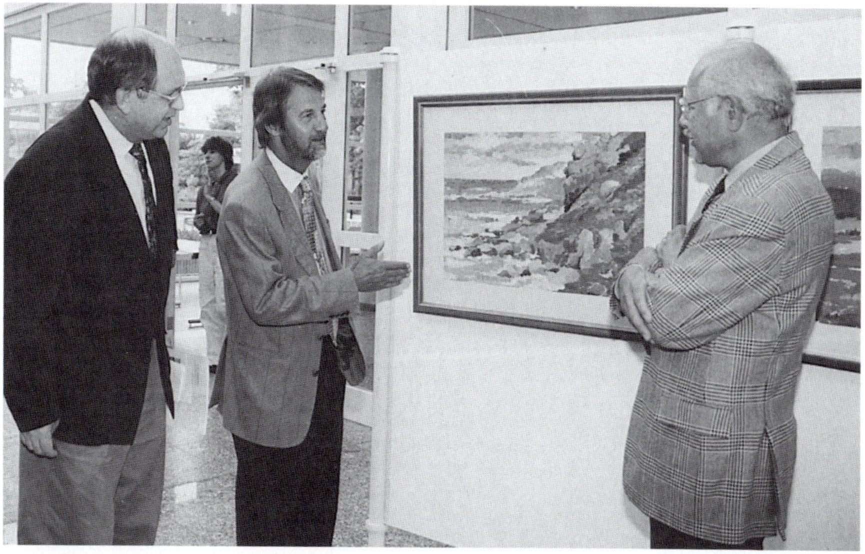

Fig. 128
Dr. Reinhard Grunwald, Administrative Member of the Management Board of the Deutsches Krebsforschungszentrum, talking to the painter Michèle Dandrieux-Werner (on the far right)

Fig. 129
African impressions by Uwe Knuth (middle), an exhibition in 1994. On the left, Prof. Dr. Werner W. Franke, Chairman of the Scientific Council; on the right, Prof. Dr. Gerhard Kaufmann, Director of the Altona Museum in Hamburg/North German State Museum

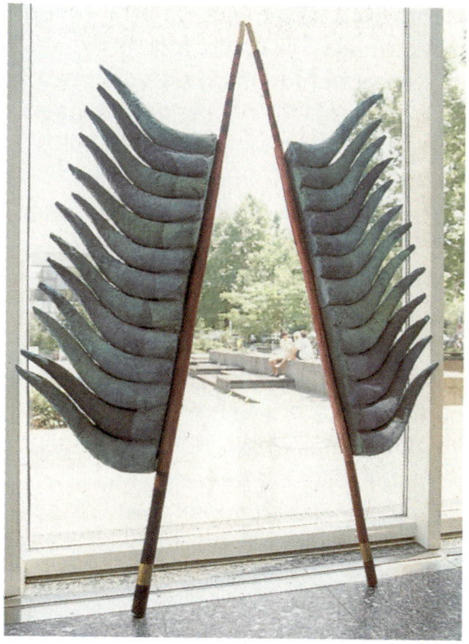

Fig. 130
A work of Bara Lehmann-Schulz

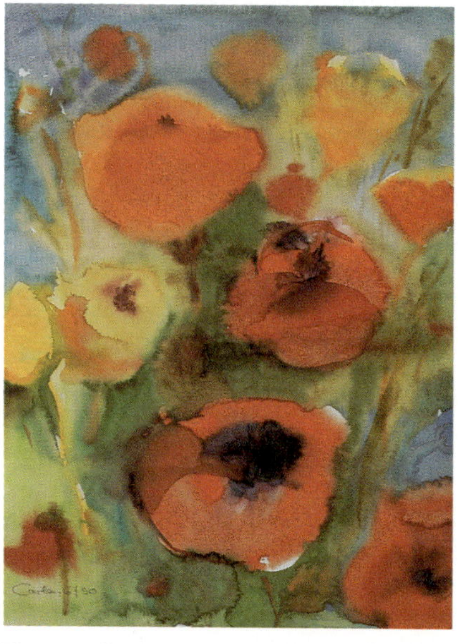

Fig. 131
Watercolor by Carla Hartmann-Obst

March 16, 1993; it was followed by the first Patients' Forum on March 18, 1993. Further forums were organized on September 7, 1993 and on September 22, 1993; on November 10, 1993 the third Pupils' Forum took place. These forums, which are geared specifically to high-school classes, particularly to advanced courses in biology, chemistry, and physics, and to patients and their families, enable the target group to be informed about new developments in a way that gives priority to its particular background and interests. Selected talks are delivered in the morning; in the afternoon these may be followed by visits to individual laboratories, which attempt to cater for the participants' wishes.

To optimize these events, an evaluation has been carried out. A survey among the participants of the second Patients' Forum in September 1993 indicated that 98% of those questioned would like another information day of this kind. At the end of the event, which lasted half a day, one-third of the participants expressed the opinion that it would be good to have even more time available in future, since "cancer is an issue one can discuss endlessly". Thus, the next patients' day was organized with a whole-day program.

More and more schools are making use of this opportunity to acquire highly concentrated information: While in 1991 and 1992 about 400 pupils visited the Center, this number doubled in 1993.

Of the individual visitors to the Deutsches Krebsforschungszentrum the politicians deserve special mention. They come in order to learn first hand about prospects for cancer research, structural and financial aspects, and issues such as animal protection, the genetic engineering law, and data protection. Among them were members of the Research Committee of the German Bundestag and the respective committees of the Landtag of Baden-Württemberg, the Federal Ministers Gerda Hasselfeldt, Horst Seehofer, Dr. Paul Krüger, and the State Ministers Brigitte Unger-Soyka (Baden-Wüttemberg) and Prof. Dr. Rolf Frick (Sachsen-Anhalt). Along with individual visitors and visitor groups, which are taken care of by the press office, frequent visits are made within the framework of scientific exchange by scientists from Germany and abroad to their colleagues at the Deutsches Krebsforschungszentrum.

All biomedical talks at the scientific institutions in Heidelberg are documented by the press office in a computer list which is available on request (current printrun: 500). This means of communication about scientific work and results provides another basis for regular contacts.

Organization of events

In the period at hand the press office has supported the organization of 24 scientific symposia, conferences, and meetings. The annual meeting of the Academia Europaea that took place September 18–21, 1991 deserves special mention. Of the appointed members of the Academia, which is an association of European researchers from all areas of science, 32 attended. The Federal Research Minister, Dr. Heinz Riesenhuber, who gave a talk entitled "Scientific Advice from the Perspective of a Minister," used the event as an opportunity to catch up with new developments in cancer research at the Deutsches Krebsforschungszentrum. Journalists from all European countries had been invited to this interdisciplinary conference, which dealt with the topics "Why we need to study the human genome," "Population migrations," "Old age: opportunities and problems," "The search for meaning in contemporary life," "Expert advice – Science and policy: Coping with uncertainty". A round-table talk was devoted to the topic of

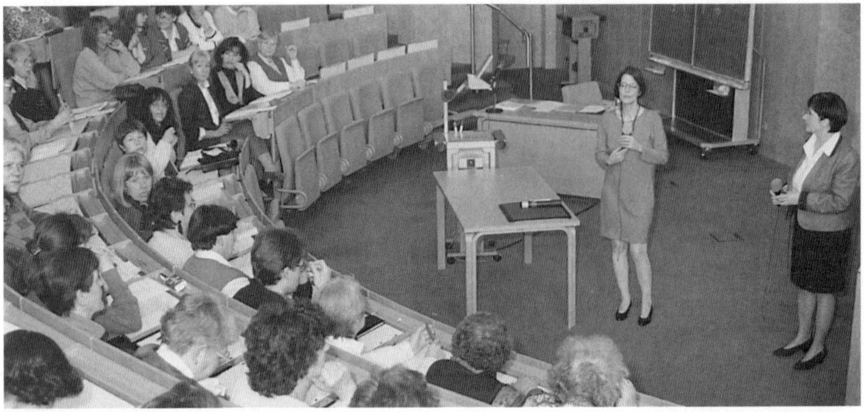

Fig. 132
Prof. Dr. Margot Zöller, head of the division "Tumor Progression and Immune Defense," and Dr. Martina Pötschke-Langer, talking to participants of the Patient's Forum

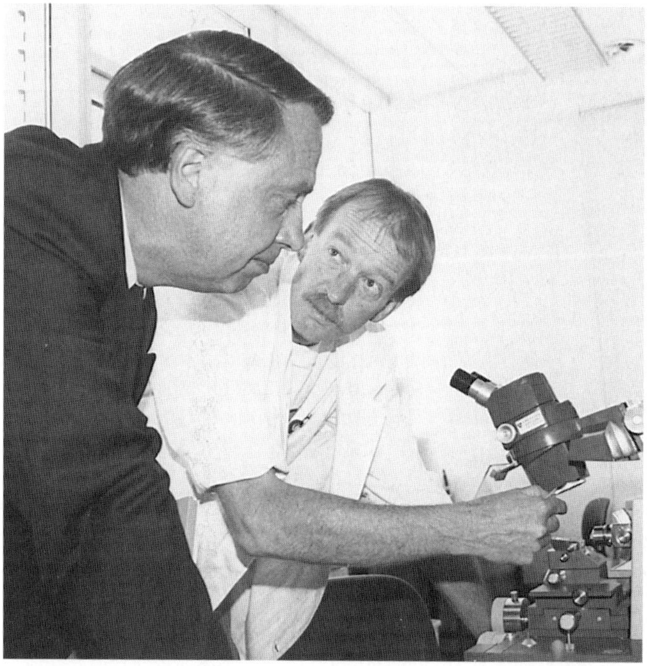

Fig. 133
Priv.-Doz. Dr. Hanswalter Zentgraf of the Research Program "Applied Tumor Virology" explaining the functioning of an ultramicrotome, which is used to cut ultrathin sections for electron microscopy, to the Parliamentary Secretary of the German Ministry for Research and Technology Bernd Neumann

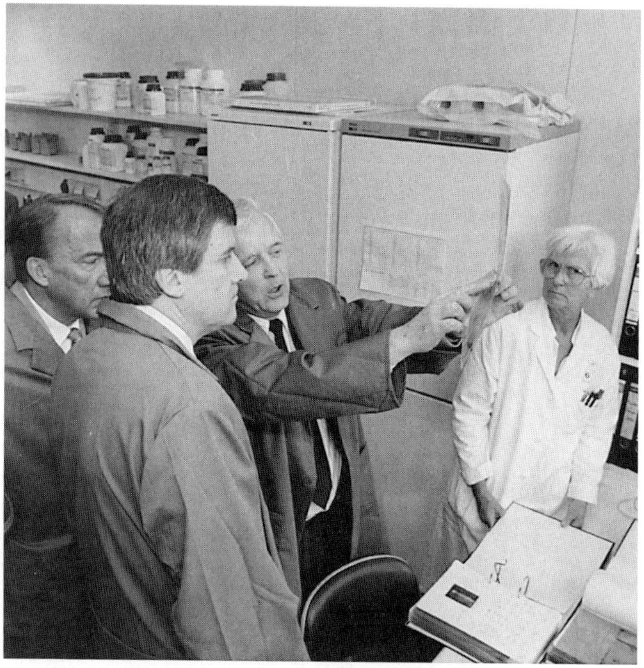

Fig. 134
The German Minister of Health Horst Seehofer learned first hand about the state-of-the-art in research on human papillomaviruses. On the right is Marion Frick, in the middle, Prof. Dr. Harald zur Hausen

"Use and abuse of expert advice: Science and politics of environment".

An important moment in 1992 was the inauguration of the new Institute for Applied Tumor Virology on 4 May. The State Secretary Dr. Gebhard Ziller from the Federal Ministry of Research and Technology, and the Science Minister of Baden-Württemberg, Klaus von Trotha, delivered speeches, and the Head of the Directorate General for Science, Research and Development of the European Union in Brussels, Prof. Dr. Paolo Maria Fasella, gave a talk on aspects of research support by the European Union.

The inauguration of the new institute also served as an occasion to arrange a symposium on human tumor viruses, which was co-organized by the General Motors Cancer Research Foundation.

The Karl Heinrich Bauer Course Laboratory, inaugurated on June 18, 1993, will play a special role in the support of young scientists at the Deutsches Krebsforschungszentrum. It will in the future enable new techniques and methods to be taught in a laboratory that is specifically geared to this purpose and will be at the courses' exclusive disposal. The establishment of this new laboratory received significant financial support from the Association for the Furtherance of Cancer Research in Germany, Heidelberg.

Protection of nonsmokers

Over the last 3 years the Deutsches Krebsforschungszentrum has been particularly active in anti-tobacco campaigns. Since 1991, the Center, together with the chairman of the medical study group "Smoking and Health," have represented the Federal Republic of Germany in the anti-tobacco working group of the European Union. In 1992, within the framework of this European collaboration and together with the Federal Union for Health and the German

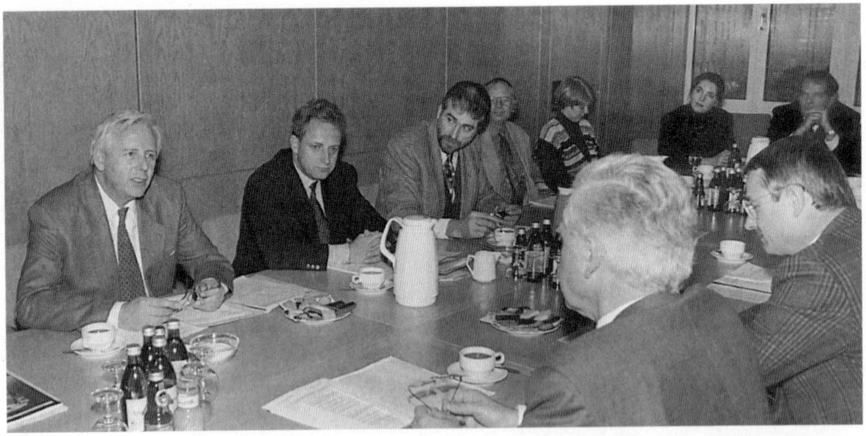

Fig. 135
Discussion at the Deutsches Krebsforschungszentrum held by the CDU working group "Science and Research" of the Regional Parliament of Baden-Württemberg about questions concerning main research objectives and the future support of cancer research. On the left, Klaus von Trotha, Minister of Science and Research of the State of Baden-Württemberg

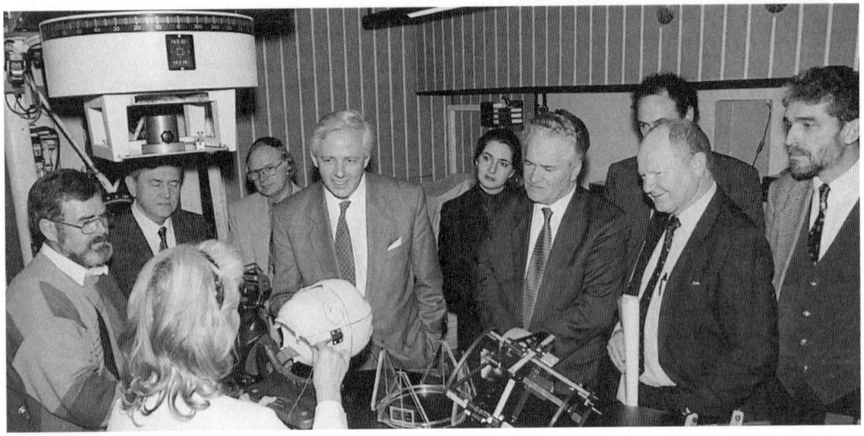

Fig. 136
The Center's cooperation with the University Radiological Hospital, here in the field of precision radiotherapy, was a subject of the visit of the CDU working group. Second from the right is Prof. Dr. Michael Wannenmacher, Managing Director of the University Radiological Hospital in Heidelberg, on the left, senior physician Dr. Rita Engenhart, University Radiological Hospital

Cancer Society, and with the support of the European Bureau for Action on Smoking and Health (BASP), Brussels, the "Coalition Against Smoking" was founded. Its aim is to translate into legal action the EU recommendations for protecting nonsmokers among other things, a ban on advertising and the prohibition of smoking in public places, for example, in Germany. At the inaugural meeting on April 29, 1992 in Bonn, 80 organizations joined the Coalition Against Smoking. Held in connection with this inaugural meeting was a symposium on the topic of "Youth Protection and Smoking" under the auspices of Prof. Rita Süssmuth, President of the German Bundestag. The second symposium was held in Bonn on October 16, 1992 and addressed the subject of "Banning Smoking in Public Buildings". Both symposia received significant financial support from the European Union's program "Europe Against Cancer". The topic of the 1994 Symposium on August 31, in Bonn was "Poverty and Smoking in Germany".

The internal agreement drawn up 6 years ago to protect nonsmokers at the Deutsches Krebsforschungszentrum now serves as a model for other health-conscious institutions that have made similar commitments, or intend to do so.

Trainees

The wide-ranging activities of the Press and Public Relations Division are only available due to the energetic efforts of the trainees who come to learn about, and gain practical experience in, the fields of scientific journalism and public relations. In the years 1991 to 1993, 20 trainees worked in the division, among them 11 biologists, a chemist, a publicist, an ecotrophologist, a social scientist, a PhD student of scientific theory, a qualified translator, a medic, and two physicists. The trainees are directly involved in the day-to-day work of the division and, whenever possible, their 3- to 6-month stay gives them the opportunity to carry out a project of their own.

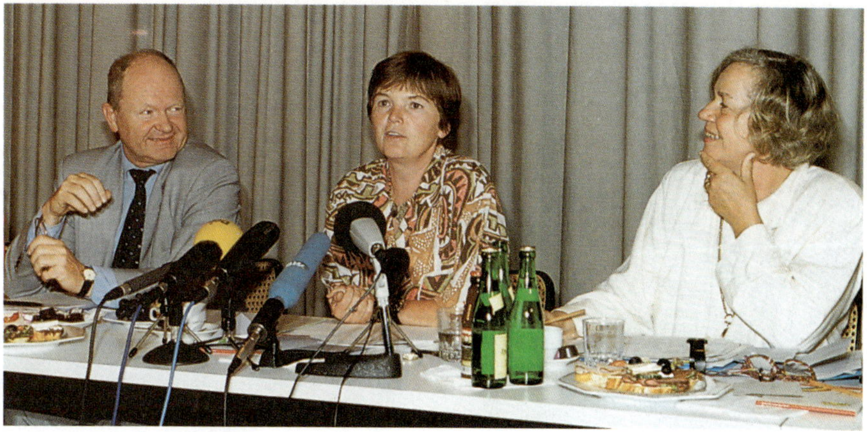

Fig. 137
Press conference of the “Coalition Against Smoking” on the occasion of a symposium on “Poverty and Smoking” in August 1994 in Bonn. On the left, Prof. Dr. Michael Wannenmacher in his function as President of the German Cancer Society. In the center, Dr. Ulrike Maschewsky-Schneider, Bremen Institute for Prevention Research and Social Medicine

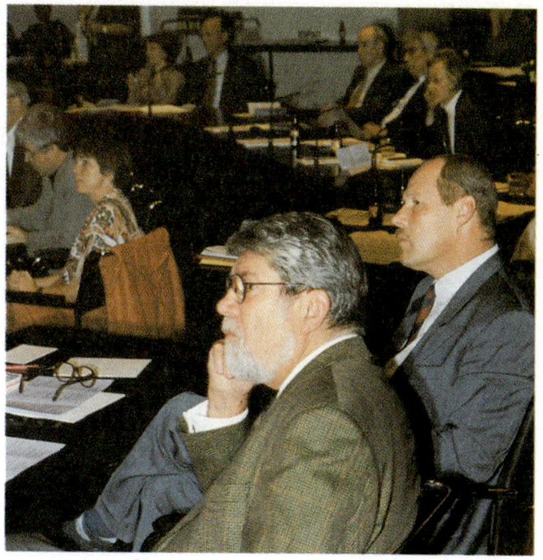

Fig. 138
Listening attentively, the President of the Federal German Association for Health, Dr. Hans-Peter Voigt, and the Executive Secretary, Gottfried Neuhaus, co-organizers of the symposium “Poverty and Smoking”

The telephone Cancer Information Service (KID: Krebsinformationsdienst)

KID is the nationwide telephone service of the Deutsches Krebsforschungszentrum which has offered free information and answers to questions on the subject of cancer since 1986. It was founded with the aim of providing objective information to enable people to cope with the disease and with the problems that it entails, to help reduce fears and prejudices, and to support the patients' own activities and those of their relatives. Thus KID – linked to the Press and Public Relations Division – serves as a bridge between the technical world of the specialists and the general public.

KID is a project of the Federal Ministry of Health, with financial support also being contributed annually by the Ministry of Employment, Health, Family, and Social Affairs of the State of Baden-Württemberg. The Tumor Center Heidelberg/Mannheim supports the service with expert information.

The motivation behind this service stems from the high level of interest shown by the general public in questions of cancer research and therapy, and from the large number of enquiries on this topic addressed to the Deutsches Krebsforschungszentrum. These demonstrate the great need for information concerning the complex, and for the layman often confusing, subject of oncology. The many threats to existence posed by cancer are as yet not counterbalanced by sufficient concrete information that is relevant to the individual. It is common knowledge that doctors and medical specialists are frequently overtaxed when it comes to dealing with problems that go beyond the primary care. Patients and their families often feel alone and unsupported in matters relating to the details of the individual treatment, the significance of various methods of diagnosis, and about how to carry on their lives, for example, with regard to nutrition. As a possible source of information the media tend to cause more problems and uncertainties than they solve, since they only publish isolated items of news that do not fit together to form a useful picture. On the other hand, numerous scientific studies have shown that relevant objective information can indeed help the afflicted to cope with the disease and the related problems.

The Cancer Information Service has thus taken up the challenge of counteracting the deficit of reliable information communicated about the causes of cancer, prevention, early detection, therapies, and related social and social-rights questions. The results of both national and international research efforts are also integrated into the available information, thus providing a novel concept which is designed to serve the needs of interested members of the public and cancer sufferers, their families and friends. The model upon which the KID is based is the Cancer Information Service of the National Cancer Institute in the USA, which has operated successfully since 1976. The special feature of this service is the personal information and the possibility of reacting to individually expressed needs. The chosen medium of communication, i.e., the telephone, facilitates the provision of direct information and answers to the individual's specific questions, and the enquirer can always remain anonymous. KID regards itself as a nerve center for up-to-date information on all aspects of oncology; it does not dispense advice, nor does it express an opinion; rather, it communicates the latest scientific knowledge and certainly also a picture of areas that are still the subject of scientific controversy. KID cannot and will not become a substitute for a consultation with the doctor, and makes this need clear to patients whilst also attempting to help answer questions that arise as a preliminary to such a consultation.

In the 8 years of its existence, KID until the end of the year 1993 has received more than 83000 enquiries. A great many more attempts to get through – in 1992 alone the number was 59 139 – were registered by the counting device but could not be connected due to lack of capacity. In 1991 and 1992 the Federal Minister of Health made special financial support available in order that the new (former Eastern German) States could be integrated into this service. These funds were used, among other things, to initiate a letter-answering service, to selectively distribute information material, and to investigate the provisions made for cancer sufferers in the new States. Contacts were made to all the newly established health facilities.

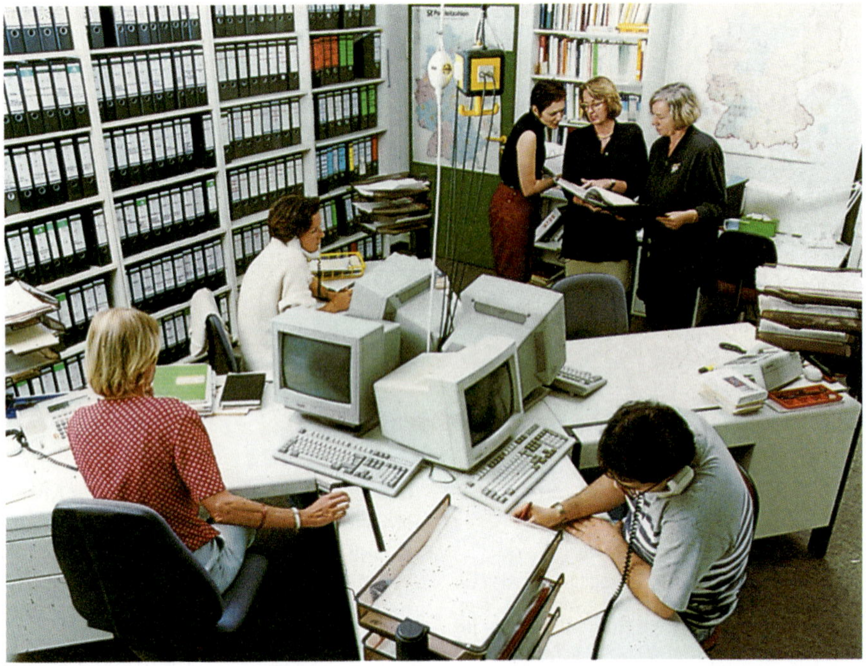

Fig. 139
The telephone Cancer Information Service KID answers approximately 11 000 questions relating to cancer every year

In the meantime, people from the eastern part of Germany have also begun to make use of KID. Some limitations remain, however, since the telephone network still has insufficient capacity.

From 8 a.m. until 8 p.m., Monday through Friday, anyone may call KID at phone number 06221-410121. No question is regarded as too "stupid" or too strange. Three times a week – on Tuesdays, Wednesdays, and Thursdays, from 6 p.m. to 8 p.m. – KID also provides information in Turkish.

The telephone service is operated by 21 freelance staff members who work in shifts and who man up to four telephone lines at one time. All these staff are health professionals: doctors, pharmacologists, chemists, nurses, psychologists, or medical-technical assistants. They thus largely avoid the use of technical jargon in their conversations. All of them have acquired basic knowledge of oncology in a comprehensive annual training program. In this, scientists and clinicians from all specialist areas instruct them in the basics of the most important oncological disciplines, explain the latest medical and methodological developments, and also discuss methods of leading a conversation. This annually repeated event, which is tailored to current requirements, is supplemented by regular internal events providing information about the latest developments.

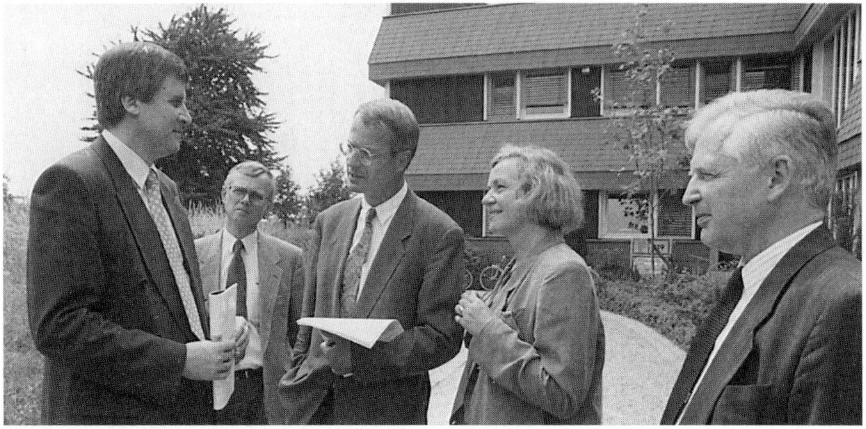

Fig. 140
The German Minister of Health Horst Seehofer on a visit to the Cancer Information Service KID, a project of his ministry. Second from the left is Dr. Konrad Buschbeck, German Ministry of Research and Technology

The information which is needed to answer the telephone enquiries is put together according to topic by the multidisciplinary team comprising the full-time staff members who form the scientific and organizational backbone of the service. A continually updated database contains the most important basic information in text form as well as about 2000 addresses of cancer-related institutions – from tumor centers and aftercare clinics through psychosocial advice centers. All this information can be accessed directly on the telephone.

Most of the enquiries received can be answered immediately with the help of the available pool of information. New questions concerning, for example, the latest research data or new methods of as yet unproven efficacy, are passed on to the investigative team, who have access to a multitude of sources of oncological information. In particular, the geographical and structural proximity to the Deutsches Krebsforschungszentrum and the hospitals of the Tumor Center Heidelberg/Mannheim means that expert knowledge is always close at hand. The necessary information is acquired in personal or telephone contact with the scientists of the Deutsches Krebsforschungszentrum, oncologists from the hospitals of the Tumor Center Heidelberg/Mannheim, experimental and clinical scientists from other research institutes in Germany or abroad, and with administrative organizations responsible for social welfare in Germany. Other sources of information are the central library of the Deutsches Krebsforschungszentrum with its roughly 68 000 volumes and international literature databases for biomedicine which can be accessed on-line from the scientific information department of the Deutsches Krebsforschungszentrum. The information which is gathered by these various means is collated and turned into readily understandable texts which are then given to the staff that man the telephone service. In answer to the most commonly asked questions and on particularly topical subjects, the scientific staff prepare written summaries which ensure that the corresponding questions are answered in a consistent manner. These texts are regularly updated. The sustained investigative work leads to a continual growth of the information pool of KID. In order to structure and manage this information, and to make it permanently available to the staff of the telephone service, KID works with a specially designed database system which runs on networked personal computers. This database system contains and manages two essential areas of information: first, the texts related to the most commonly posed questions and to currently important topics, which can be retrieved by entering relevant keywords, and, second, the addresses of about 2000 tumor centers, specialist oncological groups, aftercare facilities, psychosocial cancer advice centers, self-help organizations, and other cancer-related organizations and facilities to which the caller can turn in case of need. The databank also includes contact persons in medical centers who can help the KID staff with special investigations. In order to collect reliable and up-to-date details of cancer centers, specialist oncological groups, aftercare clinics, and psychosocial advice centers, KID carried out its own surveys.

In making available addresses, KID does not offer information “for its own benefit” but pursues the principle of comprehensive cover and integrative information: The nationwide communication of addresses should help the caller to find the necessary facilities as close as possible to his or her home.

With the assistance of this documentation of facts and addresses together

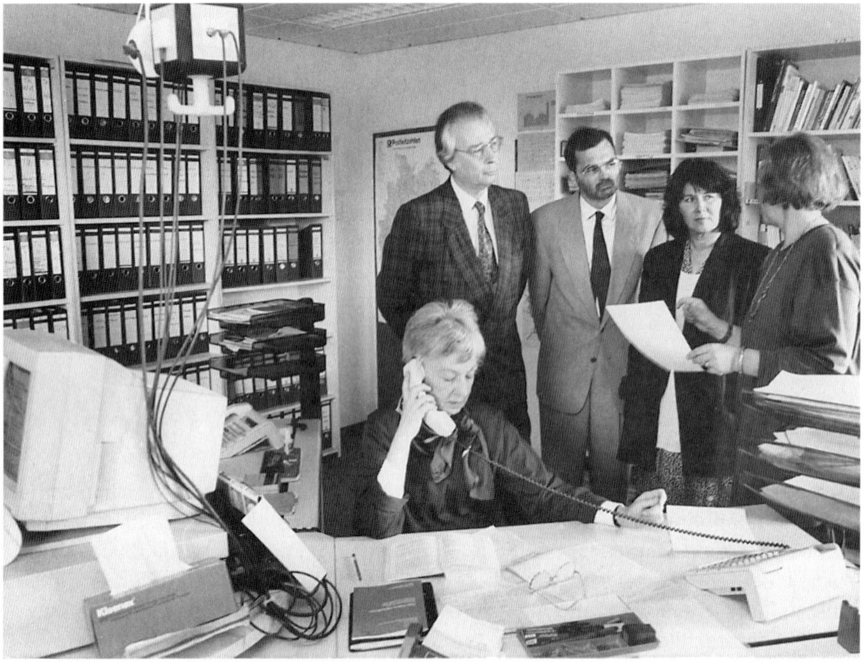

Fig. 141
The Minister for Women and the Family, Further Education and the Arts of the State of Baden-Württemberg, Brigitte Unger-Soyka, and the then Member of Parliament Prof. Dr. Hartmut Soell learning about the work of the Cancer Information Service KID and, in particular, about the possibilities and limits for its expansion. In the middle is Prof. Dr. Stefan C. Meuer, member of the Scientific Council of KID

with a reference library containing the most important oncological basics and a collection of the many cancer leaflets and brochures available from various sources (in case written information is requested), more than 85% of the enquiries can be answered immediately. The remaining 15% comprises new or complex questions which require further searching. The result of this search is communicated to the caller in a second conversation; when requested, the return call is made by KID.

That the information is both correct and up to date is guaranteed by the permanent communication with hospitals and scientists. The quality and consistent standard of the information provided by KID is also ensured by regular further training of the staff and continuous supervision under the guidance of an experienced psychologist, which includes extensive case discussions. Fundamental decisions concerning the content are the responsibility of the scientific advisory council of the Cancer Information Service. This comprises clinicians from the Tumor Center and scientists from the Deutsches Krebsforschungszentrum.

Every call is statistically evaluated with the help of a specially designed questionnaire. This records – anonymously and encoded – the most important elements of every conversation. This facilitates not only an exact appraisal of the requirements of the caller, but also the continuous evaluation, further development, and improvement of the service. In this way KID is trying to identify special information deficits in particular sections of the community and thus contribute to their alleviation.
Who calls the Cancer Information Service? Two-thirds of the callers are women. About 45% are cancer sufferers and 40% close relatives of patients. Doctors and other health service professionals also take advantage of KID, with about 7% of the enquiries coming from this sector. A further group of callers – also about 7% of the total – are interested members of the public who are neither directly nor indirectly affected by cancer. However, since prevention of cancer is also an important issue, such consultations have a high priority too.

The questions addressed to the Cancer Information Service are very wide ranging. The most common topic is therapy (about 60%), followed by aftercare, diagnostics, and cancer risk factors. Where the question is related to a particular type of cancer, for men these are intestinal cancer, and prostate and bronchial carcinomas, for women, in more than 45% of cases, breast cancer. On the other hand, in relation to their incidence, rare tumors are quite frequently the topic of enquiries. The most common occasion for calling is after the completion of the first treatment, i.e., some time after the patient has been released from hospital. This would appear to indicate that, in this situation of re-orientation, both the afflicted and their relatives find themselves in something of an information vacuum.

The group of non-afflicted callers poses questions mainly about symptoms, followed by cancer risk factors, methods of diagnosis, and early recognition.

Beyond this statistical evaluation, the experience gained in the work of KID has also thrown up a large number of new questions. These have been investigated since the beginning of 1987 within the framework of accompanying scientific studies. The topics of investigation have included, among others, "Knowledge about, and attitude to, cancer, tumor medicine, and prevention," "Information about cancer – the value of various sources and media for the public," "Requirements of KID callers for information about methods of unproven efficacy," "Knowledge and perception of cancer risks in the German population – definition of information measures that could possibly be improved" (a project within the framework of the program "Europe Against Cancer"), and "The role of information in helping patients to overcome cancer". The object of these investigations is to first determine the current situation, and thence contribute to the future development in the health services of communication and the information demand concerning cancer. In the period 1991–1993, 10 talks and 12 information booths at symposia and congresses were used by the staff of KID as a means of drawing attention to what the Cancer Information Service can offer.

In addition, in 1993 KID published a book with the title "Thema Krebs – Fragen und Antworten" (Subject Cancer – Questions and Answers) (Springer-Verlag, Heidelberg). The book presents the most common questions together with detailed answers; it also includes a list of addresses which give the reader the possibility of directly contacting centers for cancer therapy and aftercare.

Information about cancer plays an essential role in coping with the disease, both for patients and for their relatives. Enquiries about the value attributed to information from the media were made by the Cancer Information Service in supplementary telephone interviews. These show that newspapers, magazines, books, and brochures are valued second only to a consultation with the doctor. Television, on the other hand, is rated lower than a conversation with relatives and friends. However, those questioned expressed a distinctly low opinion of the quality of the information reported in the press. The main criticisms concerned lack of clarity and sensationalism. Medical programs on television are evidently an exception, and these were judged favorably. Now we have come full circle: from the work with the press, which is aimed first and foremost at the media and only indirectly at members of the public, to the Cancer Information Service, which directly provides the individual with "unfiltered" information. The latter thus serves as an essential addition to the brief reports to be found particularly in the print media, which are easily misunderstood and may awaken false hopes. A close cooperation between the two areas has proved to be exceptionally useful, for example, in enabling journalists to be provided with background information, or in that television and radio programs or press reports include in their coverage a mention of the KID telephone number. The extremely positive experience to date makes clear that there are possible courses of "concerted action" which help to ensure the provision of lively and sound cancer information.

19

Meeting, Workshops and Symposia

For many years now, the Deutsches Krebsforschungszentrum has been organizing an intensive information exchange between scientists in Germany and abroad.

The following events, which took place between 1991 and 1993, deserve special mention:

Workshop on "Biostatistical Analysis of the Micronucleus Mutagenicity Assay", organized by the working group "Chemical Pharmaceutical Research" of the German Region of the International Biometric Society in cooperation with the Deutsches Krebsforschungszentrum
February 6, 1991

6th Symposium of the Division of Experimental Cancer Research within the German Cancer Society
April 10–12, 1991

Workshop on "Bioinformatics Aspects of the European Human Genome Project" – Meeting of the European partners in the "Human Genome Network" at the Deutsches Krebsforschungszentrum
April 26, 1991

"6th A.P.I.S. Congress on Medical Computing" of the "Association pour la Promotion de l'Informatique de Santé" in cooperation with the Deutsches Krebsforschungszentrum
May 6–8, 1991

Symposium on "Genes Controlling Cell Growth and Tumorigenesis in Drosophila" of the "Human Frontier Science Program", organized in cooperation with the Deutsches Krebsforschungszentrum
September 7–9, 1991

Annual meeting of the European Academy of Sciences "Academia Europaea", organized in cooperation with the Deutsches Krebsforschungszentrum
September 18–21, 1991

4th Heidelberg Cytometry Symposium, meeting of the Society for Cytometry in cooperation with the Deutsches Krebsforschungszentrum
October 17–19, 1991

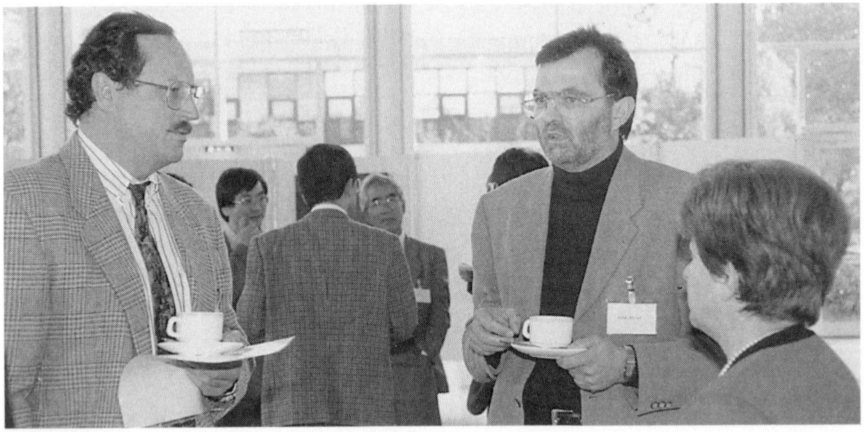

Fig. 142
At the German-Japanese workshop on specific aspects of cancer research in 1992: Prof. Dr. Bernhard Fleckenstein, Institute for Clinical Virology of the University of Erlangen-Nuremberg (left), Prof. Dr. Stefan C. Meuer, head of the Division of Applied Immunology of the Deutsches Krebsforschungszentrum and coordinator of the German-Japanese collaboration (center), Elfriede Egenlauf, head of the General Administration Department

International symposium on "Skin Carcinogenesis in Man and in Experimental Models" of the Deutsches Krebsforschungszentrum and the University of Heidelberg
October 29, 1991

"Second European Workshop on FDG in Oncology" of the European Program "Concerted Action in PET in Oncology" in cooperation with the Deutsches Krebsforschungszentrum
December 9–11, 1991

Symposium on "Molecular Biology of Aging" of the Heidelberg Academy of Sciences in cooperation with the Deutsches Krebsforschungszentrum
December 13–14, 1991

International course in "Cancer Epidemiology" of the Association for Documentation, Information and Statistics, the German Association for Social Medicine and Prevention, and the Deutsches Krebsforschungszentrum
April 6–10, 1992

International symposium on "Human Tumor Viruses" of the Deutsches Krebsforschungszentrum in cooperation with the General Motors Cancer Research Foundation
May 3–6, 1992

International symposium on "Computational Methods in Genome Research", European Data Resource for Human Genome Analysis
July 1–4, 1992

Symposium on "Neue Methoden in der Protein- und Nukleinsäure-Biochemie" (New methods in the biochemistry of proteins and nucleic acids) of the Society for Biological Chemistry in cooperation with the Deutsches Krebsforschungszentrum
September 10–12, 1992

Symposium on "Gene, Chromosomen, Krebs" (Genes, chromosomes, cancer), meeting of the working group "Molecular Genetics and Cytogenetics" of the German Cancer Society in cooperation with the Deutsches Krebsforschungszentrum
September 24–25, 1992

"3rd Indo-German Workshop on Recent Results in Cooperative Cancer Research" of the Deutsches Krebsforschungszentrum
October 4–7, 1992

Symposium on "Host Defence Mechanisms and Molecular Basis of Cancer" of the German-Japanese Collaborative Program in Cancer Research
October 18–21 1992

5th Heidelberg Cytometry Symposium of the Society for Cytometry in cooperation with the Deutsches Krebsforschungszentrum
October 22–24, 1992

Symposium on "Adhäsionsmoleküle" (Adhesion molecules) of the German Society for Immunology in cooperation with the Deutsches Krebsforschungszentrum
February 11–12, 1993

Symposium on "Dilemma – Logic Engineering in Primary Shared Care and Oncology" of the Deutsches Krebsforschungszentrum
February 13–15, 1993

Workshop on "Neue Planungsmethoden in der Strahlentherapie" (New planning methods in radiotherapy), organized by the University Radiological Hospital in cooperation with the Deutsches Krebsforschungszentrum
March 19–20, 1993

Symposium on "Molekularbiologische Ursachen der Krebsentstehung, neue Therapieformen und epidemiologische Untersuchungen" (Molecular-biological causes of carcinogenesis, new therapies and epidemiological research), 7th symposium of the Division of Experimental Cancer Research within the German Cancer Society in cooperation with the Deutsches Krebsforschungszentrum
March 23–27, 1993

Symposium on "Patenting of Human Genes and Living Organisms", organized in cooperation with the Heidelberg Academy of Sciences
July 1–2, 1993

Symposium on "Gene Diagnosis and Gene Therapy" of the Association for Clinical-Biomedical Research (KBF), organized jointly with the Deutsches Krebsforschungszentrum
October 4–6, 1993

Workshop on "Management of Clinical Research" of the Deutsches Krebsforschungszentrum
October 6–8, 1993

6th Heidelberg Cytometry Symposium of the Society for Cytometry in cooperation with the Deutsches Krebsforschungszentrum
October 21–23, 1993

International symposium on "Novel Approaches in Cancer Therapy" of the German Cancer Society in cooperation with the Deutsches Krebsforschungszentrum
December 1–4, 1993

International symposium on "Quantitative Risk Assessment" of the Deutsches Krebsforschungszentrum
December 2–3, 1993

Statutes and Articles of the Foundation Deutsches Krebsforschungszentrum

in the version according to the resolution passed by the Board of Trustees dated 21 June 1991, published in the Legal Gazette Baden-Württemberg on 9 August 1991

I. General Provisions

Section 1
Legal Form, Seat

The Deutsches Krebsforschungszentrum, a foundation under public law of the Land Baden-Württemberg, has its seat in Heidelberg.

Section 2
Purpose of the Foundation

(1) It is the purpose of the Foundation to engage in cancer research.

(2) The Foundation may undertake other tasks in this connection, inter alia further education and advanced training, and especially the promotion of young scientists.

(3) The research results are to be published.

Section 3
Non-Profit Institution

(1) As a non-profit institution the Foundation shall exclusively and directly serve the public interest, in particular scientific interests according to fiscal regulations.

(2) Any profits made may only be used for the purposes laid down in the Statutes and Articles. The Foundation may not grant benefits to any person by expenditures which run counter to the purposes of the Foundation or by disproportionately high awards.

Section 4
Assets of the Foundation

The assets of the Foundation shall consist of the goods and titles which have been or are being created or acquired with the aid of the funds placed at its disposal by the Federal Republic of Germany, hereinafter referred to as the Federal Republic, the German Land Baden-Württemberg, hereinafter referred to as the Land, or by third parties. The assets of the Foundation shall be used for the purposes laid down in section 2.

Section 5
Financing of the Foundation

(1) The Federal Republic and the Land will provide for the necessary expenditures of the Foundation in as far as this is not covered by income from other sources or by own or foreign means – with the exception of donations and investment returns therefrom – by allowances according to further agreement.

(2) The means to be provided according to paragraph 1 will be allocated to the Foundation according to the provisions of the budgetary law within the framework of the approved budgets of the Foundation and the budgets of the Federal Republic and the Land.

Section 6
Budget of the Foundation

(1) The budget of the Foundation must contain any receipts to be expected in the fiscal year, any probable expenses, and any probable authorizations to incur liabilities. Receipts and expenditures must be balanced.

(2) The budget will have to be approved by the authority controlling the Foundation.

(3) Grants made to the Foundation are to be recorded in an appendix to the Foundation's accounts.

II. Organs of the Foundation

Section 7
Executive Organs

The organs oÏf the Foundation are:

a) the Board of Trustees,
b) the Management Board,
c) the Scientific Council.

Section 8
Tasks of the Board of Trustees

(1) The Board of Trustees will supervise the legality, expediency, and economy of the conduct of the Foundation's transactions. It will decide on the aims of research and important research policy and financial affairs of the Foundation. It will determine the principles of management and those governing result control. It may give directives to the Management Board in special matters of research policy and finance as well as for the implementation of result control.

(2) The Board of Trustees sets up the annual budgets and the long- term financial plans including the programs for development and investment. It will decide on changes in the Statutes and Articles and on the dissolution of the Foundation as well as on other matters laid down in these Statutes.

(3) The following matters must be previously approved by the Board of Trustees:

a) the annual and long-term research programs;
b) taking up further tasks and discontinuing previous tasks;
c) the foundation, dissolution, and amalgamation of research programs, divisions, and central facilities, the start and termination of projects, and the extension of research programs and projects;
d) the appointment and recall of the heads of divisions, of the administrative director as well as of the directors of central facilities and projects, as well as the appointment of the coordinators of the research programs;
e) the regulations for research programs and projects;
f) the regulations for elections and the rules of procedure;
g) the regulations governing appointments;
h) principles governing the utilization of the research results of the Foundation;
i) extraordinary legal transactions and measures exceeding the framework of current business operations which may exert considerable influence upon the position and activity of the Foundation; significant agreements concerning cooperation with other German undertakings and institutions, and agreements concerning cooperation with foreign undertakings and institutions; entering into contracts which impose upon the Foundation obligations exceeding a period of one year, inasfar as they are not within the scope of normal business or provided for in the approved budget;
k) drawing up, changing or terminating employment contracts in excess of or outside the tariff, granting other benefits in excess of or outside the tariff, as well as entering into contracts exceeding an amount fixed by the Board of Trustees;
l) measures of collective tariff commitments or formation and general regulations concerning remuneration and social benefits, as well as setting up directives governing the granting of reimbursement of travel and moving costs, of separation allowances, and of expenses for the use of motor vehicles.

(4) For particular types of legal transactions and measures, the Board of Trustees may give its agreement in general.

(5) In urgent cases it is sufficient to have the prior written consent of the President and the Deputy President of the Board of Trustees. The other members of the Board of Trustees are to be immediately informed by the President about the action.

Section 9
Composition of the Board of Trustees

(1) The Board of Trustees consists of, at most, eighteen honorary members.

(2) Out of these

a) four members – one of them being the President – will be delegated and removed from office by the Federal Republic,
b) two members – one of them being the Deputy President – will be delegated and removed from office by the Land,
c) three scientists working for the Foundation and without a seat on the Management Board – at least one of them being head of a division – will be appointed by the Land in

agreement with the Federal Republic from a list of six nominees drawn up by all members of the scientific staff. Further details will be settled by election regulations to be issued by the Management Board in consultation with the Scientific Council and with the consent of the Board of Trustees. If those appointed have seats on the Scientific Council, their membership in the Scientific Council will be terminated upon acceptance of their appointment to the Board of Trustees,

d) seven external members (mainly specialists) will be appointed by the Land in agreement with the Federation upon consultation with the Management Board and the Scientific Council,

e) two members as the representatives of the University of Heidelberg, i.e. one proposed jointly by the Faculties of Medicine and Natural Sciences as well as the Rector (President) during his term of office or a professor charged by the latter, will be appointed by the Land in agreement with the Federal Republic.

(3) The members referred to in paragraph 2, items c, d and e will be appointed for a maximum period of three years. Re-appointment is permitted. After expiration of their term of office they will remain in office until the new appointments have been made according to paragraph 2, items c, d and e. Members may be removed from office for important reasons. Members leaving before their terms of office have expired must immediately be replaced from among the non-appointed applicants from the list of nominees according to paragraph 2, item c or by a new appointment according to paragraph 2, item d. Should the list of suggestions be exhausted, the procedure according to paragraph 2, item c shall be applied. Suggestion and appointment will be valid for the remaining term of office.

Section 10
Scientific Committee of the Board of Trustees

(1) The Scientific Committee prepares the decisions of the Board of Trustees in all scientific matters within the framework of section 8.

(2) The Scientific Committee bears the responsibility for the timely evaluation of the results of research programs, divisions and projects based on scientific expertise. As a rule, they set up ad hoc commissions manned by external scientists for this purpose.

(3) The Scientific Committee of the Board of Trustees consists of the external scientific members of the latter according to section 9, paragraph 2, item d. From among its members a chairman and a deputy chairman are elected. The President and the Deputy President of the Board of Trustees may take part in the sessions as guests. The Scientific Committee may set up standing rules which also determine the competence and procedures of the ad hoc commissions in greater detail.

Section 11
Standing Rules of The Board of Trustees and its Committees

(1) The Board of Trustees may set up standing rules which also determine the competence and procedure of the Committees in greater detail. Persons who are not members of the Board of Trustees may also hold a seat on the Committees; they will not take part in passing resolutions in Committees granted jurisdiction. A representative of the Federal Republic will assume the chair.

(2) The Board of Trustees may set up Committees to prepare its decisions as well as for certain matters to be decided by the Committee itself. At least one member each according to section 9, paragraph 2, items a through d must hold a seat on each Committee.

Section 12
Meetings of the Board of Trustees and its Committees

(1) The Board of Trustees will be convened by the President once in six months as a rule, but at least once every calendar year.

(2) The members of the Management Board as well as the chairman of the Scientific Council and the chairman of the staff representation or their deputies are entitled to attend the meetings of the Board of Trustees and its Committees in a consulting capacity, inasfar as the Board of Trustees or the Committee do not decide otherwise.

Section 13
Resolutions of the Board of Trustees and its Committees

(1) The Board of Trustees will constitute a quorum if two-thirds of its members are present or are represented in compliance with paragraph 2. The President or his deputy must be present. Committees holding power of decision will constitute a quorum if one member each according to section 9, paragraph 2, items a through c is present or represented.

(2) If unable to attend, the members of the Board of Trustees delegated by the Federal Republic and the Land may arrange to be represented by members of their administration, other members may be represented by a member of the Board of Trustees provided with a written limited power of attorney valid for the individual contingency.

(3) Resolutions of the Board of Trustees are passed with a majority of the valid votes cast. The President and the Deputy President have a double, transferable vote. In case of parity, the President shall have the casting vote. With important questions of research policy, in financial matters, in matters according to section 8, paragraphs 2 and 3, as well as with the appointment of the members and the release of the Management Board, resolutions may not be passed counter to the votes of members of the Board of Trustees delegated by the Federal Republic or the Land.

(4) Paragraphs 2 and 3 apply to the Committees correspondingly.

(5) In individual cases, the President, or if he is prevented, his deputy may cause resolutions to be passed in writing, by telex or by cable, insofar as no member of the Board of Trustees registers his immediate protest.

Section 14
Functions of the Management Board

(1) The Management Board directs the Foundation.

(2) The Management Board seeks the prior approval of the Scientific Council on the matters set down in section 8, paragraph 3, items a through g, as well as on

- the annual budget and long-term financial plans including the programs for development and investment;
- measures for the implementation of efficiency control of scientific work;
- measures to promote the flow of scientific information within the Foundation (work reports, colloquia, hearings);
- the co-operation with universities, other research institutions and international establishments;
- the submission of the scientific progress report to the Board of Trustees.

(3) Insofar as the Scientific Council's proposals in these matters should deviate, the Management Board will initiate a renewed joint discussion with the Scientific Council. If agreement cannot be reached, the Management Board will decide. If the Management Board makes a decision which deviates from the recommendations of the Scientific Council, it will have to supply an explanation in writing to the Scientific Council and the Board of Trustees.

Section 15
Composition of the Management Board, Scope of Authority

(1) The Management Board consists of at least one scientific and one administrative member. The administrative member shall be qualified for employment in the higher administrative service. The term of office for the members of the Management Board is limited and will, as a rule, amount to five years. Reappointment is permitted. Appointments may be revoked at any time.

(2) The chairman of the Management Board and the other members will be appointed and recalled by the Board of Trustees after consultation with the Scientific Council. The Scientific Council has the right of nomination for scientific members and for the chairman.

The members of the Management Board may not at the same time be coordinators of research programs or be members of the Scientific Council. The President of the Board of Trustees, who in this capacity represents the Foundation, will enter into, change or terminate contracts with the members of the Management Board.

(3) The chairman of the Management Board will be the scientific representative of the Foundation. Together with the administrative member he will represent the Foundation judicially and extrajudicially. In matters of current administration the administrative member may represent the Foundation on his own.

(4) The Management Board will set up standing rules which require the approval of the Board of Trustees. The standing rules will also regulate the authority according to paragraph 3, sentences 2 and 3 in the event the authorized representatives are prevented from fulfilling their function.

(5) The administrative member of the Management Board will be in charge of budget affairs in the sense of section 9 of the budget regulations of the Land Baden-Württemberg.

Section 16
Tasks of the Scientific Council

(1) The Scientific Council advises the Board of Trustees and the Management

Board in all significant matters of a scientific nature. In particular, it will offer advice concerning

a) the annual and long-term research programs;
b) appointment procedures, in particular the drawing up of appointment lists;
c) the appointment and recall of the heads of divisions as well as the directors of central facilities and projects;
d) taking up further functions and discontinuing previous functions;
e) founding, dissolving and amalgamating research programs, divisions and central facilities, starting and terminating projects, as well as extending research programs and projects;
f) issuing regulations for research programs and projects;
g) the appointments procedure;
h) principles for the utilization of the research results of the Foundation;
i) the annual budget and long-term financial plans including programs for development and investment;
k) measures for the implementation of result control of scientific work;
l) measures for the promotion of the flow of scientific information within the Foundation (work reports, colloquia, hearings);
m) the co-operation with universities, other research institutions and international establishments;
n) the scientific progress report.

In these matters the scientific Council, insofar as this is necessary according to section 14, paragraph 2, will pass resolutions about its consent with the intended decisions of the Management Board. If agreement cannot be teached, the procedure according to section 14, paragraph 3 will be applied.

(2) The Scientific Council may demand information from the Management Board on scientific matters and matters of research policy.

Section 17
Composition and Resolutions of the Scientific Council

(1) The Scientific Council consists of

a) the coordinators of research programs,
b) an equal number of representatives of the scientific staff.

(2) The members according to paragraph 1, letter b will be elected for a period of three years by the scientific staff of the Foundation in compliance with an election order. The election order is laid down by the Management Board in consultation with the Scientific Council and with the consent of the Board of Trustees.

(3) The Scientific Council elects from its midst a chairman and a deputy chairman.

(4) The members of the Management Board, the President of the Board of Trustees or a member of the Board of Trustees to be determined by the latter and a member of the staff representation may attend the meetings of the Scientific Council in a consultative capacity insofar as the Scientific Council does not decide otherwise in any individual instance.

(5) The Scientific Council will constitute a quorum if two thirds of its members including the chairman or the deputy chairman are present. Resolutions require a majority of the valid votes cast.

(6) The Scientific Council in consultation with the Management Board and with the consent of the Board of Trustees will set up standing rules governing the representation of the members.

III. Research Programs, Divisions, Projects and Central Facilities

Section 18
Research Programs and Divisions

(1) Research programs are the thematically defined and temporary collaboration of divisions.

(2) Divisions are scientifically independent research units co-operating within research programs. There are temporally limited and unlimited divisions. They are headed by heads of divisions who are appointed for an unlimited or limited period of time.

Being organizational units, the divisions serve the purpose of the Foundation. Within the divisions, working groups may be organized.

(3) The management of a research program consists of the heads of the divisions of that research program. It coordinates the scientific work of the divisions of that research program and makes all necessary decisions.

(4) The management of the research program nominates, with the consent of the Scientific Council and the Management Board, a coordinator from among its members. After approval from the Board of Trustees, the coordinator will be appointed by the Management Board. The term of office will amount to three years; re-appointment is possible. The tasks of the coordinators of the research programs are laid down in the standing order of the research programs, which also provides a research program committee and a research program assembly.

(5) The Management Board sets up standing rules for the divisions and the research programs after approval by the Scientific Council and the Board of Trustees.

Section 19 Projects

(1) The Foundation may carry out part of the research program in the form of projects. A project is understood to be a research activity largely structured in detail which is temporally and financially limited, bound towards a certain aim, and which exceeds the framework of a research program and which, due to its size and scientific importance, requires an independent organizational structure.

(2) The organization and implementation of projects are laid down in a project order which the Management Board will issue with the approval of the Scientific Council and the Board of Trustees.

Section 20 Central Facilities

(1) Central facilities shall serve to fulfill tasks of the entire Deutsches Krebsforschungszentrum or of several research programs and projects. They are reporting directly to the Management Board.

(2) The participation of the scientific staff in the elections to the Scientific Council and the Board of Trustees is regulated by the Management Board in the respective election orders with the approval of the Board of Trustees and the Scientific Council.

IV. Administration and Personnel Affairs

Section 21 Accounting, Auditing and Acceptance of the Accounts

(1) Accounts must be rendered annually by the Management Board concerning the income and expenditure as well as the assets and liabilities of the Foundation. Notwithstanding the legal auditing rights of the Federal Audit Office and the Audit Office of Baden-Württemberg, the annual accounts must be audited by a chartered accountant or auditing establishment. The Board of Trustees will decide who is to be entrusted with this task.

(2) At the end of the calendar year a business report and a statement of account is to be submitted to the Board of Trustees, the authority in control of the Foundation and the auditing authorities.

(3) Section 109, paragraph 3 of the budget regulations of Baden-Württemberg is applicable to the release. Organ for decision making is the Board of Trustees.

Section 22 Scientific Staff

The scientific staff as defined in these Statutes and Articles consists of all employees of the Foundation who are either university graduates or who carry out corresponding activities in the scientific field on the basis of equivalent abilities and experience and who have entered into an employment contract with the Foundation.

Section 23 Personnel Affairs

(1) Prior to the appointment of heads of divisions and the employment of scientific staff according to section 8, paragraph 3, item d, an appointment procedure is to be carried through pursuant to further regulations laid down in an appointment order to be issued by the Management Board in consultation with the Scientific Council and with the consent of the Board of Trustees.

(2) Decisions concerning the legal status of civil servants employed by the Found-ation will be made by the competent authorities according to the legal regulations of the Land on the basis of appli-cations which are decided upon by the competent organs of the Foundation.

Section 24 Changes Affecting the Statutes and Articles and Dissolution of the Foundation

Resolutions concerning changes affecting the Statutes and Articles and the dissolution of the Foundation may not be passed without the votes of the members of the Board of Trustees delegated by the Federal Republic and the Land who have a double vote in such matters. The Management Board and the Scientific Council are to be previously consulted. The resolutions will not take effect until they have been approved by the authority in control of the Foundation.

Section 25 Accumulation of Assets

(1) In the event of the dissolution of the Foundation, the Foundation's assets

will pass to the Federal Republic and the Land in proportion to the value of the grants made by each of them, insofar as these assets do not exceed the value of the grants awarded and any contributions made in kind at the time of dissolution. Any balance then remaining will, in agreement with the Federal Republic, be used on a non-profit basis in the sense of the paragraph titled „tax-privileged purposes“ of the tax code.

Section 26

Effective Date and Transitional Provisions

(1) These Statutes and Articles will go into effect on the day following their announcement in the Law Gazette of Baden-Württemberg.

(2) With the enactment of these Statutes and Articles, the Statutes and Articles of February 7, 1983 (Law Gazette, p. 86) and July 9, 1986 (Law Gazette, p. 278) become ineffective.

(3) The membership of the acting directors of the institutes and the scientific staff members of the Scientific Council continues in the framework of their term of office until the coordinators of the research programs are appointed and new scientific staff members have been elected.

(4) The terms of office of the acting directors of the institutes will be terminated upon the enactment of these Statutes and Articles.

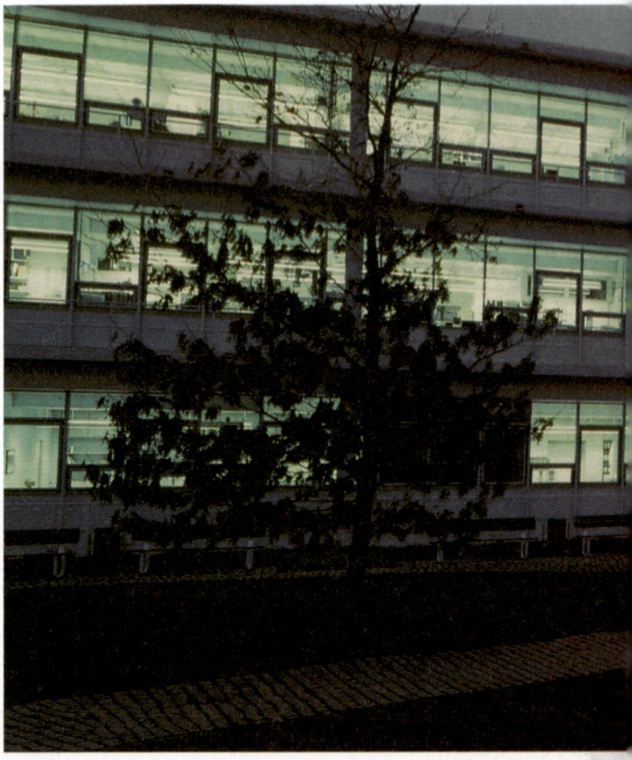

Fig. 143
The new laboratories of the Research Program "Applied Tumor Virology"

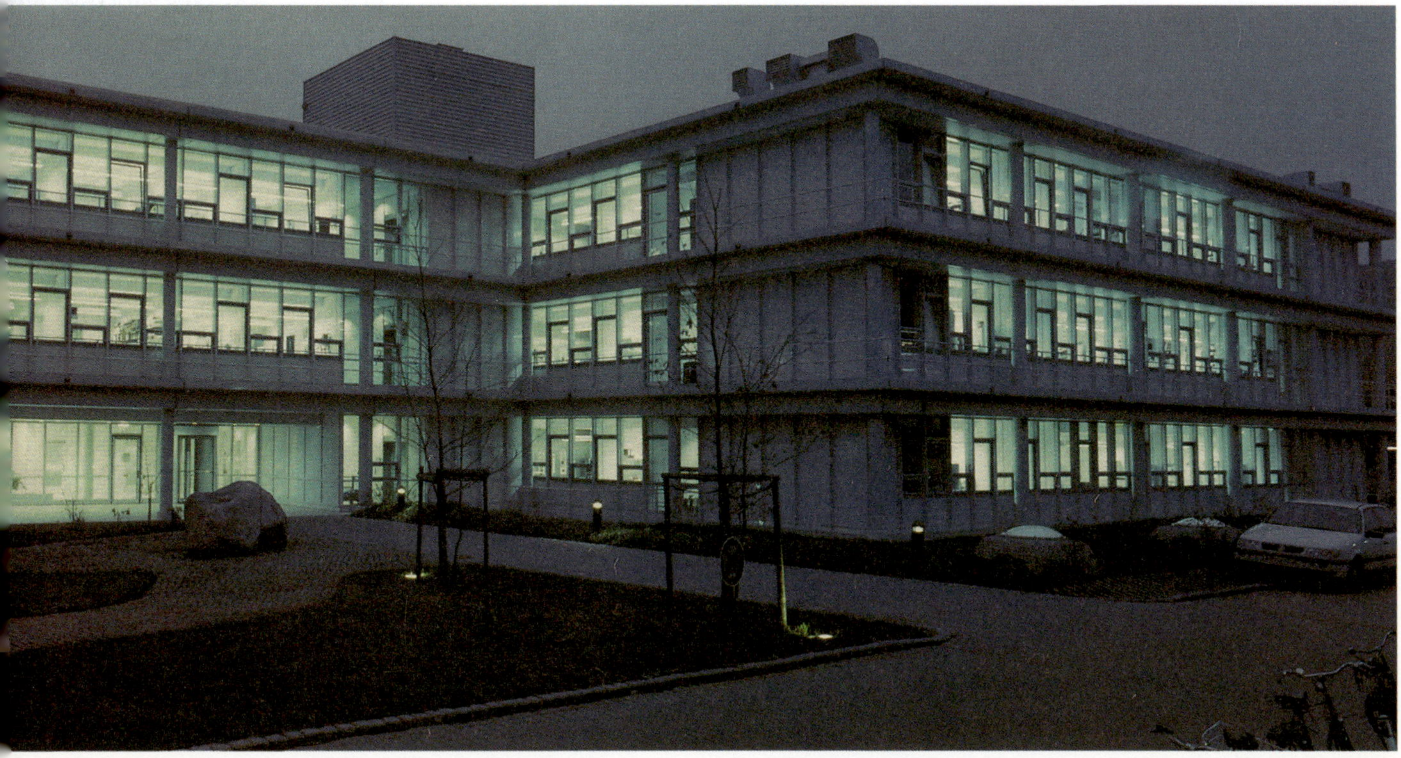

21

Index